Review of Histology

Michael Bruce Ganz, M.D.

Medical Resident at

The University of Illinois Hospital

Chicago, Illinois

Donald Lee Levick, M.D.

Pediatric Resident at

St. Christopher's Hospital for Children

Philadelphia, Pennsylvania

James W. Lash, Ph.D.

Professor of Anatomy at

The University of Pennsylvania

School of Medicine

Philadelphia, Pennsylvania

Review of Histology

A Self-Instructional Guide

J. B. Lippincott Company

Philadelphia

London   Mexico City   New York

St. Louis   São Paulo   Sydney

Acquisitions Editor: William Burgower
Sponsoring Editor: Sanford J. Robinson
Manuscript Editor: Elizabeth P. Lowe
Indexer: Julia Schwager
Design Director: Tracy Baldwin
Design Coordinator: Earl Gerhart
Designer: Arlene Putterman

Production Supervisor: Kathleen P. Dunn
Production Coordinator: George V. Gordon
Compositor: Monotype Composition Company, Inc.
Color Separations: Frantz Lithographic Services, Inc.
Printer/Binder: The Lancaster Press, Inc.
Cover Printer: Algen Press Corp.

6 5 4 3 2 1

Library of Congress Cataloging in Publication Data

Ganz, Michael Bruce.
    Review of histology.

    Includes index.
    1. Histology—Programmed instruction.   I. Levick, Donald Lee.
II. Lash, James W., DATE
III. Title
QM551.G36   1985   611′.018   83-26802
ISBN 0-397-50471-3

The authors and publisher acknowledge permission to reproduce the following: Figs. 1-4, 1-5, 1-8 through 1-11, 1-15, 1-19, 2-6, 2-7, 2-13, 3-3, 4-4, 6-7, 6-17, 6-18, 7-19 through 7-22, 8-3 through 8-5, 8-7, 8-8, 9-1, 9-5, 9-6, 9-16 through 9-18, 10-3, 10-15, 11-2, 13-8 through 13-12, 14-1, 14-7, 14-9, 14-16, 14-20, 14-23, 14-25, 14-28, 15-2, 15-8, 16-9 through 16-11, 18-5, 18-7, and 18-8 from Ham AW, Cormack DH: Histology, 8th ed. Philadelphia, JB Lippincott, 1979; Fig. 1-3 from Farquhar MG, Palade GE: J Cell Biol 17:375, 1963; Fig. 1-7 from Wilgram GF, Weinstock A: Arch Dermatol 94:456, 1966; Fig. 1-13 from Cardell R: Anat Rec 180:309, 1974; Fig. 1-16 from Cardell R: Int Rev Cytol 48:221, 1977; Figs. 1-18 and 9-3 from Paterson JA, Leblond CP: J Comp Neurol 175:373, 1977; Fig. 4-7 from Steer HW: J Anat 121:385, 1976; Fig. 5-2 from Bloom W, Fawcett DW: Textbook of Histology, 10th ed. Philadelphia, WB Saunders, 1975; Fig. 6-8 from Holtrop ME, King GJ: Clin Orthop 123:177, 1977; Fig. 8-12 from Somlyo AP, Devine CE, Somlyo AV et al: Philos Trans R Soc Lond [Biol] 265:223, 1973; Fig. 9-10 from Barr ML: The Human Nervous System. New York, Harper & Row, 1972; Fig. 10-13 from Fawcett DW: J Histochem Cytochem 13:75, 1965; Fig. 11-1 from Nichols BA, Bainton DF, Farquhar MG: J Cell Biol 50:498, 1971; Fig. 15-11 from Collet A: Arch Ital Anat Istol Pathol 39:119, 1965; Fig. 15-12 from Collet AJ, Chevalier G: Am J Anat 148:275, 1977; Fig. 16-4 from Tisher CC: Anatomy of the kidney. In Brenner BM, Rector FC (eds): The Kidney, vol 1. Philadelphia, WB Saunders, 1976; and Fig. 17-3 from Farquhar MG: Mem Soc Endocrinol 19:97, 1971.

This book is dedicated to our families and friends,
whose patience and persistent support enabled us to turn dream into reality.

M.G. and D.L.

Foreword

Most instructors of histology have experienced the situation where their favorite textbook, whatever its merits, is scorned by the students. But considering that every class comprises individuals with different study patterns and different specialty desires, is it any wonder that no one text satisfies an entire class?

When Michael Ganz and Donald Levick first approached me about their concept of a book based on the student's motivations and desires, I hesitated because I was unsure that I would use such a book. I soon reconsidered, thinking that not only should students learn what their instructors think they should learn, but also they should have the opportunity to learn in a manner that is comfortable to them. This is especially important during the stress-ridden first year of professional school, or in preprofessional school.

Review of Histology: A Self-Instructional Guide represents the very type of study guide Drs. Ganz and Levick would like to have used in their own histology class. Its unique format makes it ideal for use outside the laboratory as a teaching aid. For my part, I have given advice and counsel in the selection and presentation of material, and I have checked for possible errors. The organization and choice of examples, however, are largely theirs.

It is hoped that this book will be especially useful to students, for it is put together from a student's perspective on what should be learned in order to understand fully the structures, functions, and ideas of histology.

James W. Lash, Ph.D.

Acknowledgments

We should like to thank Dr. Chandrasekaran Nagaswami, whose magic in the darkroom is responsible for a great many of the black-and-white light photomicrographs contained herein. His many hours of work are deeply appreciated.

We wish to express our sincere and heartfelt appreciation to Dr. Arthur W. Ham and Dr. David H. Cormack, who have graciously consented to allow us to reproduce a great many superb illustrations from the eighth edition of *Histology*. By their exceptional kindness and generosity they have enabled us to produce a book that is far superior to what it would otherwise have been, and for this we are deeply grateful.

Our thanks to the staff members of the J. B. Lippincott Company who were involved in this project. Their hard work, and especially their patience, was essential in the completion of this very difficult undertaking. Special thanks to Sanford Robinson, Susan Caldwell, Rosanne Hallowell, and Betsy Lowe.

Lastly, and mostly, we offer our thanks to Dr. James Lash for his wisdom and guidance, and for coming through when we needed him the most. Thanks, Jay.

M.G. and D.L.

Contents

Introduction

The purpose of this atlas-text is twofold. *Review of Histology: A Self-Instructional Guide* will function to teach rapid identification of, first, organelles in electron micrographs, then simple cells, the numerous tissues, and, finally, organs.

The textual portion will present a basic explanation of organelle function, cellular function, tissue arrangement and physiological importance, and organ structure and function.

Each chapter builds on knowledge acquired in the previous chapters, so it is essential to READ THIS BOOK IN ORDER AND READ EVERYTHING CAREFULLY. Several types of questions are presented throughout the book, and EACH question is numbered individually.

The most common type of question is that of *text blanks*, _____. These blanks represent either facts, descriptions, or names that have been explained earlier in the text. Often the blanks can be answered by studying the adjacent light or electron micrograph. Small blanks, __ __ __, are sized appropriately; each of these blanks stands for a single letter, for example, _r_ _E_ _R_.

Illustration blanks are those blanks directly associated with an illustration. These blanks can be text blanks, part of an illustration caption, or an arrow pointing to a certain part of the illustration. All of these are numbered and are best answered in sequence, just like the text blanks. REMEMBER, you will find that you will be referring back to the illustration at appropriate times in the text, where the illustration blanks should then be filled in.

The last type of blank encountered will be that of the *multiple choice*. This is similar to that of a text blank, except that we give alternatives from which to choose.

Review of Histology

1

Cytology

After completing this chapter, you should be able to identify the following:

1 Mitochondria
2 Golgi apparatus
3 Ribosomes
4 Rough and smooth endoplasmic reticulum

5 Nuclei
6 Nucleoli
7 Plasma membranes

Also, after completing this chapter, you should understand the following:

1 The specific function(s) of each organelle
2 The importance of each organelle in staining in a routine light micrograph

3 The interrelationships between organelles
4 The importance of electron microscopy

Organelles are structures that form parts of the cell. They may be found within the cytoplasm or may make up the cell boundary. Different classes of organelles generally have different functions.

Cell Membrane

The cell membrane is the outer limit of the living cell and its interface with the environment. The cell membrane is composed of a continuous layer of lipids with individual protein and glycoprotein molecules embedded or anchored in this **(1)** _____ matrix. Also called the plasmalemma or plasma membrane, the **(2)** _____ _____ acts as a selective permeability barrier and therefore regulates the **(3)** _____ of substances into and out of the cell.

From the electron micrograph, the **(4)** _____ _____ is seen to be composed of **(5)** _____ layers; the outer, inner, and middle lamellae (Fig. 1-1). The **(6)** _____ (*bi, tri*)laminar cell membrane is composed of carbohydrates, proteins, and lipids. Because cell membranes exist in a fluid state, there is movement of the components, such as **(7)** _____, **(8)** _____, and **(9)** _____, within each lamella. Ranging from 95 A to 110 A in thickness, the **(10)** _____ _____ may not always appear as a trilaminar structure due to the angle of section. (You should finish #13 at this point.)

1 *glycoprotein*
2 *cell membrane*
3 *passage or exchange*

4 *plasma (cell)*
  membrane
5 *three*
6 *tri*
7 *lipid*
8 *glycoprotein*
9 *protein*
10 *plasma (cell)*
  membrane

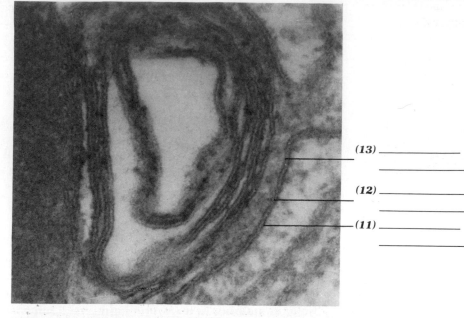

(13) _____

_____

(12) _____

_____

(11) _____

_____

11 outer lamella
12 middle lamella
13 inner lamella

FIG. 1-1. EM of human splenic red pulp (original magnification ×200,000). (Courtesy of Robert M. Powell, University of Pennsylvania School of Veterinary Medicine)

Intercellular Junctions

Where the cell membrane from one cell meets that of another, various types of intercellular junctions may form. These junctions are characteristic of epithelial cells.

One type is the *zonula* ("girdle") *occludens*, also called the tight junction. From the electron micrograph (Fig. 1-2) it can be inferred that the *(14)* _____ (*outer, inner, middle*) lamellae of the cell membranes of the neighboring cells are fused. The junction encircles the entire cell and allows no particulate matter to pass through; therefore, this is an excellent *(15)* _____ barrier. The *(16)* _____ _____ also functions in holding adjacent cells together.

14 outer

15 permeability
16 zonula occludens

(17) _____

_____

17 zonula occludens

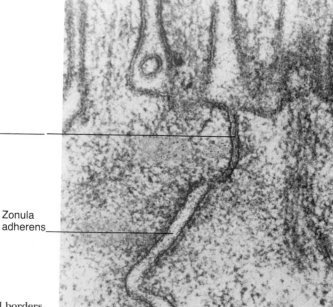

Zonula
adherens

FIG. 1-2. EM of lateral cell borders.

Cell Membrane

The *zonula adherens* serves primarily as a firm adhesion between neighboring cells. Between the neighboring membranes is a protein and glycosaminoglycan matrix that serves as an intercellular glue. The *zonula adherens* also consists of an electron-dense area in the cytoplasm next to the **(18)** _____ lamellae. This serves to anchor fine cytoplasmic filaments. A *zonula adherens* is similar to a *zonula* **(19)** _____ _____ in that both are beltlike zones encircling entire cells.

The zonula adherens and the *zonula occludens* together make up the terminal bar, which is a junctional structure found in apical regions between cells.

18 *inner*

19 *occludens*

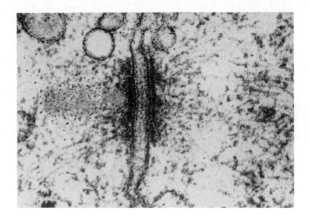

FIG. 1-3. EM of macular adherens.

A third type of intercellular junction is the *macula* ("spot") *adherens* or *desmosome* (Fig. 1-3). Unlike the **(20)** _____ _____ and the **(21)** _____ _____, the macula adherens does not encircle the cell. Yet there are structural and functional similarities between the **(22)** _____ adherens and the **(23)** _____ adherens. The electron-dense area located **(24)** _____ _____ _____ is more pronounced in the macula adherens. Tonofilaments (to be discussed later) course through this electron-dense area. The gluelike glycosaminoglycan matrix in between the **(25)** _____ _____ is more pronounced, and an intermediate line can be seen between the two halves of the macula adherens or **(26)** _____ (Fig. 1-4). A hemidesmosome is a junction between an epithelial cell and a noncellular supporting structure.

20 *zonula adherens*
21 *zonula occludens*

22 *zonula*
23 *macula*

24 *in the cytoplasm next to the inner lamella*

25 *neighboring cell membranes*
26 *desmosome*

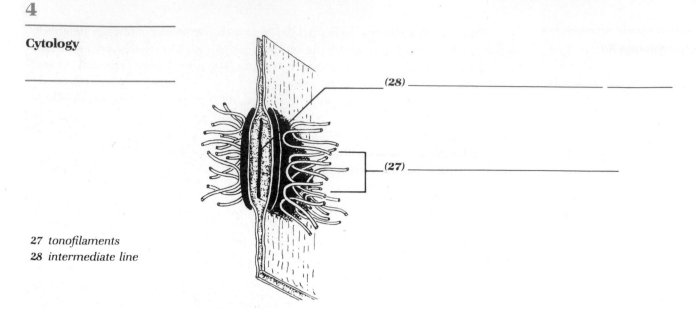

27 tonofilaments
28 intermediate line

FIG. 1-4. Diagram of a desmosome.

The final intercellular junction is called the nexus (gap junction). The nexus is formed by structures that are embedded on both sides of the junction in the cell membranes involved. These structures, packed in a hexagonal array, have central pores; therefore, two cells can **(29)** _____ with each other by allowing the passage of small ions and molecules (Fig. 1-5).

29 communicate

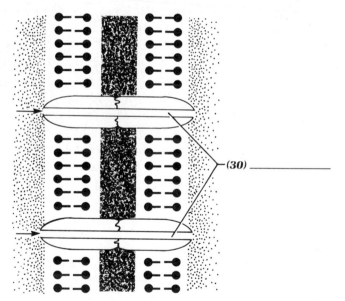

30 pores

FIG. 1-5. Diagram of a gap junction (longitudinal section).

The distance between adjacent cell membranes in a gap junction is 2 nm. Do any of the other intercellular junctions have any type of intercellular communication, and if so, which ones? **(31)** _____ (Fig. 1-6)

31 no

Cell Membrane

(32) _____

(33) _____

(34) _____

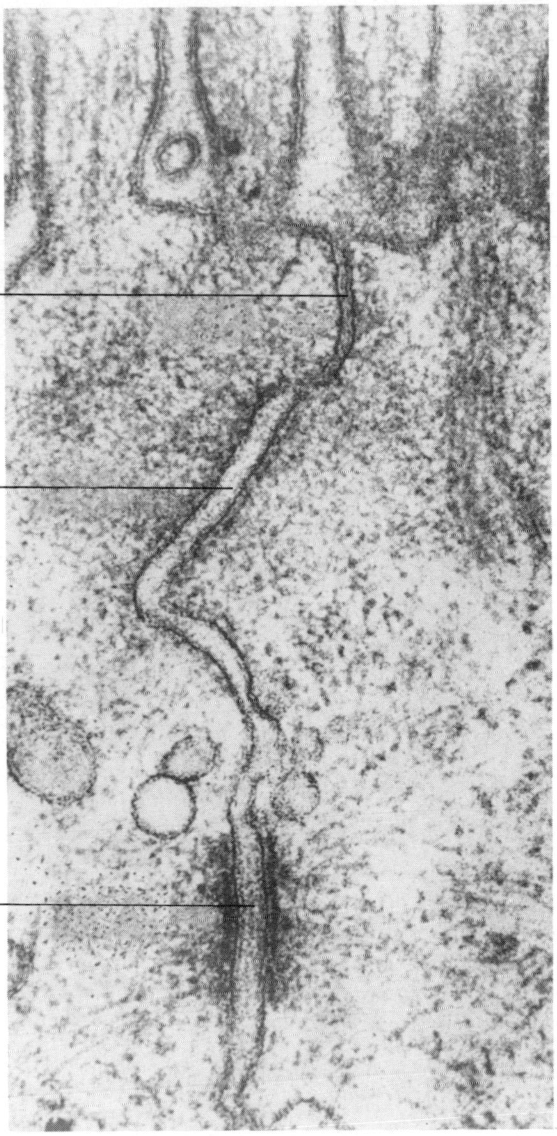

FIG. 1-6. EM of the three intercellular junctions that make up the junctional complex.

32 *zonula occludens*

33 *zonula adherens*

34 *macula adherens*

Cellular Filaments

There are two populations of filamentous strands in the cytoplasm of most cells. One type of microfilament is termed a tonofilament. These tonofilaments are found interlacing the electron-dense area of the (35) _____ _____ _____
_____, and confer mechanical stability to this intercellular junction

35 *macula adherens*

36 *tonofilaments*

37 *macula adherens*

38 *tonofilaments*

39 *zonula adherens*

40 *Fine cytoplasmic*

(Fig. 1-7). These *(36)* _____ are also scattered singly throughout the cytoplasm, providing support for the entire cell structure. The diameter of the tonofilaments ranges from 9 nm to 12 nm, and their length is variable.

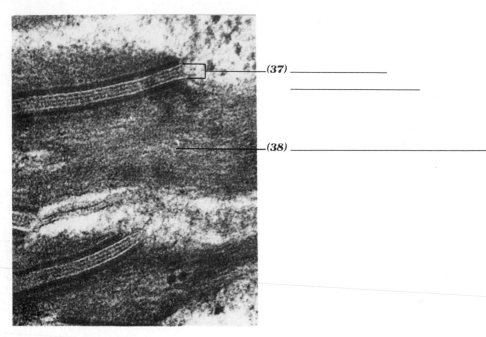

(37) _____
_____

(38) _____

FIG. 1-7. EM of epithelial cells (original magnification ×114,000).

The second type of microfilament is approximately 7 nm in diameter (Fig. 1-8). These fine cytoplasmic filaments are found anchored in the electron-dense area of the *(39)* _____ _____ and in the terminal web. The terminal web is formed by the interlacing of cytoplasmic filaments from apical specializations (that is, microvilli) and the filaments of the *zonula adherens*. *(40)* _____ _____ filaments are found throughout

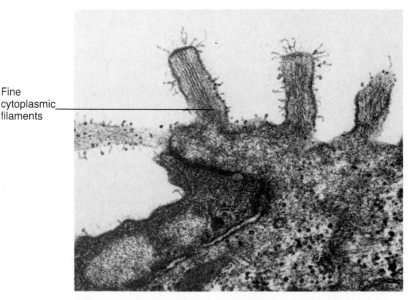

Fine cytoplasmic filaments

FIG. 1-8. EM of epithelial cells (original magnification ×60,000).

Cellular Filaments

41 cytoplasmic filaments
42 tonofilaments

43 fine cytoplasmic
   filaments
44 tonofilaments

45 microtubules
46 cytoskeleton
47 microtubules

48 larger
49 hollow

the cytoplasm and function in both cell movement and stability. Both types of microfilaments, the fine *(41)* _____ _____ and the *(42)* _____ are part of the framework of the cell called the cytoskeleton.

Also present in the cytoplasm are microtubules (Fig. 1-9). These are tubular rather than solid filamentous structures as in the *(43)* _____ _____ _____ and *(44)* _____. Microtubules are 25 μm in diameter and are of variable length. Important in maintaining cell shape, *(45)* _____ constitute part of the cell framework, the *(46)* _____. Microtubules also function in the movement of organelles within cells. Complexes of *(47)* _____ form components of other organelles, including the shaft of motile apical specializations (such as cilia) and the mitotic spindle that forms during cell division. Microtubules have a *(48)* _____ *(larger, smaller)* diameter than tonofilaments and appear as a *(49)* _____ *(hollow, solid)* structure in cross section.

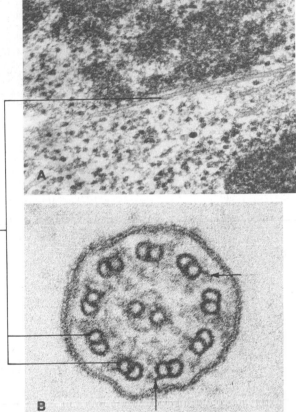

Microtubules

FIG. 1-9. *(A)* EM (original magnification ×50,000). *(B)* EM of a cilium (original magnification ×220,000). Arrows point to short arms, involved in releasing energy for movement.

Mitochondria

Organelles are the functional components of the cell. Termed the "power-house" of the cell, the mitochondria are responsible for energy production (Fig. 1-10). Although the general shape varies, all mitochondria are surrounded by two unit membranes, each one being *(50)* _____ laminar. The *(51)* _____ *(outer, inner)* membrane is thrown into folds called cristae. Cristae can either be tubular or shelflike in appearance. There is no direct correlation between the shape of the mitochondria and the shape of their cristae. The number of cristae per

50 tri

51 inner

52 cristae

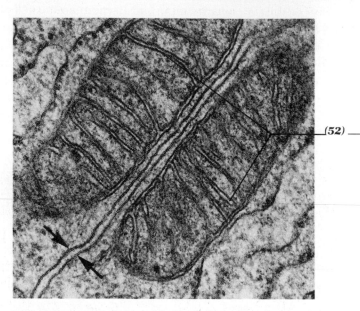

(52) _____

FIG. 1-10. EM of mitochondria (original magnification ×86,000). Arrows point to cell membranes.

mitochondrion and the number of individual mitochondria will increase with the cell's need for energy. Cells whose energy requirement are low usually have relatively *(53)* _____ *(small, large)* numbers of mitochondria, each containing fewer *(54)* _____ than normal. The converse is also true.

The matrix of the mitochondria is usually *(55)* _____ *(more, less)* electron dense than the cytoplasm. Within the matrix are prominent electron-dense *(56)* _____, composed of calcium and other ions (Fig. 1-11).

53 small

54 cristae

55 more

56 granules (dots)

57 cristae

58 granules

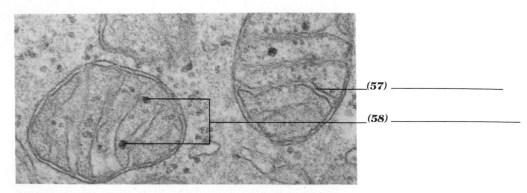

(57) _____

(58) _____

FIG. 1-11. EM of mitochondria (original magnification ×80,000).

Ribosomes

Ribosomes

Ribosomes are cytoplasmic organelles essential for protein synthesis. They appear free in the cytoplasm or attached to a membranous structure. Free ribosomes are found scattered as small, inactive electron-dense particles or inactive clusters (3–30 ribosomes). These free small clusters are called polyribosomes (or polysomes) and are responsible for the synthesis of **(59)** _____ to be used by the cell (e.g., enzymes). Clusters of ribosomes called **(60)** _____ can also be found attached to a membranous structure called the rough endoplasmic reticulum (rER). The attached polysomes primarily synthesize proteins to be secreted or used by the cell membrane. A cell which has **(61)** _____ (*few, many*) polysomes is probably actively engaged in protein synthesis, while a cell in which individual **(62)** _____ predominate should have a relatively **(63)** _____ (*high, low*) rate of protein synthesis. Therefore, in examining a cell that was actively secreting proteins, you would expect attached polysomes to be more numerous than **(64)** _____ ribosomes.

59 protein

60 polyribosomes
   (polysomes)

61 many

62 ribosomes
63 low

64 free

65 mitochondria

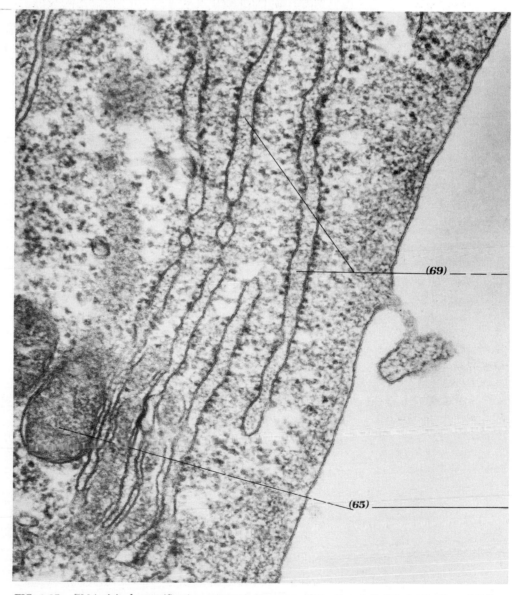

FIG. 1-12. EM (original magnification ×60,000). (Courtesy of Dr. George E. Palade, Section of Cell Biology, Yale University School of Medicine)

Rough Endoplasmic Reticulum

The rER consists of membranes arranged in a parallel formation forming hollow membranous structures called cisternae ("flattened sacs"; Fig. 1-12). The membranes of the rER have a structure similar to the *(66)* _____ arrangement of the plasma membrane. Studded with *(67)* _____, the *(68)* _____ endoplasmic reticulum is involved in protein synthesis. Ribosomes synthesize *(70)* _____ and secrete it through the membranes into the lumina of the cisternae. The proteins released from the ribosomes may be abundant enough to make the lumen appear electron dense. Transitional vesicles carrying these secretions bud off the membranes of the *(71)* __ __ __. The rER synthesizes protein used by the cell membrane or for *(72)* _____ into the extracellular space. The rough *(73)* _____ _____ is continuous with the nuclear membrane.

66 trilaminar

67 ribosomes
68 rough
69 rER
70 protein

71 rER
72 secretion
73 endoplasmic reticulum

Smooth Endoplasmic Reticulum

Smooth endoplasmic reticulum (sER), less commonly called the agranular endoplasmic reticulum, closely resembles the rough, except that the

(74) _____ _____

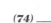

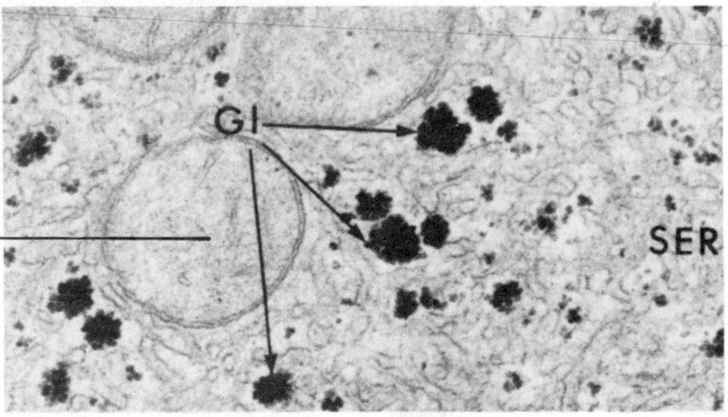

74 mitochondria

FIG. 1-13. EM of a liver cell. GI = glycogen granules. (Original magnification ×38,000.)

(75) _____ are absent (Fig. 1-13). The sER is often continuous with the rER. Most of the membranes of the smooth *(76)* _____ _____ are in the form of tubules, which branch and anastomose freely with one another. Parallel stacks of cisternae are generally *(77)* _____ (*more, less*) commonly found in the smooth endoplasmic reticulum. The smooth *(78)* _____ _____ is involved in lipid synthesis, steroid formation, and the detoxification of certain drugs.

75 ribosomes

76 endoplasmic reticulum

77 less
78 endoplasmic reticulum

Golgi Complex

The membrane-bound saccules of the Golgi complex are arranged in slightly curved stacks forming convex and concave surfaces (Fig. 1-14). The membranous

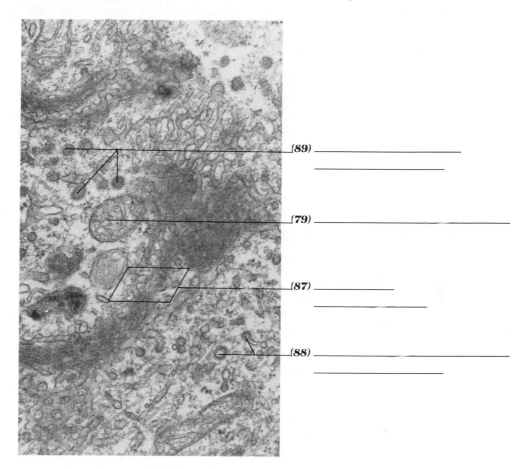

(89) _____

_____

(79) _____

(87) _____

_____

(88) _____

_____

FIG. 1-14. EM of portion of human melanoma cell (original magnification ×35,000). (Courtesy of Dr. Gerd Maul, Wistar Institute, Philadelphia, Pennsylvania)

79 *mitochondria*

80 *sER*

81 *rough*
82 *transitional*
83 *rER*
84 *Golgi*
85 *protein*

86 *larger*
87 *Golgi complex or Golgi saccules*
88 *transitional vesicles*
89 *secretory vesicles*

wall of the Golgi complex closely resembles that of the *(80)* __ __ __. There are generally three to eight saccules making up each Golgi apparatus. The convex, or forming, face of the Golgi receives numerous small transitional vesicles from the *(81)* _____ endoplasmic reticulum. There is no direct physical continuity between the membrane systems, therefore *(82)* _____ vesicles are the only means of communication between the *(83)* __ __ __ and the *(84)* _____ complex. These transitional vesicles fuse with the membrane of the Golgi and thus transfer the *(85)* _____ they are carrying to the Golgi complex, where it is modified and packaged.

At the maturing, or concave, face of the Golgi, the final product is released in membrane-bound secretory granules. Are the secretory granules generally larger or smaller than the transitional vesicles? *(86)* _____. A single cell may contain more than one stack of Golgi saccules. Often these multiple Golgi complexes are grouped together in an area close to the nucleus. In routine light microscopy, this area stains very poorly. (You should finish #89 at this point.)

Lysosomes

Lysosomes are membrane-bound sacs containing hydrolytic enzymes that enable the cell to degrade ingested material. Their diameter ranges from 5 nm to 8 nm and in electron micrographs (EM) appear with varying electron density (Fig. 1-15).

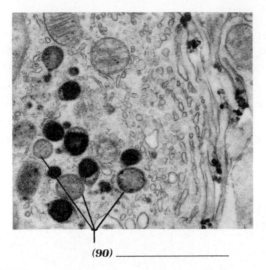

FIG. 1-15. EM of part of a macrophage (original magnification ×18,000).

(90) _____

90 lysosomes

These differences are due to the contents and degree of activity of the lysosome. If lysosomes are considered specialized secretory granules that do not leave the cell, what two organelles would be involved in their production? *(91)* __ __ __ and *(92)* _____ _____.

91 rER
92 Golgi complex

Cellular Inclusions

Cellular inclusions are usually accumulations of stored metabolites or cell products such as protein, lipid, carbohydrate, or pigment. Inclusions may be amorphous, particulate, or crystalline in nature. Glycogen, one such inclusion, appears diffusely distributed in the cytoplasm or in coarse clumps (Fig. 1-16).

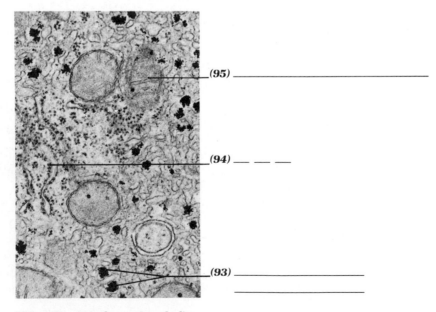

(95) _____

(94) __ __ __

(93) _____

_____

FIG. 1-16. EM of a portion of a liver cell (original magnification ×27,000).

93 glycogen granules
94 rER
95 mitochondria

Cellular Inclusions

How can one differentiate between glycogen inclusions and lysosomes?
(96) _____

96 glycogen granules are smaller and aggregated into clumps; lysosomes are homogeneous and membrane bound

Nucleus

The most prominent feature in most cells is the nucleus. The nuclear membrane (or envelope) is composed of two unit membranes that enclose a space known as the perinuclear cisterna (Fig. 1-17). What other organelle has a double membrane? *(97)* _____. Nuclear pores are formed at points where the inner and outer nuclear membranes are continuous. The nuclear pore is 70 nm in diameter and serves as a point of exchange between the nucleus and the cytoplasm. The exchange of materials is somewhat restricted by a thin diaphragm covering the pore.

97 mitochondria

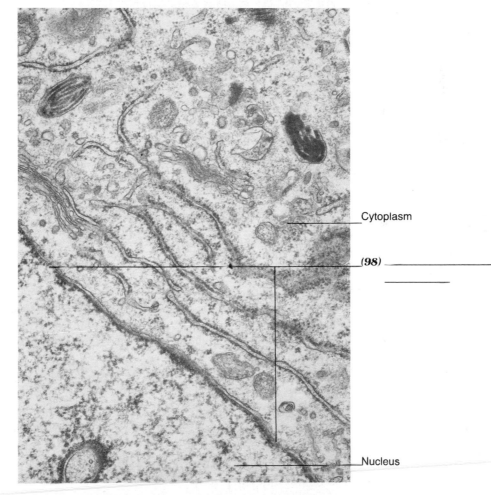

Cytoplasm

(98) _____

Nucleus

FIG. 1-17. EM of human melanocyte cell (original magnification ×30,000). (Courtesy of Gerd Maul, Wistar Institute, Philadelphia, Pennsylvania)

98 nuclear pore

The outer nuclear membrane is studded with ribosomes so that it is structurally and morphologically similar to the *(99)* __ __ __. Is the outer nuclear membrane continuous with the rER? *(100)* _____.

99 rER
100 yes

Nucleolus

Within the nucleus is a large discrete electron-dense structure called the nucleolus (Fig. 1-18). Nucleoli (often more than one per cell in humans) may lie against the inside of the **(101)** _____ envelope or may appear to be free in

101 *nuclear*

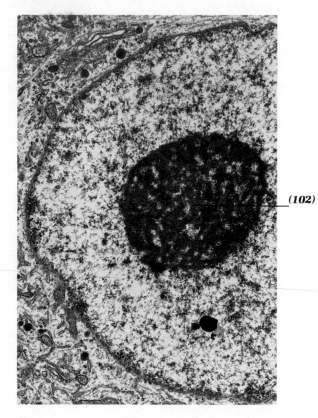

(102) _____

102 *nucleolus*

FIG. 1-18.   EM of a nucleus (original magnification ×15,000).

the nucleoplasm. There is no membrane around the nucleolus. Hence, these **(103)** _____ are in direct contact with the rest of the nucleoplasm. The nucleolus is the site of ribosomal ribonucleic acid (RNA) synthesis. When requirements for protein are increased, the number of cytoplasmic **(104)** _____ should increase, and this should be reflected by an increase in the number and activity of **(105)** _____.

103 *nucleoli*

CHROMATIN   The chromosomes of the nucleus contain the genetic material and are visible as compact individual structures during certain stages of cell division (Fig. 1-19). During most of the cell cycle, the genetic material is found uncoiled in the form of threadlike chromatin. Chromatin that is actively participating in deoxyribonucleic acid (DNA) replication or RNA transcription is called euchromatin. Euchromatin is highly uncoiled, and areas of the nucleus rich in **(106)** _____ stain very lightly in both light and electron microscopy. Less active **(107)** _____ is called heterochromatin. This is more highly coiled or condensed than **(108)** eu_____, and appears as dark-staining patches scattered throughout the nucleoplasm.

104 *ribosomes*
105 *nucleoli*

106 *euchromatin*
107 *chromatin*
108 *chromatin*

Nucleus

109 heterochromatin

110 euchromatin

(109) —————————————————

(110) —————————————————

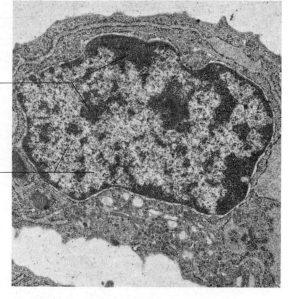

FIG. 1-19. EM of a chondrocyte.

Consequently, if the nucleus is pale staining with a few dark patches, it consists mostly of *(111)* _____ and you would assume that a large part of the genome is *(112)* _____ (*active, inactive*). Patterns of euchromatin and heterochromatin within any cell will change as the activity of the cell's genome changes.

111 euchromatin
112 active

2   Epithelia

After completing this chapter, you should be able to identify the following:

1 All types of epithelia

2 Surface modifications of
   epithelia

3 Stratified epithelia

Also, after completing this chapter, you should understand the following:

1 The function of each type of
   epithelia

2 The functional differences
   between the different types of
   epithelia

3 The importance of surface
   modifications

Epithelial tissue, found both internally and externally, functions to protect the body from the environment, is involved in the transport of molecules, and acts to delineate boundaries and create fluid compartments. It is classified according to the number of cell layers and the shape of the most superficial cells. An epithelium composed of one cell layer is called a simple epithelium. If there is more than one layer of cells, it is referred to as a stratified epithelium.

Simple Squamous Epithelia

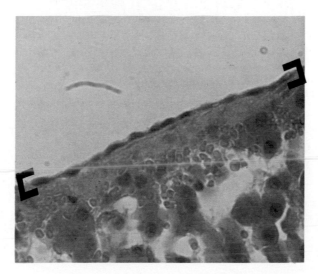

FIG. 2-1. Photomicrograph of simple squamous epithelia, hematoxylin-eosin (H and E) stain (original magnification ×125).

Epithelia

1 *one*
2 *simple*
3 *squamous*

4 *simple squamous*

5 *simple squamous*
  epithelium
6 *Endothelium*
7 *mesothelium*

8 *zonula occludens*
9 *zonula adherens*

10 *endothelium*
11 *simple squamous*

The brackets in Figure 2-1 enclose a layer of epithelial cells. This epithelium is *(1)* _____ layer(s) thick; therefore it is a *(2)* _____ epithelium. These cells are shaped like thin flat plates. Another name for this shape is squamous. This epithelium is therefore classified as a simple *(3)* _____ epithelium.

Simple squamous epithelium is found lining many surfaces including the following: the luminal border of blood vessels, lymph vessels, and the heart; the serous body cavities; the cornea; the inner tympanic membrane; the renal capsule; and the alveolar surface of the lung.

The simple squamous epithelium found lining the walls of blood vessels, lymph vessels, and the heart is called endothelium. Endothelium is morphologically identical to other *(4)* _____ _____ epithelia under the light microscope. When found lining the serous body cavities such as the pleural, pericardial, and peritoneal cavities, the *(5)* _____ _____ _____ is called mesothelium. *(6)* _____ and *(7)* _____ are simple squamous epithelia that are specially named according to their specific location.

In some endothelia, terminal bars may be found between the cells close to the luminal edge. What components are found in a terminal bar? *(8)* _____ _____ and *(9)* _____ _____ .

The epithelium lining the lumen of the vessel is called an *(10)* _____, or a *(11)* _____ _____ epithelium (Fig. 2-2). It is so thin that the cytoplasm is barely visible and the

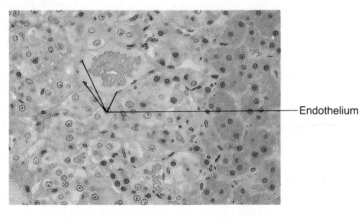

— Endothelium

FIG. 2-2. Photomicrograph of an arterial blood vessel, H and E stain (original magnification × 125).

dark-staining *(12)* _____ protrude outward. This is often the case with other examples of *(13)* _____ _____ epithelium as well. Where is mesothelium found? *(14)* _____ _____ Where is endothelium found? *(15)* _____ _____

12 *nuclei*
13 *simple squamous*
14 *lining serous body*
   cavities
15 *lining the walls of blood*
   vessels, lymph vessels,
   and the heart

Simple Cuboidal Epithelium

Simple Cuboidal
Epithelium

Simple cuboidal epithelium, as the name suggests, is *(16)* _____ layer(s) thick. In a longitudinal section of these cells, the length is *(17)* _____ *(equal to, greater than, less than)* the width (Fig. 2-3). The nuclei usually appear to be located *(18)* _____. Simple cuboidal cells are found in the distal renal tubule, thyroid, ovary, lens, and retina.

16 one
17 equal to

18 centrally

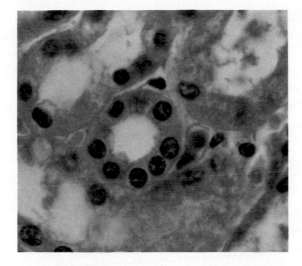

FIG. 2-3. Photomicrograph of a collecting tubule, H and E stain (original magnification ×500).

Certain cuboidal cells will stain more eosinophilic. The eosinophilic nature is often due to an increased number of mitochondria in the cytoplasm. Therefore, any cell with *(19)* _____ *(high, low)* energy requirements, such as those involved in active transport of ions across the plasma membrane, will stain *(20)* _____ due to large numbers of *(21)* _____.

A surface specialization found in some simple cuboidal epithelia is the microvillus. Microvilli are apical extensions of the cell that are usually cyclindrical in shape. They are 0.5 μm to 1.0 μm long, and are composed of a covering plasma membrane and cytoplasm containing fine cytoplasmic filaments. These filaments interlace with the filaments of the zonula *(22)* _____, forming the *(23)* _____. They are present in the greatest number (as many as 2000 microvilla per cell) on cells whose principal function is absorption. This is because microvilli serve to increase *(24)* _____, thus increasing the opportunity for absorption.

19 high

20 eosinophilic
21 mitochondria

22 adherens
23 terminal web

24 surface area

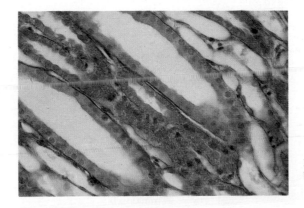

FIG. 2-4. Photomicrograph of a renal tubule, H and E stain (original magnification ×125).

In a light micrograph, microvilli appear as a fuzzy border on the (25) _____ (*apical, basal*) surface. This is usually referred to as a *brush* or *striated* border (Fig. 2-4). Simple cuboidal epithelia with microvilli are found in the proximal renal tubule, choroid plexus, and intercalated ducts of salivary glands.

25 apical

Simple Columnar Epithelium

Taller than the cuboidal cells are the columnar cells (Fig. 2-5). The nuclei of

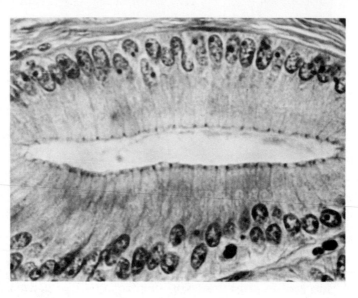

FIG. 2-5. Photomicrograph of simple columnar epithelium (original magnification ×300).

simple columnar epithelia are usually located somewhat basally and have an elongated oval shape. Relative to each other, how are the nuclei arranged? (26) _____ Simple columnar cells are found lining the stomach, large intestine, and apocrine sweat glands.

26 in a row, at the same level

27 microvilli

(27) _____

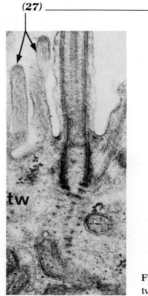

FIG. 2-6. Electron micrograph (EM) of the surface of a ciliated cell. tw = terminal web.

Simple Columnar Epithelium

Apical specializations of simple columnar cells are microvilli and cilia (Figs. 2-6 and 2-7). Cilia, 5 μm to 15 μm in length, have a highly ordered internal arrangement of microtubules, while the **(28)** _____

_____ filaments of microvilli are not orderly arranged. Both cilia and microvilli are directly continuous with the cytoplasm of the cell and are therefore covered by a **(29)** _____

_____. Cilia are **(30)** _____ (*much longer, much shorter*) than normal microvilli. The microtubules of the **(31)** _____ arise from a dense elongate granule called the basal body, which is located at the base of the cilia. The principal function of the cilia is to propel a fluid or mucous film over the surface of the epithelium by rapid coordinated beating movements. These movements are aided by the **(32)** _____ within the cilia.

28 *fine cytoplasmic*

29 *cell (plasma) membrane*
30 *much longer*
31 *cilia*

32 *microtubules*

(33) _____

33 *cilia*

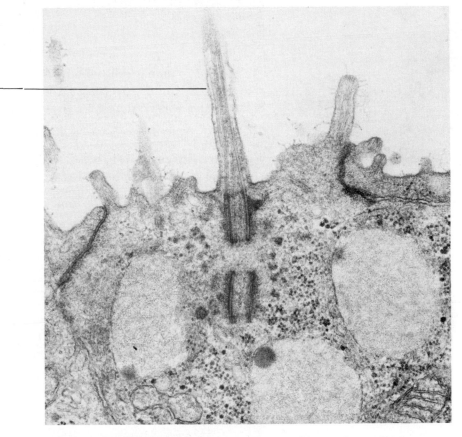

FIG. 2-7. EM of the apical surface of a mucous cell (original magnification ×40,000).

Ciliated simple columnar epithelium is found in the uterus, oviducts, small bronchi, some paranasal sinuses, and central canal of the spinal cord (Fig. 2-8). Cilia can also be found in fewer number on individual cells of most types of epithelia.

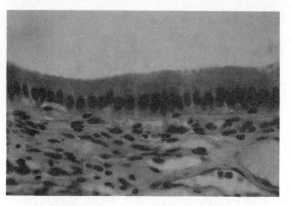

FIG. 2-8. Photomicrograph of simple columnar epithelium with microvilli (gallbladder), H and E stain (original magnification ×250).

Simple columnar cells with microvilli whose function is **(34)** _____ are found in the small intestine, appendix, gallbladder, and striated ducts of salivary glands.

34 absorption

Nonkeratinized Stratified Squamous Epithelium

Stratified squamous epithelium is **(35)** _____ (*one, greater than one*) cell layer thick (Fig. 2-9). What is the shape of cells in the

35 greater than one

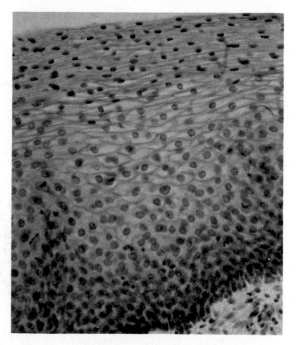

FIG. 2-9. Photomicrograph of the vagina, H and E stain (original magnification ×250).

most apical layer of a stratified squamous epithelium? **(36)** _____ _____ There is a gradual flattening of the cells from the basal polyhedral cell layer to the apical cell layer. This epithelium is found on surfaces subjected to "wear and tear"; thus it serves a **(37)** _____ (*protective, transportive*) function. Stratified squamous epithelium lines the buccal cavity, part of the epiglottis, esophagus, vagina, female urethra, conjunctiva, and cornea.

36 flattened plates

37 protective

Keratinized Stratified
Squamous Epithelium

Keratinized Stratified Squamous Epithelium

Where stratified squamous epithelium occurs on the exposed outer surface of the body, the superficial layers are modified for increased protection and water impermeability (Fig. 2-10). The cells have lost their usually prominent (38) _____, and their cytoplasm has been largely replaced by a sclero-protein, keratin. Are these superficial cells alive? (39) _____. Such a keratinized (40) _____ _____ epithelium comprises the outer layer of the skin, known as the epidermis.

38 nuclei
39 no
40 stratified squamous

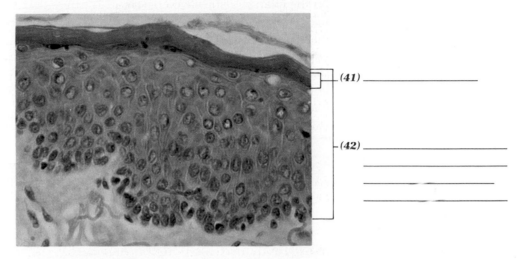

(41) _____

41 keratin

(42) _____

_____

_____

_____

FIG. 2-10. Photomicrograph of the skin, H and E stain (original magnification ×200).

42 keratinized stratified
squamous epithelium

Stratified Cuboidal Epithelium

Stratified cuboidal or stratified columnar epithelium is relatively rare and is most often found in a narrow zone where a stratified squamous epithelium meets either a simple or a transitional epithelium. This epithelium is generally found in the largest ducts of the salivary glands; in the fornix of the conjunctiva; in areas of the pharynx, epiglottis, and urethra; in the recto-anal junction; and in the cavernous portion of the male urethra (Fig. 2-11).

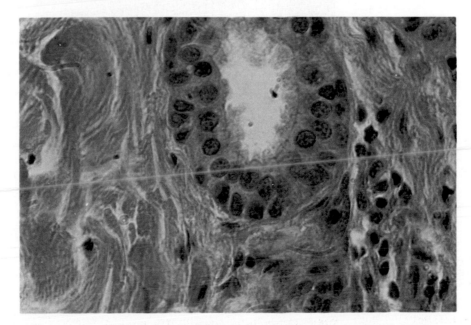

FIG. 2-11. Photomicrograph of a salivary gland duct, H and E stain (original magnification ×500).

Transitional Epithelium

A unique type of stratified epithelium whose superficial cell layers change shape in response to distension is the transitional epithelium. Usually seven to ten cell layers thick, the basal layer of transitional epithelium is columnar in shape, while the middle layers assume a polyhedral shape. Can the basal and middle cell layers change shape with distension? *(43)* _____ (Figs. 2-12 and 2-13). When not under tension, the superficial cell layer consists of large cells with a characteristic rounded free surface. When distended, these cells become flattened and take on the characteristic shape of *(44)* _____ cells, while the underlying layers remain mostly unchanged. Occasionally, cells of the superficial layer may be binucleate. *(45)* _____ epithelium is well adapted to lining tubes and hollow organs that are subjected to frequent *(46)* _____ and contraction. This type of epithelium is found lining the excretory urinary system: major renal calices, urinary bladder, ureters, and prostatic urethra.

43 no

44 squamous

45 Transitional

46 distension

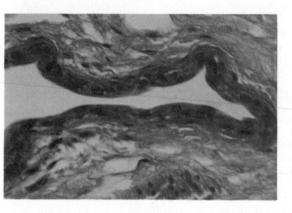

FIG. 2-12. Photomicrograph of the ureter, H and E stain (original magnification ×600). Is this distended or contracted transitional epithelium? *(47)* _____
_____
_____

47 distended transitional epithelium

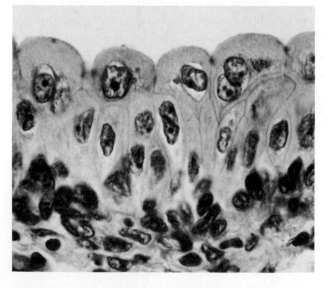

FIG. 2-13. Photomicrograph of the bladder, H and E stain (original magnification ×500). Is this distended or contracted transitional epithelium? *(48)* _____
_____
_____

48 contracted transitional epithelium

Pseudostratified Epithelium

Pseudostratified
Epithelium

In a pseudostratified epithelium, all cells are in contact with an underlying basement membrane, but not all reach the apical surface of the epithelium. By

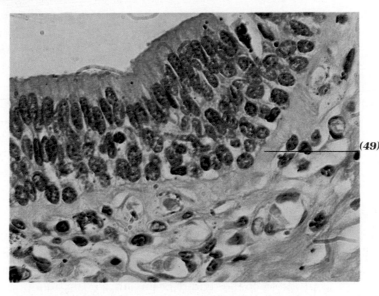

49 basement membrane

FIG. 2-14. Oblique section of the penile urethra, H and E stain (original magnification ×600).

light microscopy, a *(50)* _____ stratified epithelium appears to be composed of columnar cells, which extend through the entire thickness of the epithelium, and shorter rounder cells, which rest on the basement membrane and do not reach the surface of the epithelium (Fig. 2-14). Because of the varying heights of the cells, the dark-staining *(51)* _____ appear at different levels and thus give the appearance of a *(52)* _____ _____ (*simple, stratified*) epithelium.

50 pseudo

A basement membrane is an extracellular specialization located on the *(53)* _____ (*apical, basal*) surface of epithelia. The *(54)* _____ membrane is a supporting structure composed of a glycoprotein matrix in which are embedded collagen fibers. The thickness of the basement membrane varies. The basement membrane beneath the pseudostratified epithelium of the trachea is the most prominent in the body.

51 nuclei
52 stratified

53 basal
54 basement

At the electron microscope level, the basement *(55)* _____ can often be subdivided into a basal lamina and a reticular lamina. The basal lamina appears as a relatively homogeneous sheet, 50 nm to 1000 nm thick, that is in direct contact with the *(56)* _____ membrane of the most basal layer of epithelial cells. These epithelial cells produce both the *(57)* _____ matrix and the fine fibers that make up the *(58)* _____ lamina. The reticular lamina, located beneath the basal lamina, is produced by underlying connective tissue cells and not by the *(59)* _____ cells. It is composed of a glycoprotein *(60)* _____ and reticular fibers that are considered thicker than those of the overlying *(61)* _____.

55 membrane

56 plasma (cell)

57 glycoprotein
58 basal

59 epithelial
60 matrix
61 basal lamina

Pseudostratified epithelium is found lining the interlobar ducts of the salivary glands and the membranous portion of the male urethra.

Pseudostratified epithelium with cilia is located in the respiratory tract, part of the tympanic membrane, and the lacrimal sac.

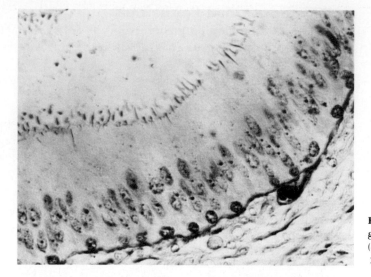

FIG. 2-15. Photomicrograph of the epididymis (original magnification ×300).

A surface modification unique to pseudostratified epithelium is stereocilia. Stereocilia lack the characteristic inner component of true cilia, *(62)* _____. Stereocilia are actually very long microvilli, but they lack the rigidity of the latter owing to a poorly developed supporting network of fine cytoplasmic filaments. Like that of microvilli, the function of stereocilia is to increase the *(63)* _____ capacity of the cell. Pseudostratified epithelium with stereocilia is found lining the vas deferens and epididymis (Fig. 2-15).

62 microtubules

63 absorptive

Exocrine Glands

After completing this chapter, you should be able to identify the following:

1 Glands   4 Goblet cells

2 Mucous cells   5 Ductal cells

3 Serous cells

Also, after completing this chapter, you should understand the following:

1 Secretory processes in multi-cellular glands   3 The function of ductal cells

2 The differences between uni-cellular and multicellular glands

---

The epithelia discussed in the preceding chapter are found covering an external or internal surface. Most glands of the body are also composed of an epithelium that has differentiated from such a covering epithelium. Cells and associations of cells specialized for secretion are called glands. There are two major categories of glands, defined according to the type of channel used to convey the **(1)** _____ _____ of the gland to its destination. Those that release their products into the blood or lymph system are called endocrine glands and will be discussed in Chapter 17. Glands that secrete either directly or by way of a system of excretory ducts onto an external or internal surface are called exocrine glands.

1 secretion

Exocrine Secretion

Merocrine

There are three mechanisms of exocrine secretion. Merocrine secretion is the most common method by which exocrine **(2)** _____ secrete. This process involves fusion between the membrane of the secretory granule and the plasma membrane. When this occurs, will there be any loss of cytoplasm during secretion? **(3)** _____. Merocrine secretion is also called exocytosis.

2 glands

3 no

Exocrine Glands

4 secretory granules

5 Golgi complex

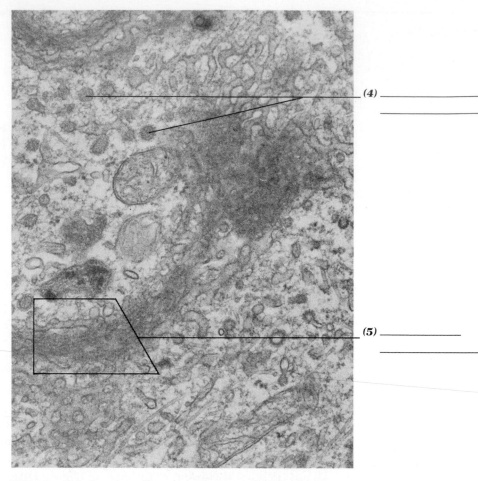

(4) _____

_____

(5) _____

_____

FIG. 3-1. EM of portion of human melanoma cell (original magnification ×35,000). (Courtesy of Dr. Gerd Maul, Wistar Institute, Philadelphia, Pennsylvania)

Production and release of a merocrine secretion involves polysomes, rough endoplasmic reticulum (rER), Golgi apparatus, and secretory granules (Fig. 3-1). The protein synthesized by the *(6)* _____ is secreted into the rER. Transitional vesicles bud off from the *(7)* __ __ __ and congregate at the *(8)* _____ or *(9)* _____ (*convex, concave*) face of the Golgi. A carbohydrate moiety is bound to the protein within the Golgi apparatus. The final product for secretion is released from the *(10)* _____ or *(11)* _____ (*convex, concave*) face of the Golgi as secretory granules. These secretory granules move through the cytoplasm with the aid of *(12)* _____. The secretory granule's membrane fuses with the *(13)* _____ _____, enabling it to release its secretory product. This process of expulsion of materials from cells is called *(14)* _____, also known as *(15)* _____ secretion.

6 polysomes
7 rER
8 forming
9 convex

10 maturing
11 concave

12 microtubules
13 plasma (cell) membrane

14 exocytosis
15 merocrine

Apocrine
In the mechanism of apocrine secretion, the plasma membrane fuses with itself rather than with a secretory granule, thus releasing a membrane-bound body containing varying amounts of *(16)* _____ (*cytoplasm, nucleus*) in addition to the secretory product. It therefore differs from *(17)* _____ secretion in that during the latter process there is no loss of cytoplasm. Mammary glands and apocrine sweat glands secrete by this method and by merocrine secretion.

16 cytoplasm

17 merocrine

Exocrine Secretion

Holocrine

Holocrine secretion consists of the release of whole cells into excretory ducts, or the total discharge of the contents of cells leading to their complete destruction. Sebaceous glands and the seminiferous tubules exhibit *(18)* _____ secretion.

18 holocrine

Goblet Cells

Exocrine glands may be unicellular or multicellular. Goblet cells are the only form of unicellular *(19)* _____ (*exocrine, endocrine*) glands (Fig. 3-2). The main body of the goblet cell is *(20)* _____ (*oval, flat*) and contains the secretory granules. Directly below the secretory granules is the *(21)* _____ and a thin expanse of cytoplasm. The secretory granules contain a protein–polysaccharide substance called mucin. Because mucin stains

19 exocrine
20 oval

21 nucleus

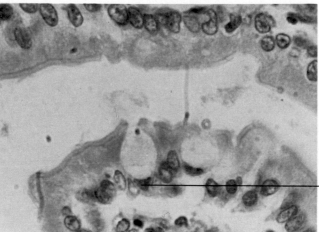

(22) _____
_____ _____ _____
_____

FIG. 3-2. Photomicrograph of the intestinal wall showing a goblet cell, hematoxylin-eosin (H and E) stain (original magnification ×500).

22 nucleus of goblet cell

poorly with hematoxylin-eosin (H and E) or is removed by fixation and embedding, the apical ends of goblet cells appear light. The secretory granules are released by exocytosis, also called *(23)* _____ secretion. Upon release, mucin is hydrated and forms mucus, a lubricating substance.

23 merocrine

Multicellular Glands

Multicellular glands have a variety of morphologies. The simplest form of multicellular *(24)* _____ gland is a sheet of epithelial cells that have become secretory in function. The gastric mucosa is an example of a secretory sheet. Slightly more complex than the secretory *(25)* _____ are intra-epithelial glands. These are small accumulations of *(26)* _____ cells that form their own lumen. Intra-epithelial glands can be found in the nasal mucosa and in the urethra. Like the goblet cells, the secretory sheets and *(27)* intra _____ glands usually secrete *(28)* _____ .

24 exocrine

25 sheet
26 secretory

27 epithelial
28 mucus

All other multicellular glands empty into a duct system that may be lined by either secretory or, in most cases, non-secretory epithelial cells. Glands in which the terminal, or secretory, portion(s) secrete into an unbranched common excretory duct are called simple exocrine glands. Glands that secrete into a branched duct system are called compound *(29)* _____ _____ (Fig. 3-3).

29 exocrine glands

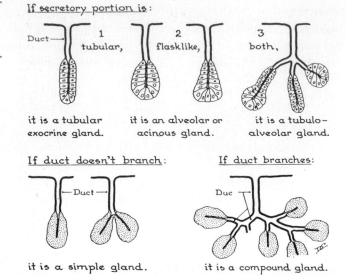

If secretory portion is:

1 tubular,

2 flasklike,

3 both,

it is a tubular exocrine gland.

it is an alveolar or acinous gland.

it is a tubulo-alveolar gland.

If duct doesn't branch:

If duct branches:

it is a simple gland.

it is a compound gland.

FIG. 3-3. Diagram showing the different kinds of secretory units of the exocrine glands and the difference between simple and compound glands.

Simple Glands

Simple glands have a *(30)* _____ *(branched, unbranched)* excretory duct. They are classified solely on the basis of the morphology of the terminal or *(31)* _____ portion.

If the secretory cells are grouped to form tubules, the gland is a simple *(32)* _____ gland. The intestinal glands of Lieberkühn, Brunner's glands of the duodenum, and the eccrine sweat glands are examples of this type.

If the secretory cells of the gland form a saclike or spherical unit rather than a slender *(33)* _____, then the gland is called an alveolar or acinar gland. Examples of simple alveolar glands are the common sebaceous glands and the meibomian glands of the eyelid, which are specialized sebaceous glands. Are the ducts of sebaceous glands branched? *(34)* _____

Compound Glands

A compound gland can be thought of as many simple glands all leading into a common excretory duct. As a result, the excretory duct system appears *(35)* _____ *(branched, unbranched)*. The secretory portion can be all tubular, that is, a compound *(36)* _____ gland *(e.g.,* renal tubules); all alveolar, that is, a *(37)* _____ _____ gland *(e.g.,* salivary glands); or mixed tubular and alveolar, that is, a compound tubulo-alveolar gland *(e.g.,* pancreas).

Mucous Glands

Within the secretory portion of any type gland, individual cells can also be classified according to the type of product they secrete (Fig. 3-4). These cells are said to be either serous or mucous. Mucous glands, as we have seen, secrete *(38)* _____, a protein–polysaccharide complex that becomes hydrated after secretion to produce *(39)* _____, a lubricating or protective material. Unicellular mucous glands are referred to as *(40)* _____ cells. Mucous cells, when they compose the *(41)* _____ portion of a gland, have distinct cell borders and a relatively wide glandular lumen.

30 *unbranched*

31 *secretory*

32 *tubular*

33 *tubule*

34 *no*

35 *branched*
36 *tubular*
37 *compound alveolar*

38 *mucin*
39 *mucus*
40 *goblet*
41 *secretory (terminal)*

Mucous Glands

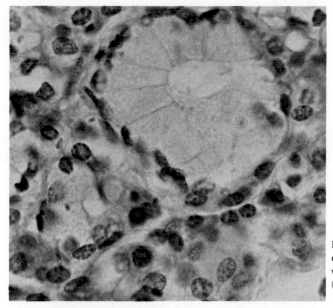

FIG. 3-4. Photomicrograph of mucous cells from a salivary gland, H and E stain (original magnification ×500).

Serous Glands

Serous cells secrete a watery fluid that is often rich in proteins, especially enzymes (Fig. 3-5). Serous cells are found most commonly in compound exocrine

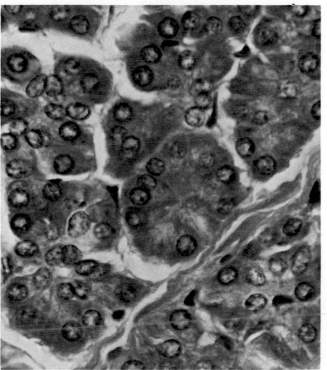

FIG. 3-5. Photomicrograph of serous cells from a salivary gland, H and E stain (original magnification ×500).

glands. Do serous cells stain darker or lighter than mucous cells in an H and E preparation? *(42)* _____. The intense basophilia of serous cells is caused by the abundance of *(43)* _____ located on the *(44)* _____ endoplasmic reticulum. The nucleus is usually spherical, rather

42 darker
43 polysomes (ribosomes)
44 rough

Exocrine Glands

45 *mucous*

46 *difficult*

47 *indistinguishable*

48 *distinct*

than greatly flattened as it is in *(45)* _____ cells. The serous cell nucleus is situated in the basal half of the cell. The apex of the cell may stain somewhat eosinophilic because of the relative absence of organelles and the extraction of secretory material.

When serous cells make up the secretory portion of a gland, it is *(46)* _____ (*easy, difficult*) to see a lumen. The lateral cell borders of serous cells in a gland are relatively *(47)* _____ (*distinguishable, indistinguishable*). This is in contrast to glands composed of mucous cells where the lumen is often quite visible and the lateral cell borders are more *(48)* _____.

Mucoserous Glands

Some exocrine glands deliver both serous and mucous secretions through their ducts (Fig. 3-6). These are called mucoserous or mixed glands. Morphologically,

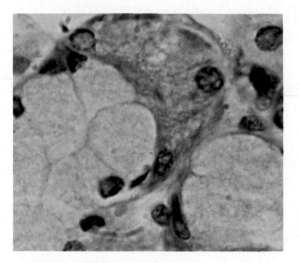

FIG. 3-6. Photomicrograph of mucous cells and serous demilunes, H and E stain (original magnification ×500).

these glands often consist of mucous secretory units capped by crescent-shaped groups of serous cells. These crescent-shaped caps are called *(49)* _____ (*mucous, serous*) demilunes.

49 *serous*

Excretory Ducts

The excretory duct system of exocrine glands is usually lined with nonsecretory

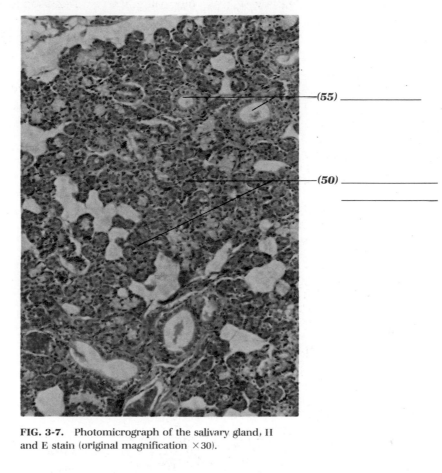

(55) _____

(50) _____

_____

FIG. 3-7. Photomicrograph of the salivary gland, H and E stain (original magnification ×30).

50 *serous glands*

cells and conveys the *(51)* _____ to the epithelial surface (Fig. 3-7). The duct cells often modify the secretion by resorbing fluid or ions or both. Such cells might be expected to stain more eosinophilic than the secretory cells because of the presence of greater numbers of *(52)* _____ in their cytoplasms. What surface specializations would you expect to see in such absorptive cells? *(53)* _____. The largest ducts have a simple or stratified *(54)* _____ epithelium, while smaller ducts have varying heights of cuboidal epithelium.

51 *secretion*

52 *mitochondria*

53 *microvilli*
54 *cuboidal (columnar)*
55 *ducts*

4

Connective Tissue

After completing this chapter, you should be able to identify the following:

1 Loose connective tissue
2 Dense connective tissue
3 Dense irregular connective tissue
4 Elastic fibers

5 Reticular fibers
6 Collagen fibers
7 Mast cells
8 Macrophages
9 Plasma cells

Also, after completing this chapter, you should understand the following:

1 The importance of all three types of fibers
2 The importance of ground substance

3 The function of different connective tissues

Connective tissues are composed of fixed or wandering cells (or both) embedded in large amounts of extracellular materials. Are epithelia embedded in large amounts of extracellular materials? *(1)* _____. Among their many functions, connective tissues provide support for the other body tissues. They are subdivided into the *specialized connective tissues* and *connective tissue proper*, according to the types of fixed or wandering *(2)* _____ present and the nature of the

1 no

(3) _____ material. Specialized connective tissues include adipose tissue, cartilage, bone, and blood, while

2 cells

3 extracellular

(4) _____ _____ _____ occupies the regions between all other organs and tissues, and thus provides support for them. Specialized connective tissues will be discussed in separate chapters.

4 connective tissue proper

All connective tissues are derived from a primordial embryonic tissue called mesenchyma. The characteristics of mesenchyma are similar to those of connective tissue, in that it is composed of cells embedded in

(5) _____ materials. The differentiation of mesenchyma will result in the formation of the various types of

5 extracellular

(6) _____ _____ previously listed. Mesenchymal cells will develop into the cells specific for each variety of connective tissue.

6 connective tissues

Connective tissue proper consists of extracellular fibers embedded in an amorphous ground substance, plus wandering and fixed *(7)* _____. The function of connective tissue *(8)* _____ is related to both its structure and location. The subclassification of connective tissue proper is determined by whether the *(9)* _____ fibers are loosely woven or

7 cells

8 proper

densely packed. There are three categories of *(10)* _____ _____

9 extracellular

_____ _____: loose (or areolar), dense irregular, and dense regular connective tissue. Bear in mind that this classification is not exact and the various types of connective tissue proper grade into one another through

10 connective tissue proper

transitional forms.

11 *areolar*
12 *fibers*

13 *connective*

14 *extracellular*

Loose Connective Tissue

Loose connective tissue, also called **(11)** _____ connective tissue, consists of loosely interwoven **(12)** _____ embedded in a ground substance along with various cell types. Generally, loose connective tissue is found beneath all covering epithelia and between muscles. In these locations it is usually referred to as a fascia. Loose **(13)** _____ tissue is also diffusely located throughout the body. As in all connective tissues, both fibers and ground substance are **(14)** _____ (*intracellular, extracellular*). In most preparations, the ground substance is not visible and the most obvious component is the extracellular fibers (Fig. 4-1).

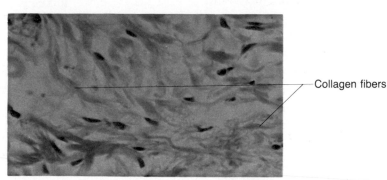
Collagen fibers

FIG. 4-1. Photomicrograph of loose connective tissue, hematoxylin-eosin (H and E) stain (original magnification ×200).

Fibers

COLLAGENOUS FIBER There are three types of fibers: collagenous, elastic, and reticular. Collagenous fibers are found in virtually all connective tissues in varying amounts. In loose connective tissue, collagenous fibers appear as wavy structures of various diameters, staining **(15)** _____, and having a **(16)** _____ (*random, organized*) arrangement with respect to one another. Collagenous fibers are somewhat flexible and impart a great tensile strength and resistance. They are composed of the protein collagen.

15 *eosinophilic*
16 *random*

ELASTIC FIBERS Elastic fibers can stretch longitudinally and can recoil after stretching, returning connective tissue to its original shape. Can collagen fibers do this? **(17)** _____. Elastic fibers appear as branching networks and are thicker than most **(18)** _____ fibers. The components of elastic fibers are bundles of microfilaments and an amorphous protein, elastin. Within a fiber, elastin molecules are less organized than the **(19)** _____ molecules that make up collagenous fibers. Elastic fibers are not as abundant as collagenous fibers in loose connective tissue.

17 *no*
18 *collagenous*

19 *collagen*

RETICULAR FIBERS Reticular fibers are composed of collagen, yet are thinner than both **(20)** _____ and **(21)** _____ fibers (Fig. 4-2). Reticular fibers are arranged to form a delicate meshwork. Reticular fibers and collagen fibers have a similar composition: Both are composed of the protein, **(22)** _____.

20 *collagenous*
21 *elastic*

22 *collagen*

Loose Connective Tissue

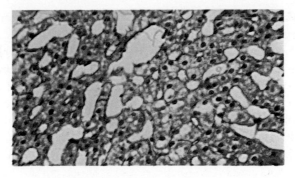

FIG. 4-2. Photomicrograph of a liver, H and E with reticular stain (original magnification ×250).

Ground Substance

The other extracellular component beside the fibers is *(23)* _____ _____. Also called the matrix, it is composed of glycosamino-glycans (GAGS) and glycoprotein. The chemical composition of ground substance is responsible for a thin gellike property that allows for the passage of nutrients. How does the ground substance appear in most preparations? *(24)* _____ _____.

23 *ground substance*

Fibroblasts

24 *not visible in most*
preparations

There are fixed and wandering cells embedded in the *(25)* _____ _____ (Fig. 4-3). The most common fixed cells in connective

25 *ground substance*

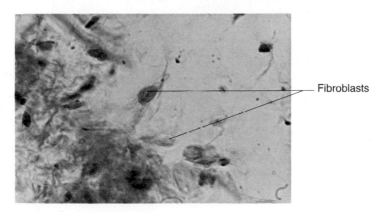

Fibroblasts

FIG. 4-3. Photomicrograph of a loose connective tissue, H and E stain (original magnification ×125).

tissue are the fibroblasts (Fig. 4-4). They are fusiform in shape; however, the cytoplasm and cell outline are difficult to delineate. Fibroblasts are usually identified by their oval *(26)* _____ and prominent nucleolus. The shape of the nucleus will very often appear irregular because of the plane of section.

26 *nucleus*

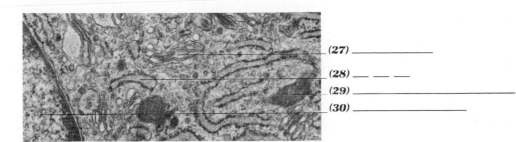

(27) _____

(28) __ __ __

(29) _____

(30) _____

FIG. 4-4. Electron micrograph (EM) of a part of an active fibroblast (original magnification ×42,000).

27 *Golgi*
28 *rER*
29 *mitochondrion*
30 *nucleus*

Connective Tissue

31 *fibers*
32 *ground substance*
33 *protein*
34 *basophilic*
35 *fibroblast*
36 *eosinophilia*
37 *branching*

38 *fibroblasts*

The fibroblasts are responsible for the production of both extracellular components, the (31) _____ and the (32) _____ _____. When actively synthesizing (33) _____ (*lipid, protein, phosphate*) for the extracellular components, fibroblasts stain (34) _____. Another feature of an active (35) _____ is extensive cytoplasmic branching. An inactive fibroblast will have a tendency toward (36) _____ (*eosinophilia, basophilia*) and exhibit less (37) _____ of the cytoplasm.

Macrophages

The only other fixed cells in connective tissue besides the (38) _____ are the fixed macrophages (Fig. 4-5). Also called

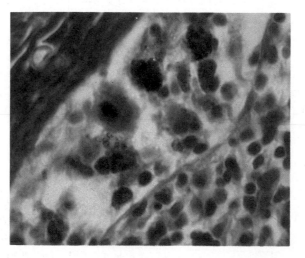

FIG. 4-5. Photomicrograph of macrophages, Mallory's triple stain (original magnification × 125).

39 *macrophage (histiocyte)*

40 *eccentric*

41 *plasma (cell) membrane*

42 *cytoplasm*
43 *lysosome*
44 *phagosomes*
45 *lysosomes*

histiocytes, macrophages are irregular in shape and have a pale-staining cytoplasm. The nucleus of the (39) _____ stains dark, and is smaller than the nucleus of the fibroblast. Usually, the macrophage's nucleus is (40) _____ (*central, eccentric*) in location, and may appear indented. The main function of macrophages is phagocytosis and destruction of debris and bacteria from the extracellular environment. Phagocytosis is the process of engulfing particles from the environment; therefore, the process involves invaginations of the (41) _____ _____. As a result of this invagination, saclike structures containing the extracellular substance are formed in the (42) _____. These saclike structures, called phagosomes, fuse with the digestive organelles of the cell, the (43) _____. Thus, a very active macrophage has many (44) _____ and (45) _____ in its cytoplasm. When activated, fixed macrophages become wandering macrophages and are extremely phagocytic. By light microscopy, less active macrophages may be difficult to distinguish from fibroblasts unless they have previously ingested some type of visible particulate matter.

Mast Cells

Most of the wandering cells of loose connective tissue (monocytes, lymphocytes, and granulocytes) are of the blood series and will be discussed in Chapter 7. Mast cells are wandering cells that develop from the cells of the primordial embryonic tissue, *(46)* _____. Mast cells typically contain large round granules that can be made to stain bright (Fig. 4-6). These character-

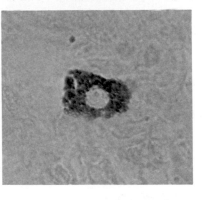

46 mesenchyma

FIG. 4-6. Photomicrograph of a mast cell (original magnification ×500).

istic granules, like secretory granules, are each surrounded by a *(47)* _____ and contain potent pharmacologic mediators involved in the inflammatory response. The appropriate stimulus triggers the release of the granules by the process of *(48)* _____ (Fig. 4-7). The nucleus of the mast cell is located *(49)* _____ and is surrounded by the numerous *(50)* _____. (You should finish #52 at this point.)

47 membrane

48 exocytosis
49 centrally
50 granules

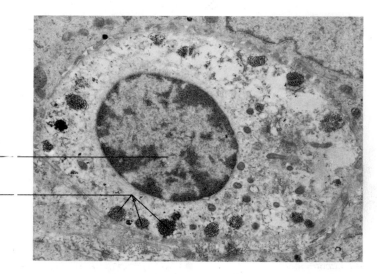

(51) _____

(52) _____

51 nucleus

52 granules

FIG. 4-7. EM of a partially degranulated mast cell.

Plasma Cells

A cell type that is relatively uncommon in typical connective tissue is the plasma cell (Fig. 4-8). Plasma cells themselves do not emigrate from the blood but they

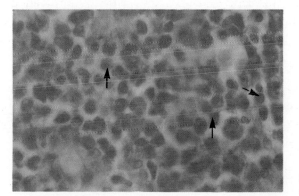

FIG. 4-8. Photomicrograph of plasma cells (*arrows*).

53 *connective tissue*

54 *eccentric*
55 *basophilic*

56 *rER*

57 *protein*
58 *loose (areolar)*

59 *covering*

60 *dense*
61 *dense*
62 *loose*
63 *loose*

64 *loose*

65 *greater*

differentiate in the *(53)* _____ _____ from the lymphocytes that have done so. The nucleus of the plasma cell is *(54)* _____ (*central, eccentric*) in position, and the chromatin is arranged in a cartwheel pattern. The *(55)* _____ (*eosinophilic, basophilic*)-staining cytoplasm is occupied by an extensive system of rER and a great number of voluminous Golgi complexes. Beside the ribosomes on the *(56)* __ __ __, there are a great number of free ribosomes in the cytoplasm. The abundant ribosomes and the highly developed rER are involved in the synthesis of a special *(57)* _____ that aids in the body's humoral defenses.

All the components of *(58)* _____ connective tissue have been discussed. Note that this type of connective tissue can be found beneath any layer of *(59)* _____ epithelium.

Dense Irregular Connective Tissue

Dense irregular connective tissue has the same elements as loose connective tissue, but in different proportions. For each component of connective tissue, check the tissue type in which it is more abundant:

Extracellular fibers *(60)* _____ (*dense, loose*)
Fiber bundles *(61)* _____ (*dense, loose*)
Ground substance *(62)* _____ (*dense, loose*)
Cells *(63)* _____ (*dense, loose*)

The fibers of dense irregular connective tissue, like those of *(64)* _____ connective tissue, are randomly oriented (Fig. 4-9). Because of the

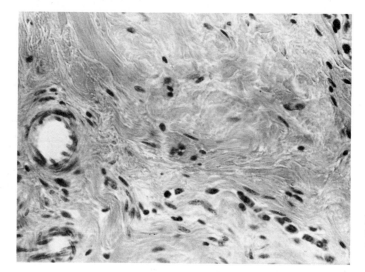

FIG. 4-9. Photomicrograph of dense irregular connective tissue (original magnification ×200).

(65) _____ (*greater, lesser*) number of collagen fibers, dense irregular connective tissue is far less flexible and is extremely resistant to stretch. This type of connective tissue is found forming the capsules of organs; sheaths of tendons; the outer wrapping of tubular organs, nerves, and muscles; and beneath the loose connective tissue of the skin.

Dense Regular Connective Tissue

Dense Regular
Connective Tissue

Dense regular connective tissue offers the greatest resistance to stretch (Fig. 4-10).

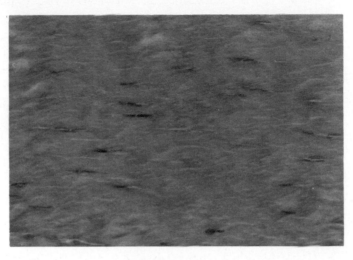

FIG. 4-10. Photomicrograph of dense regular connective tissue, H and E stain (original magnification ×125).

Virtually the only cells present in dense regular connective tissue are the cells that produce the extracellular substances, the *(66)* _____. The fiber bundles, most of which are collagenous, are oriented parallel to one another, and may appear either straight or wavy. Between the fiber bundles appear the dark and flattened *(67)* _____ of the fibroblasts. Tendons consist solely of dense regular connective tissue, but have a covering sheath of *(68)* _____ _____ connective tissue. Dense regular connective tissue is found in aponeuroses and is the major component of ligaments.

66 *fibroblasts*

67 *nuclei*

68 *dense irregular*

Elastic Connective Tissue

A special type of connective tissue proper that has elastic fibers as its primary component is elastic connective tissue. What are the properties of elastic fibers? *(69)* _____
_____
_____. Elastic connective tissue is found in the walls of hollow organs that undergo distension. The elastic fibers are often arranged in concentric lamellae, as in the largest arteries and parts of the heart. As in other connective tissues, the elastic fibers are embedded in *(70)* _____ _____. The components of both fibers and ground substance are produced by *(71)* _____.

69 *can stretch and recoil; thicker fiber bundles, forming branching networks*

70 *ground substance*
71 *fibroblasts*

Reticular Connective Tissue

Reticular connective tissue, another type of connective tissue proper, consists mainly of reticular fibers. How are reticular fibers organized? *(72)* _____ What type of protein are reticular fibers composed of? *(73)* _____. There are a large number of free cells found in reticular connective tissue. This type of connective tissue is found around the sinusoids of the liver (see Fig. 4-2) and forms the stroma of lymphatic and hematopoietic organs.

72 *form a delicate meshwork*
73 *collagen*

5   Adipose Tissue

After completing this chapter, you should be able to identify the following:
1 Adipocytes   2 Brown adipose tissue

Also, after completing this chapter, you should understand the following:
1 The distribution of adipose tissue   2 The function of both white and brown fat

---

Adipose tissue, commonly referred to as fat, is considered a specialized type of connective tissue. Adipose tissue is composed primarily of lipid-filled cells called adipocytes enclosed in a fine mesh of reticular fibers. There are two distinct types of *(1)* _____ tissue that differ in color, distribution in the body, and vascularity. The two types are white *(2)* _____ _____, which under gross observation appears white or yellow, and brown *(3)* _____ _____, which appears *(4)* _____.

1 adipose
2 adipose tissue

White Adipose Tissue

3 adipose tissue

4 brown

White adipose tissue is far more abundant than *(5)* _____ adipose tissue (Fig. 5-1). The cells of adipose tissue, which are called *(6)* _____, are large (as great as 120 μ in diameter in mature white fat), and assume either a spherical shape or, by mutual deformation, a polyhedral shape. In mature white adipose tissues, the nucleus of the *(7)* _____ is displaced to the *(8)* _____ (*periphery, center*) of the cell by a large single droplet of lipid filling the cytoplasm.

5 brown

6 adipocytes

7 adipocyte
8 periphery

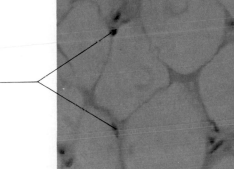

(9) _____

9 nuclei

FIG. 5-1. Photomicrograph of white adi pose tissue, hematoxylin-eosin (H and E) stain (original magnification ×250).

Adipose Tissue

The lipid, consisting of triglycerides, exists as a single droplet, and thus adipose cells of this kind are described as *(10)* _____ (*unilocular, multilocular*). The lipid is extracted by most fixation procedures; therefore, in a normal hematoxylin-eosin (H and E) stain, it will appear empty.

10 unilocular

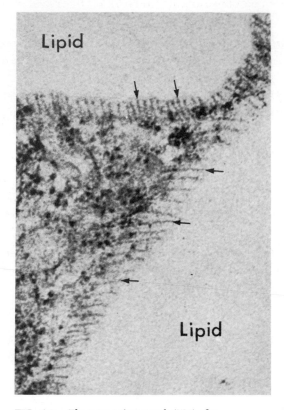

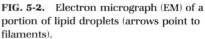

FIG. 5-2. Electron micrograph (EM) of a portion of lipid droplets (arrows point to filaments).

The droplet of *(11)* _____ is not enclosed by a membrane, but is often separated from the surrounding cytoplasm by 5-μ diameter filaments arranged around its periphery in an orderly array (Fig. 5-2). Each adipocyte is surrounded by a layer of glycoprotein that corresponds both functionally and morphologically to the boundary layer of epithelia, the basal *(12)* _____.

11 lipid

Adipocytes, or *(13)* _____ cells, are held together by a delicate meshwork of recticular fibers that form the stroma or supporting elements of the tissue. Reticular fibers are made of the protein *(14)* _____. Between adipocytes are capillaries that course through the network of *(15)* _____ _____ that support the tissue.

12 lamina
13 adipose (fat)

White adipose tissue, consisting of adipocytes that have an eccentric *(16)* _____, a thin rim of *(17)* _____, and which are enmeshed in *(18)* _____ _____, is found throughout the body. White adipose tissue serves as a padding and provides resistance to shock for the internal organs it surrounds. Also, white *(19)* _____ _____ is important as a store of metabolizable lipid. Either deposition or mobilization of the *(20)* _____ composing the lipid can occur in response to the energy demands of the person.

14 collagen

15 reticular fibers

16 nucleus
17 cytoplasm
18 reticular fibers
19 adipose tissue

20 triglyceride

21 *brown*

22 *white adipose*

Brown Adipose Tissue

Brown adipose or brown fat, as its name implies, is *(21)* _____ in color under gross observation. Its adipocytes are approximately one half the size of those found in *(22)* _____ _____ tissue and have proportionately more cytoplasm per cell (Fig. 5-3). The nuclei of brown fat adipocytes are

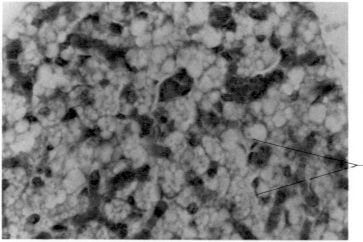

— Capillary

FIG. 5-3. Photomicrograph of brown adipose tissue, H and E stain (original magnification ×125).

less eccentric than those in mature white fat. The cytoplasm of brown *(23)* _____ _____ contains a greater number of spherical mitochondria in addition to a normal complement of the other organelles. Electron micrographs (EMs) show that the mitochondria occupy a very large part of the *(24)* _____ (*nucleoplasm, cytoplasm*) and have numerous cristae. Mitochondria, which usually function to produce *(25)* _____, are modified in brown adipocytes to generate heat.

23 *adipose tissue*

Usually polygonal in shape, the adipocytes of brown *(26)* _____ _____ contain *(27)* _____ (*more than one, one*) lipid droplet of *(28)* _____ glycerides and therefore are *(29)* _____ locular cells (Fig. 5-4). As with white adipose tissue, the

24 *cytoplasm*
25 *energy*

26 *adipose tissue*
27 *more than one*
28 *tri*
29 *multi*

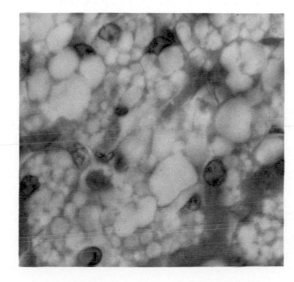

FIG. 5-4. Photomicrograph of brown adipose tissue, H and E stain (original magnification ×300).

Adipose Tissue

30 smaller
31 reticular

32 white adipose

33 heat
34 mitochondria
35 polyhedral

36 adipose

(30) _____ (smaller, larger) adipocytes of brown adipose tissue are held together by (31) _____ fibers. The supporting meshwork contains a rich supply of capillaries; the adipocytes of brown adipose tissue are therefore in a more intimate association with the capillaries than those of the (32) _____ _____ tissue. This close association with a rich blood supply enables the adipose cells to warm up the blood easily by generating (33) _____ through the action of the modified (34) _____.

Brown adipocytes, usually (35) _____ (spherical, polyhedral) do not develop in new areas after birth. New deposits of white (36) _____ tissue may however develop during postnatal life. The new deposits are usually located in loose connective tissue. Identifiable brown fat is very uncommon in human adults, but in fetuses and newborns it may occur in the axillae, in the nape and posterior triangle of the neck, near the thyroid, along the carotid sheath, and at the hilus of the kidney.

6

Bone and Cartilage

After completing this chapter, you should be able to identify the following:

1 Cartilage: hyaline, elastic, and fibrocartilage
2 Chondroblasts
3 Bone
4 Osteoblasts
5 Osteocytes
6 Osteoclasts
7 Periosteum

Also, after completing this chapter, you should understand the following:

1 The differences between cartilage and bone
2 The remodeling of bone
3 The process of intramembranous bone formation
4 The process of endochondral bone formation

Bone and cartilage are specialized connective tissues. Other specialized connective tissues include (1) _____ _____ and (2) _____. Connective tissue is characterized by specialized cells embedded in (3) _____ _____.

    The cells of cartilage and bone are found in spaces called lacunae ("small pits"), and thus are separated from the surrounding extracellular material. The extracellular component is composed of the matrix, also called the (4) _____ _____, and the extracellular fibers such as (5) _____ or (6) _____. These components are present in both bone and cartilage. As with all connective tissues, bone and cartilage are derived from a primordial embryonic tissue called (7) _____.

    Bone differs from cartilage in various ways. Bone is calcified but cartilage is not. The extracellular materials of bone have an increased proportion of fibers in relation to the (8) _____ _____ or matrix. Because (9) _____ is not calcified, nutrients can diffuse through the (10) _____ to reach the cells. Is this true of connective tissues? (11) _____. As a result of the large diffusion capacity, capillaries are not found within the cartilage matrix but only within the covering tissue, the perichondrium. Because bone is calcified, nutrients cannot reach the cells by (12) _____, and must be carried by blood vessels that traverse the bone substance. The cells of bone, which lie in spaces called (13) _____, must exist within 0.1 mm to 0.3 mm of a capillary or free surface in order to receive nutrients.

1 adipose tissue
2 blood
3 extracellular material (ground substance)

4 ground substance
5 collagen
6 elastin

7 mesenchyma

8 ground substance
9 cartilage
10 matrix
11 yes

12 diffusion

13 lacunae

Cartilage

Cartilage is essential for the growth of long bones, both before and after birth. It also functions to separate soft tissues and to provide a smooth sliding surface for joints (Fig. 6-1).

The mature cartilage cells, which exist in spaces called lacunae, are called chondrocytes. The cells that synthesize the matrix and fibers are called *(14)* _____ blasts. The ground substance, or chondromucoprotein, is composed of *(15)* glycos _____ and *(16)* _____ protein. Differences in the types and proportions of extracellular fibers determine the type of cartilage: hyaline, elastic, or fibrocartilage. Covering the cartilage in most cases is a layer of dense irregular connective tissue, the *(17)* peri _____.

14 chondro
15 aminoglycans
16 glyco

17 chondrium

18 lacunae with chondrocytes

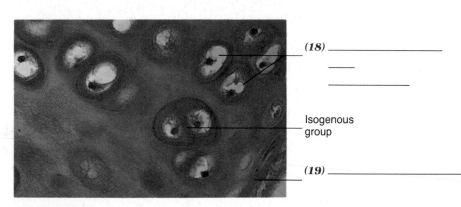

(18) _____
_____
_____

Isogenous group

(19) _____

FIG. 6-1. Photomicrograph of hyaline cartilage (original magnification ×200).

19 perichondrium

Chondroblasts

Chondroblasts, like all connective tissue cells, differentiate from embryonic *(20)* _____ cells. These cells are usually located in the inner layer of the covering tissue, the *(21)* _____, and are *(22)* _____ *(elliptic, round)*. Like the principal cells of loose connective tissue, the *(23)* _____, *(24)* chondro _____ are responsible for synthesizing both the extracellular fibers and the *(25)* _____ _____. Consequently, chondroblasts show well-developed *(26)* _____ _____ _____ and Golgi apparatus. The plasma membrane has numerous invaginations that function to increase *(27)* _____ _____, facilitating metabolic exchange in these active cells. In a hematoxylin-eosin (H and E) preparation, these cells stain *(28)* _____ *(basophilic, eosinophilic)*.

20 mesenchymal
21 perichondrium
22 elliptic
23 fibroblasts
24 blasts
25 ground substance
26 rough endoplasmic reticulum (rER)

27 surface area

28 basophilic

Cartilage

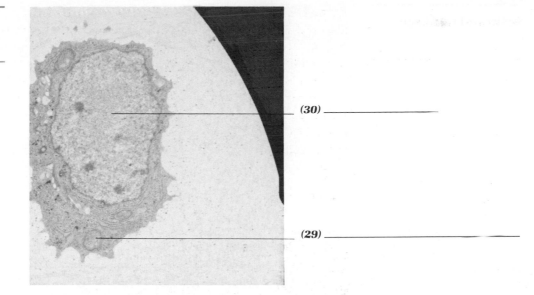

(30) _____

(29) _____

29 *mitochondrion*
30 *nucleus*

FIG. 6-2.   EM of a chondrocyte.

The chondroblasts eventually become surrounded by the extracellular materials they have synthesized and secreted. These cells are now referred to as mature cartilage cells, or *(31)* _____ _____ (Fig. 6-2). *In vivo,* these cells entirely fill the spaces or *(32)* _____. Chondrocytes take on a *(33)* _____ (*round, linear*) shape and have a rounded nucleus. One or more nucleoli may be observed. Because these cells are also actively synthesizing extracellular materials, their cytoplasm will stain *(34)* _____. Groups of two or more chondrocytes that exist closely apposed are called isogenous groups.

31 *chondrocytes*
32 *lacunae*
33 *round*

34 *basophilic*

Matrix
The matrix is mainly composed of collagen fibers and fibrils embedded in the ground substance. Collagen exists predominantly as submicroscopic fibrils and thus does not stain. The ground substance of cartilage, also called
(35) _____, appears
(36) _____ (*lighter, darker*) staining in areas surrounding lacunae. These areas of matrix are referred to as the capsules or territorial matrices. They contain freshly synthesized matrix with a high concentration of chondromucoprotein. This constitutes one mechanism of cartilage growth, called interstitial growth (growth from within). The chondrocytes divide, forming small groups of cells called *(37)* _____ groups. These cells will then synthesize and secrete fresh matrix, which will push the cells apart and expand the width of cartilage.

35 *chondromucoprotein*
36 *darker*

37 *isogenous*

Perichondrium
The layer found covering cartilage in most places is called the
(38) _____ (Fig. 6-3). It is subdivided into two layers: an outer layer of dense *(39)* _____ connective tissue and the inner layer, the chondrogenic layer, which contains cells capable of differentiating into chondroblasts. This provides for a second and more important means of cartilage growth, appositional growth. Appositional growth involves differentiation

38 *perichondrium*
39 *irregular*

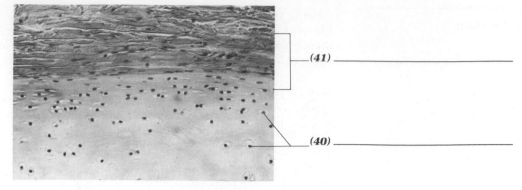

(41) _____

(40) _____

FIG. 6-3. Photomicrograph of hyaline cartilage (original magnification ×125).

40 *chondrocytes*
41 *perichondrium*

of the chondrogenic cells of the *(42)* _____ (*outer, inner*) layer of the perichondrium into *(43)* <u>chondro</u>_____, which synthesize the ground substance and fibers, increasing the width of the cartilage. Because blood vessels are only located in the inner layer of perichondrium and not within the cartilage matrix, the chondrocytes must receive their nutrients through the process of *(44)* _____. This limits the appositional growth capabilities of cartilage, since the diffusion capacity is limited.

42 *inner*
43 *blasts*

Hyaline Cartilage

Hyaline cartilage is the most common type in the body. In the embryo, it serves as a temporary skeleton and is replaced by bone in most places during growth and development, both before and after birth. Hyaline cartilage is essential for the growth of long bones, and in the adult provides a smooth surface (the articular surface) to facilitate movement in the *(45)* _____ (Fig. 6-4). Hyaline

44 *diffusion*

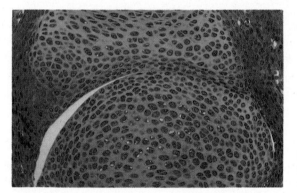

FIG. 6-4. Photomicrograph of articular cartilage, hematoxylin-eosin (H and E) stain (original magnification ×30).

45 *joint*

(46) _____ is found in parts of the larynx, trachea, and bronchi; the anterior end of the nose; and the ventral ends of the ribs. Perichondrium covers hyaline cartilage in all places listed, except the smooth surface of the joints, the *(47)* _____ surface.

Hyaline cartilage is the prototype cartilage and is representative of all the components previously described.

46 *cartilage*

47 *articular*

Cartilage

48 hyaline
49 collagenous

Elastic Cartilage

Elastic cartilage differs from *(48)* _____ cartilage in that two types of fibers, elastic and *(49)* _____ fibers, are synthesized by the chondroblasts of elastic cartilage (Fig. 6-5). The abundant network of elastic fibers

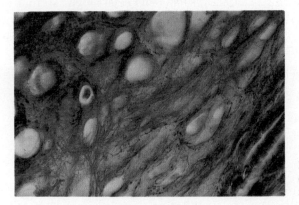

FIG. 6-5. Photomicrograph of elastic cartilage, Kornhauser quad stain (original magnification ×125).

within the matrix are continuous with the perichondrium. Elastic fibers are composed of the protein *(50)* _____. Elastic cartilage is more flexible and resilient than hyaline cartilage, and is found in areas where this is required. It is located in the auricles of the ear, in the walls of the internal auditory canal and eustachean tube, in the epiglottis, and in some of the laryngeal cartilages.

50 elastin

Fibrocartilage

Fibrocartilage may be considered a transitional form between hyaline cartilage and the component of tendon, *(51)* _____ connective tissue. It is found in intervertebral disks, in the attachments of certain ligaments, and in the symphysis pubis. Fibrocartilage is extremely resistant to stretch, because of the great amount of *(52)* _____ fibers and the scarcity of *(53)* _____ fibers. The fibers can be oriented randomly or in columns aligned with rows of chondrocytes. There is very little ground substance in fibrocartilage, as it is located mostly around lacunae in an area called the *(54)* _____ matrix. There is no perichondrium associated with fibrocartilage.

51 dense regular

52 collagenous
53 elastic

54 territorial

Bone

Bone also differentiates from embryonic *(55)* _____. Unlike cartilage, bone is *(56)* _____. This imparts tremendous rigidity and makes bone the strongest tissue in the body. As a result of this rigidity, bone can only grow by the appositional method and not by the *(57)* _____ method, both of which are employed by cartilage. Bone is the main component of the skeleton, supporting fleshy structures and protecting vital organs, such as those in the cranial and thoracic cavities. Bone marrow cavities, the site of differentiation of the blood cells, are located within bone.

55 mesenchyma
56 calcified

57 interstitial

Bone and Cartilage

The extracellular matrix of bone is calcified, containing both organic and inorganic components (Fig. 6-6). The organic materials are synthesized by *(58)* osteo _____; once these cells are surrounded by the matrix, they are referred to as *(59)* osteo _____ and exist in spaces called *(60)* _____. The cells exist singly, so that unlike cartilage there are no *(61)* _____ groups. Osteoclasts are multinucleate cells that participate in the remodeling of bone. The connective tissue covering the surface of

58 *blasts*
59 *cytes*
60 *lacunae*
61 *isogenous*

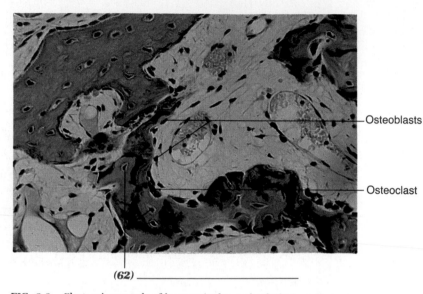

Osteoblasts

Osteoclast

(62) _____

FIG. 6-6. Photomicrograph of bone spicules and calcified cartilage, H and E stain (original magnification × 125).

62 *osteocytes*

bone is called the *(63)* _____ osteum. Because bone contains marrow cavities, there is a lining for the internal surface called the endosteum.

Osteoblasts

63 *peri*

The osteoblast is similar to the chondroblast in that it also synthesizes and secretes collagenous fibers and *(64)* _____ _____. These cells are usually located along the surface of the forming bone and are arranged side by side. The nucleus is large and rounded, and the *(65)* _____ (*basophilic, acidophilic*) cytoplasm indicates active protein synthesis. Osteoblasts have numerous long cell processes that contain longitudinally arranged actin filaments (Fig. 6-7). Secretion occurs from all cell

64 *ground substance*

65 *basophilic*

Bone

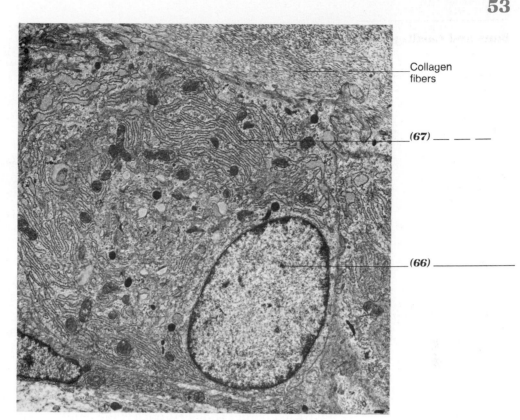

Collagen fibers

(67) —— —— ——

(66) _____

FIG. 6-7. EM of an osteoblast (original magnification ×9000).

66 nucleus
67 rER

surfaces, and both the cell body and processes become surrounded by the extracellular materials. Osteoblasts may be in contact with each other through their cell processes, which are joined by a tight junction, or **(68)** _____ ___ _____. The spaces occupied by the processes are called canaliculi.

68 zonula occludens

Osteocytes

Osteocytes are **(69)** _____ (*more, less*) basophilic than osteoblasts and have a **(70)** _____(*rounded, elongate*) shape. *In vivo*, the osteocytes occupy the entire lacuna. Is this true of chondrocytes? **(71)** _____. The cell processes, located in the **(72)** _____, enable the osteocytes to communicate with each other and spread to within **(73)** _____ mm to **(74)** _____ mm of a capillary or free surface.

69 less
70 elongate
71 yes
72 canaliculi
73 0.1
74 0.3

Osteoclasts

Osteoclasts are very large motile cells with **(75)** _____ (*one, more than one*) nucleus. They appear on the surface of bone where the normal remodeling process occurs, and are found within shallow pits in the matrix called Howship's (absorption) lacunae. Osteoclasts function by first decalcifying the bone (removing the inorganic material), and then breaking down and resorbing the **(76)** _____ (*collagen, elastic*) fibers and ground substance. This is accomplished through the elaboration of enzymes. Where decalcification has occurred, the **(77)** _____ fibers that remain may appear as a "brush border" along the bone–osteoclast interface. This is a different brush border than is found on simple cuboidal epithelium, which is composed of **(78)** _____. Osteoclasts are now thought to be derived from blood-borne monocytes (see Chap. 7).

75 more than one

76 collagen

77 collagen

78 microvilli

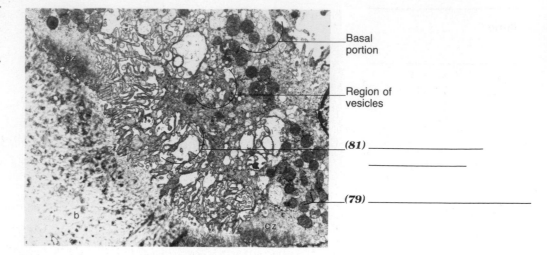

Basal portion

Region of vesicles

(81) _____

_____

(79) _____

FIG. 6-8. EM of a part of an osteoclast (*b:* bone; *CZ:* clear zone; original magnification ×8500).

The plasma membrane of osteoclasts is thrown into folds that serve to increase *(80)* _____ _____; this area is referred to as the ruffled border and is in direct contact with the bone (Fig. 6-8). This interface between the ruffled border and bone is the site of bone resorption. The cytoplasm beneath the *(82)* _____ border is called the clear zone; it surrounds the ruffled border and also contacts the bone. It probably functions to anchor the *(83)* <u>osteo</u> _____ to the bone. Deeper into the cytoplasm is the region of vesicles, which may be deep invaginations of the *(84)* _____ border that appear as vesicles owing to the plane of section. The region of vesicles may represent new secretory vesicles that have budded off from the *(85)* _____ (*Golgi, nucleus*) and traveled to the plasma membrane containing enzymes responsible for the breakdown of the matrix. The organelles and nuclei (6–50 in number) are located in the basal portion of the cell. Because of the high energy demand, an increased number of *(86)* _____ are found. The Golgi apparatus is also very prominent.

Bone contains both organic and *(87)* _____ components. The organic material is similar to that of cartilage, containing *(88)* _____ fibers and an amorphous ground substance. However, bone has a higher percentage of *(89)* <u>glyco</u> _____ than cartilage does. The inorganic material, or minerals, is mostly calcium and phosphorus organized into hydroxyapatite crystals $[(Ca_{10}PO_4)_6(OH)_2]$. The mineral is deposited after the *(90)* <u>osteo</u> _____ has secreted the *(91)* _____ (*organic, inorganic*) material, and it is located along and within the collagen fibers.

79 mitochondria

80 surface area
81 ruffled border

82 ruffled

83 clast
84 ruffled

85 Golgi

86 mitochondria

87 inorganic

88 collagenous
89 protein

90 blast
91 organic

Bone

92 periosteum

93 outer

94 perichondrium
95 dense irregular

96 osteoclasts

97 osteum

98 no

99 osteocytes

Periosteum

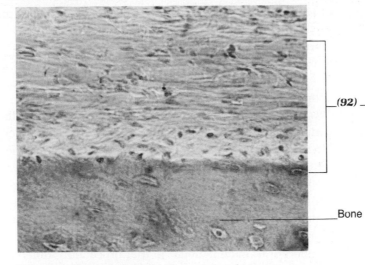

(92) _____

Bone

FIG. 6-9. Photomicrograph of bone and periosteum (original magnification ×200).

The periosteum is the layer covering the *(93)* _____ (*inner, outer*) surface of the bone (Fig. 6-9). What is its counterpart in cartilage? *(94)* _____. It is composed of an outer fibrous layer of *(95)* _____ _____ connective tissue and an inner cellular layer of osteogenic cells and blood vessels. The osteogenic cells can differentiate into osteoblasts, and may also be the progenitor cells of the multinucleated *(96)* _____. Connective tissue fibers, which bind the outer periosteal layer to the bone surface, are called Sharpey's fibers. The layer lining the inner surface of bone is the *(97)* end_____. It has the same components as the periosteum but is much thinner. The blood vessels of the periosteum and endosteum travel through the matrix to nourish the osteocytes within. The tunnels through which the vessels travel are called Volkmann's canals. Do the blood vessels of cartilage travel through the matrix? *(98)* _____.

Immature Bone

Immature bone (also called primary or woven bone) is the first bone produced by osteoblasts (Fig. 6-10). The collagen fibers are irregularly arranged, and there

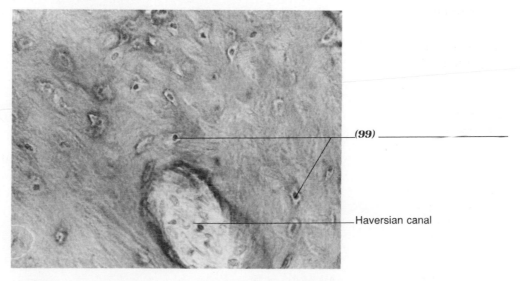

(99) _____

Haversian canal

FIG. 6-10. Photomicrograph of woven bone (original magnification ×200).

appear to be *(100)* _____ (*very few, numerous*) osteocytes. In most cases, woven bone is replaced by mature bone, although it remains at the sockets of teeth and near the sutures of flat bones of the head.

Mature Bone

Mature bone (also called lamellar or secondary bone) is the result of the continued remodeling of immature or *(101)* _____ bone by the two most active bone cells, the *(102)* _____ and the *(103)* _____ (Fig. 6-11). The collagen fibers are arranged in concentric rings called lamellae around a central vascular channel containing blood vessels, nerves, and loose connective tissue. The central canal is called a haversian canal. Osteocytes, within *(104)* _____, are found between the lamellae, and can be seen communicating through *(105)* _____. This entire structure of haversian canal and concentric *(106)* _____ is called an osteon or haversian system. The collagen fibers are arranged parallel within a lamella, but the angle of fibers is different in each lamella, so that on section, different views of the collagen fibers can be seen (Fig. 6-12).

(112) _____
_____
(107) _____
_____

FIG. 6-11. Photomicrograph of a dry ground preparation of mature bone (original magnification ×30).

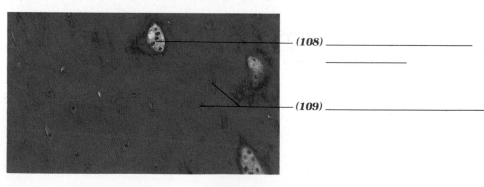

(108) _____
_____
(109) _____

FIG. 6-12. Photomicrograph of mature bone, H and E stain (original magnification ×200).

The central or *(110)* _____ canals communicate with the marrow cavity located in the center of the bone, with each other, and with the periosteum through the canals that carry the blood vessels into the matrix, the *(111)* _____ canals.

100 numerous

101 primary (or woven)
102 osteoblasts
103 osteoclasts

104 lacunae

105 canaliculi
106 lamellae

107 haversian canal

108 haversian canal

109 osteocytes

110 haversian

111 Volkmann's
112 intermediate systems

Bone

Because bone is continuously being remodeled and rebuilt, osteons will be destroyed and new ones synthesized to replace them. The remnants of osteons, called intermediate systems, appear as irregularly shaped groups of parallel lamellae between two complete osteons. The outer circumferential system is located beneath the periosteum, and the inner

(113) _____ system is located around the marrow cavity. These layers are produced by the osteoblasts that have differentiated from the **(114)** _____ cells of the **(115)** _____ (*inner, outer*) portions of the periosteum and endosteum.

113 circumferential

Compact Bone

114 osteogenic
115 inner

Grossly, bone is classified as being either compact or spongy. Compact bone has complete osteons with both an inner and outer

(116) _____ system. The intermediate systems exist as a result of the process of **(117)** _____. This type of bone is very dense and can be found as the most superficial bone in a long bone (Fig. 6-13). It contains very little marrow cavity, and thus is not very active in the formation of blood cells.

116 circumferential
117 remodeling

Spongy Bone

Spongy bone (also called trabecular or cancellous bone) is composed of numerous spicules or trabeculae of bone with a large amount of marrow space between the trabeculae. Thus, spongy bone is the primary site for **(118)** _____ _____ formation. The trabeculae, or **(119)** _____, are much thinner than compact bone so that complete haversian systems are not required. **(120)** _____ (*Osteocytes, Osteoblasts*) will be found along the surface of the trabeculae. (You should finish #121 to 123 at this point.)

118 blood cell
119 spicules

120 Osteoblasts

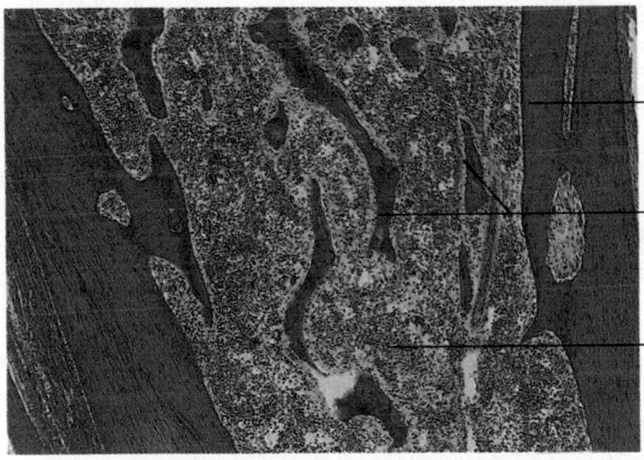

(121) _____ _____

(122) _____ _____

121 compact bone

122 spongy bone

(123) _____

_____

_____

FIG. 6-13. Photomicrograph of a part of a long bone, H and E stain (original magnification ×30).

123 bone marrow space

Bone Formation

There are two types of bone formation: intramembranous and endochondral (or osteochondral) ossification.

Intramembranous Ossification

Intramembranous bone formation involves the formation of bone directly from the embryonic connective tissue, the *(124)* _____. The primitive connective tissue cells differentiate into osteoblasts, which then line up along the mesenchymal fibers (Fig. 6-14). Secretion of extracellular materials ensues

124 mesenchyma

(125) _____

125 osteoblasts

FIG. 6-14. Photomicrograph of intramembranous bone formation, H and E stain (original magnification ×200).

from the entire cell surface, with formation of lacunae around the cell body, and *(126)* _____ around the cell processes. When this ossification process is finished, and before the bone is calcified with *(127)* _____, this prebone is referred to as osteoid (uncalcified bone). The first bone that is formed, once ossification takes place, is *(128)* _____ (*woven, lamellar*) bone and is in the form of spicules, or *(129)* _____. In between the spicules, as in *(130)* _____ (*spongy, compact*) bone, are large spaces containing the bone marrow. Lining the spicules are *(131)* osteo_____.

126 canaliculi
127 mineral

128 woven
129 trabeculae
130 spongy
131 blasts
132 appositional

Continued growth of the spicules is by the *(132)* _____ (*appositional, interstitial*) method. If the location of this new bone formation requires compact bone, as in the flat bones of the head, the osteoblasts become very active and the spicules become thicker, thus decreasing the size of the *(133)* _____ _____ cavity. The result will be mature or *(134)* _____ bone, with fully developed *(135)* _____ systems.

133 bone marrow
134 lamellar (secondary)
135 haversian

Endochondral Ossification

Endochondral bone formation involves the hypertrophy, or degeneration, and calcification of cartilage and its replacement by bone (Fig. 6-15). It is the most

Perichondrium/Periosteum _____

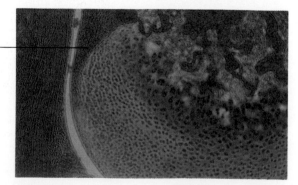

FIG. 6-15. Photomicrograph of an end of a forming bone, H and E stain (original magnification ×30).

Bone Formation

common method of the growth and development of long bones of the body. The first change is seen in the perichondrium surrounding the **(136)** _____ (*hyaline, elastic*) cartilage that serves as the temporary skeleton in the embryo. Along the shaft, or diaphysis, of the forming bone, the chondrogenic cells differentiate into osteogenic cells, and the perichondrium becomes a **(137)** _____. The osteogenic cells differentiate into **(138)** _____ and a small rim of compact bone is formed around the cartilage by the intramembranous method. Note that all endochondral bone formation is accompanied by some **(139)** _____ bone formation. The reverse is not true.

A periosteal bud, containing osteogenic cells and capillaries, grows into the cartilage matrix and forms the primary center of ossification. The periosteal bud develops from the **(140)** _____. Simultaneously, the cartilage undergoes changes to facilitate its replacement by bone (Fig. 6-16). The area farthest from the periosteal bud, and apposed to the widened end (called the epiphysis) of the forming bone, is the zone of resting cartilage. This serves to anchor the developing bone to the overlying widened area, the **(141)** _____. The adjacent area closer to the center is the zone of proliferating cartilage. In this area the cells are actively dividing and are arranged **(142)** _____ (*randomly, in columns*).

The zone of maturing cartilage is next closest to the center. Here, the cells are much **(143)** _____ (*smaller, larger*) and are beginning to degenerate. Their cytoplasm is **(144)** _____ (*pale, dark*) staining because of the presence of glycogen. The fourth area, the zone of calcified cartilage, contains chondrocytes that have totally degenerated and osteoblasts from the **(145)** _____ bud in contact with the remaining cartilage matrix. The cartilage matrix has become calcified as a result of factors released by the degenerating chondrocytes. The **(146)** _____ line up along the bands of calcified cartilage and begin to produce bone similar in shape to the **(147)** _____ of cancellous bone. As the spicules mature, the space between them develop into the **(148)** _____ cavity. (You should finish #149 to 151 at this point.)

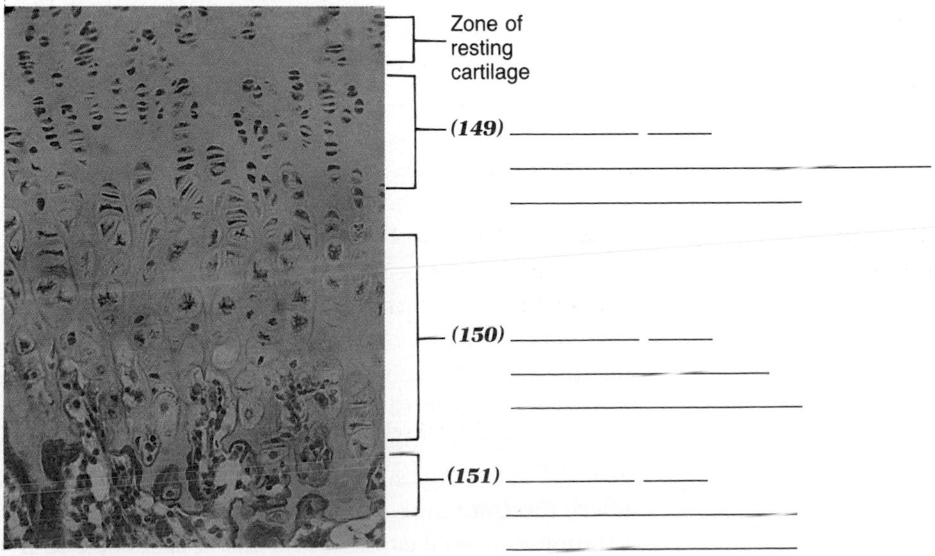

136 hyaline

137 periosteum
138 osteoblasts

139 intramembranous

140 periosteum

141 epiphysis

142 in columns

143 larger
144 pale

145 periosteal

146 osteoblasts

147 spicules (trabeculae)

148 bone marrow

149 zone of proliferating cartilage

150 zone of maturing cartilage

151 zone of calcified cartilage

Zone of resting cartilage

(149) _____ _____
_____
_____

(150) _____ _____
_____
_____

(151) _____ _____
_____

FIG. 6-16. Photomicrograph of the primary center of ossification, H and E stain (original magnification ×125).

Bone and Cartilage

The first periosteal bud grows into the shaft, or (152) _____, and develops into the (153) _____ center of (154) _____ (Fig. 6-17). Another periosteal bud grows into the widened end, or (155) _____, of the forming bone and develops into the secondary (156) _____ of ossification. The end of the forming bone remains covered by (157) _____ cartilage to serve as the articular surface. Bone development in the epiphysis remains limited,

152 *diaphysis*
153 *primary*
154 *ossification*
155 *epiphysis*
156 *center*
157 *hyaline*

158 *epiphyseal disk*

(158) _____   Secondary center
_____   of ossification

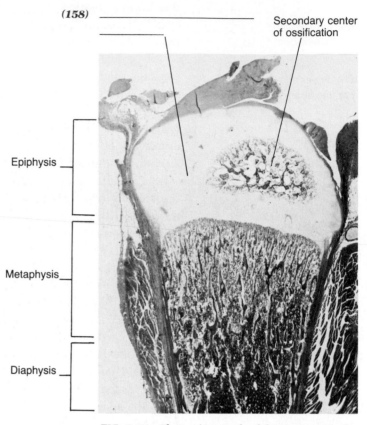

Epiphysis

Metaphysis

Diaphysis

FIG. 6-17. Photomicrograph of the upper end of a tibia.

and will not come in contact with the bone developing in the shaft until total bone growth is complete. The cartilage beneath the secondary center of ossification is referred to as the epiphyseal plate (or disk). The epiphyseal plate thickens by the (159) _____ (*appositional, interstitial*) method to provide new cartilage for the endochondral process.

Therefore, as the (160) _____ plate is thickened by growth, it is thinned on its (161) _____ (*diaphyseal, epiphyseal*) surface as it becomes part of the four zones and is replaced by advancing bone formation. Covering this growing bone is the rim of (162) _____ (*compact, spongy*) bone, which developed first. This area must also grow to accommodate the changing length of the bone, and must thicken to support the increasing weight. Growth occurs by the (163) _____ method and remodeling of the changing epiphysis involves (164) osteo _____ and (165) osteo _____. Once growth is finished, the (166) _____ plate will stop proliferating and the advancing osteoblasts will overtake it and replace it with bone, thus fusing the primary and (167) _____ centers of ossification.

159 *interstitial*

160 *epiphyseal*
161 *diaphyseal*

162 *compact*

163 *appositional*

164 *blasts*
165 *clasts*
166 *epiphyseal*
167 *secondary*

Articulations

Articulations

A joint or articulation is the structural arrangement that connects two or more bones at their site of meeting. Movement between the bones may or may not be possible, depending upon the type of joint. The joint that provides the greatest amount of movement and is the most common in the body is called the synovial joint. It consists of an articular surface, lined by *(168)* _____ cartilage, and a joint capsule.

The articular cartilage, located at the end of the bone, lies over the *(169)* _____ *(primary, secondary)* center of ossification. The cartilage is modified and *(170)* _____ *(is, is not)* covered by a perichondrium. There are three zones to the articular cartilage (Fig. 6-18). In the most

168 hyaline

169 secondary
170 is not

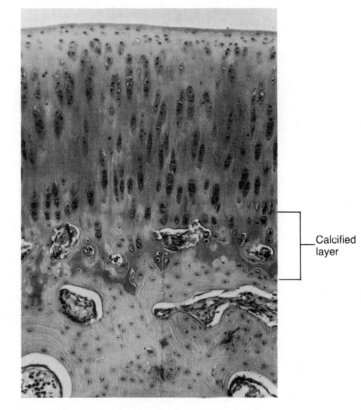

Calcified layer

FIG. 6-18. Photomicrograph of articular cartilage and subchondral bone.

superficial zone, the cells appear *(171)* _____ *(small, large)* and somewhat flattened. During development and growth, the chondrocytes in this layer divide, and growth of the area occurs by the *(172)* _____ method. In the middle layer, the chondrocytes are arranged in *(173)* _____. The *(174)* _____ fibers are also arranged in columns to provide support and to increase the weight-bearing capacity of the joint. The deepest layer appears *(175)* _____ *(calcified, hypertrophied)* and is continuously being replaced by bone as the epiphysis grows. This process is similar to that occurring on the diaphyseal end.

171 small

172 interstitial

173 columns
174 collagenous
175 calcified

Joint Capsule

The joint capsule is composed of two layers: an outer fibrous layer referred to as the fibrous capsule, and an inner layer referred to as the synovial membrane. The

Bone and Cartilage

176 outer

177 dense irregular

178 Sharpey's

179 inner

180 fibrous capsule

fibrous capsule is continuous with the **(176)** _____ (*inner, outer*) fibrous layer of the periosteum, and is composed of **(177)** _____ _____ connective tissue. As with the periosteum, there are collagenous fibers that attach the fibrous layer to the underlying bone, called **(178)** _____ fibers.

The synovial membrane lines the joint everywhere but over the articular cartilage. The inner surface is smooth and may be thrown into folds called villi. The synovial membrane, like the **(179)** _____ (*inner, outer*) layer of the periosteum, contains numerous blood vessels and nerves. The cells lining this membrane are relatively undifferentiated cells called synovial cells. The synovial membrane may lie directly on the outer layer, the **(180)** _____ _____, or it may lie on a bed of fibrous, areolar, or adipose tissue.

Blood

After completing this chapter, you should be able to identify the following:

1 Bone marrow
2 Erythrocyte
3 Pronormoblast (proerythroblast)
4 Erythroblast: basophilic, polychromatic, and orthochromatic
5 Granular leukocytes: polymorphonuclear, basophilic, and
  eosinophilic

6 Myeloblast
7 Promyelocyte
8 Myelocyte
9 Metamyelocyte
10 Nongranular leukocyte: lymphocyte and monocyte
11 Thrombocyte
12 Megakaryocyte

Also, after completing this chapter, you should understand the following:

1 The histologic changes in bone
  marrow
2 Erythropoiesis

3 Granulopoiesis
4 Thrombopoiesis

Blood is the viscous fluid that is pumped throughout the body. It is composed of a liquid component, plasma, and cellular components. The cellular components found in blood are erythrocytes (red blood corpuscles; RBCs), leukocytes (white blood corpuscles, WBCs), and thrombocytes (platelets). These cells are involved in oxygen transport and protection against infection, and are important in coagulation.

Knowledge of the histology of the mature blood elements found in an ordinary peripheral blood smear plus their formation (poiesis) in bone marrow is essential to medical practice.

Bone Marrow

Bone marrow is the major poietic organ in the normal adult. The bone marrow functions in producing RBCs, hematopoiesis; WBCs, (1) myelo_____; and platelets, (2) thrombo_____ Occupying the central cavities of the long bones of the skeleton, the spongiosa of the vertebral bodies, ribs, and sternum, and the flat bones of the pelvis, bone marrow is capable of WBC production, (3) _____poiesis, RBC production, (4) _____poiesis, and platelet production, (5) _____poiesis.

1 poiesis
2 poiesis

3 myelo
4 hemato
5 thrombo

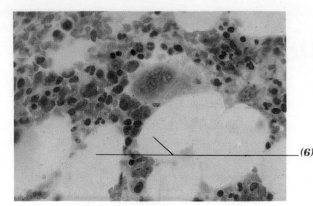

_____(6) _____

FIG. 7-1. Bone marrow, Wright's stain (original magnification ×125).

6 adipocytes

Varying in cellular proportions at various stages of life, bone marrow will usually consist mainly of blood-forming elements with an increase in adipocytes with age (Fig. 7-1). The adipose cells, *(7)* _____, in color can reflect the activity of the bone marrow: *(8)* _____ *(red, yellow)* if active or hyperactive, and *(9)* _____ *(red, yellow)* if hypoactive.

In addition to the cell precursors of *(10)* __ __ __, *(11)* __ __ __, and platelets plus *(12)* _____, the histology of bone marrow consists of a stromal network of reticular cells. The reticular cells form a loose meshwork that functions in holding together all cells; it is most difficult to see in a routine preparation.

Release of all mature blood cells is through bone marrow sinusoids. These sinusoids are composed of the *(13)* _____ fibers that make up the stroma of the bone marrow. Not routinely visible in a light micrograph, the sinusoids act as one means to regulate the number of cells released into the blood stream.

Last, in addition to the precursors of blood cellular elements are the highly phagocytic cells, the macrophages. Among other phagocytic functions, these cells help in phagocytizing extruded nuclei of developing erythrocytes. One should be able to identify the macrophages in the same manner as one would in connective tissue.

Erythrocytes

Erythrocytes, or *(14)* __ __ __ __, are the components of circulating blood that impart the *(15)* _____ color to it (Fig. 7-2). Most numerous of all cellular elements in blood, *(16)* <u>erythro</u>_____ normally range in number from 4.8 million/m² in women to 5.4 million/m² in men.

Characteristically, the RBCs, whose primary function is *(17)* _____ transport, are biconcave in shape, highly elastic in nature, and unique in that in the mature state in blood they have *(18)* _____ *(no, one, two)* nucleus(ei). Roughly 7.5 μm in diameter, the RBC is a *(19)* ____<u>concave</u>, *(20)* _____ *(highly, slightly)* elastic, *(21)* _____ *(a, multi) nucleated* cell. Easily identified by its *(22)* _____ *(lighter, darker)*-staining *(23)* _____ *(concave, convex)* center, the RBC has a small amount of the usual complement of organelles. It is the hemoglobin, an oxygen-carrying protein found in the cytoplasm, that imparts the *(24)* _____ color to the cell. (You should finish #26 at this point.)

7 adipocytes
8 red
9 yellow
10 WBC
11 RBC
12 adipocytes

13 reticular

14 RBCs
15 red
16 cytes

17 oxygen

18 no
19 bi
20 highly
21 a
22 lighter
23 concave

24 red

Erythrocytes

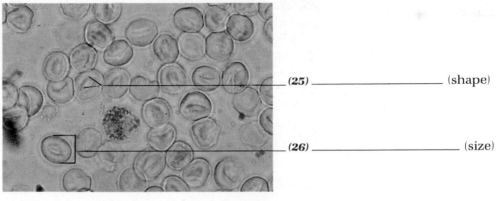

(25) _____ (shape)

25 *biconcave*

(26) _____ (size)

26 *7.5 μm*

FIG. 7-2. Erythrocyte, Wright's stain.

Erythropoiesis

Erythropoiesis, the formation of **(27)** _____ in **(28)** _____, begins with a pluripotential stem cell. The pluripotential stem cell is capable of differentiating into any of the cell lines. With the proper hormonal stimulation, the pluripotential **(29)** _____ will differentiate into the first cell of the erythrocyte cell line, the pronormoblast (proerythroblast; Figs. 7-3, 7-4, and 7-5).

27 *erythrocytes*
28 *bone marrow*

29 *stem cell*

Proerythroblast

Ranging from 14 μm to 19 μm in diameter, the pronormoblasts are the **(30)** _____ (*first, second*) true cell of the erythrocyte cell line and differentiate from the **(31)** _____.
Having a centrally placed nucleus with one or two faint nucleoli, the proerythroblast is homogeneously **(32)** baso_____. All organelles normally found in a cell are also evident here.

30 *first*
31 *pluripotential stem cell*

Basophilic Erythroblast

Slightly smaller than its precursor the **(33)** proerythro_____, the basophilic erythroblast also has a **(34)** _____ (*central, eccentric*) nucleus, **(35)** _____ (*three to five, one or two*) nucleoli and very coarse chromatin in the nucleus. Slightly **(36)** _____ (*larger, smaller*) than the **(37)** proerythro_____, the basophilic **(38)** erythro_____ is best differentiated by its even deeper and more royal blue **(39)** baso_____-staining cytoplasm; hence its name (see Fig. 7-3).

32 *philic*

33 *blast*
34 *central*
35 *one or two*
36 *smaller*
37 *blast*
38 *blast*
39 *philic*

Polychromatic Erythroblast

Progeny of the basophilic **(40)** _____ lead to the polychromatic erythroblasts (see Fig. 7-4). These cells are smaller (8 μm–12 μm) and also have a smaller nucleus with no evidence of any nucleoli. Its distinguishing feature is evident by its name, polychromasia.
The deep basophilia of the polychromatic erythroblast's precursors, the **(41)** _____ and **(42)** _____, is due to the numerous ribosomes in the cytoplasm and on the rough endoplasmic reticulum, **(43)** ___ ___ ___. The bluish gray-staining slowly disappears in the polychromatic **(44)** erythro_____ as the ribosomes decrease in number. Concomitant with this change in the number of

40 *erythroblast*

41 *proerythroblast*
42 *basophilic erythroblast*

43 *rER*
44 *blast*

ribosomes is the increased production of hemoglobin, which increases the eosin-ophilia of the cell. The tinctural-staining affinities of the cell reflect the true proportion of the ribosomes to the amount of hemoglobin. Therefore, as the cell matures, the bluish color, **(45)** ___ilia___, **(46)** _____ (*decreases, increases*), and the pinkish color, **(47)** _____ilia, **(48)** _____ (*decreases, increases*) as the production of the oxygen-carrying **(49)** _____ (*protein, lipid*) **(50)** _____ **(51)** _____ (*decreases, increases*). (You should finish #53 at this point.)

45 *baso*
46 *decreases*
47 *eosino*
48 *increases*
49 *protein*
50 *hemoglobin*
51 *increases*

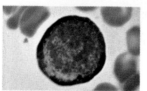

FIG. 7-3. Basophilic erythroblast, Wright's stain.*

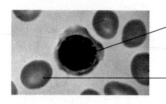

(52) _____

(53) _____

_____

52 *nucleus*

FIG. 7-4. Polychromatic erythroblast, Wright's stain.

_____

53 *red blood cell*

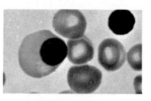

FIG. 7-5. Orthochromatic erythroblast, Wright's stain.

Orthochromatic Erythroblast

Also called normoblasts, orthochromatic erythroblasts mature from the **(54)** _poly_____ **(55)** _erythro_____ and, as one would expect, these cells have a more **(56)** _____philic color with only a slight **(57)** _____philic tint due to some free **(58)** _____ left in the cytoplasm. (See Fig. 7-5.) The nucleus in this cell is smaller and highly irregular in size, and starts to assume a(n) **(59)** _____ (*central, eccentric*) position rather than the usual **(60)** _____ (*central, eccentric*) position of its precursors.

The nucleus of the orthochromatic erythroblast is pinched off with some cytoplasm and a covering plasma membrane. The extruded nucleus, by way of exocytosis, is then digested by phagocytic cells in the bone marrow, the **(61)** _____. The newly formed **(62)** __ __ __ is released into the blood through the **(63)** _____.

Newly released erythrocytes still retain a slight bluish green tint due to left-over **(64)** _____ in the **(65)** _____ (*nucleus, cytoplasm*). Ordinarily called polychromaphilic erythrocytes, if stained with cresyl

54 *chromatic*
55 *blasts*
56 *eosino*
57 *baso*
58 *ribosomes*
59 *eccentric*
60 *central*

61 *macrophages*
62 *RBC*
63 *sinusoids*
64 *ribosomes*
65 *cytoplasm*

* Figs. 7-3 to 7-5, 7-7, 7-9 to 7-12, 7-14 and 7-15 from Bloom W, Fawcett DW: Textbook of Histology, 10th ed. Philadelphia, WB Saunders, 1975

Erythropoiesis

blue the ribosomes will clump together and one will see a bluish skein. These uniquely stained cells are called reticulocytes and are used clinically to reflect the activity of the bone marrow.

Control of Erythropoiesis

As stated before, the *(66)* pluri _____ _____ _____ is under hormonal control and can differentiate into *(67)* _____ (*one, any*) cell line. If properly stimulated, the stem cell will differentiate first into the *(68)* pro _____, which matures into the *(69)* _____ _____, then to the *(70)* _____ _____, and then to the *(71)* _____ _____. Finally, the nucleus is extruded and *(72)* _____ by macrophages in the *(73)* _____ (*blood stream, bone marrow*). The stimulating factor in erythropoiesis is erythropoietin, and it is produced by the kidney.

66 *potential stem cell*
67 *any*

68 *erythroblast*
69 *basophilia erythroblast*
70 *polychromatic erythroblast*
71 *orthochromatic erythroblast*
72 *phagocytized*
73 *bone marrow*

Leukocytes

Leukocytes are nucleate *(74)* __ __ __s that circulate in the blood. Produced in the *(75)* _____ _____ by *(76)* _____, leukocytes are divided into granulocytes (those with granules in their cytoplasm) and nongranulocytes (without granules). Further subdivision of the granulocytes reveals three distinct, easily identifiable cell types: polymorphonuclear leukocytes (PMNL, neutrophils, or "polys"), eosinophilic leukocytes (eosinophils), and basophilic leukocytes (basophils). The nongranular leukocytes consist of two distinct and not so easily identifiable cell types: monocytes and lymphocytes.

Totally anywhere from 5,000 to 10,000 cell/m^2 in a normal adult, leukocytes are *(77)* _____ (*equivalent, much lesser, much greater*) in number to erythrocytes. The physiological importance of leukocytes is that of controlling infection, not of transporting oxygen, like that of the *(78)* _____.

74 *WBCs*
75 *bone marrow*
76 *myelopoiesis*

77 *much lesser*

78 *erythrocytes*

Granular Leukocytes

Polymorphonuclear Leukocytes

Polymorphonuclear leukocytes or *(79)* _____ are *(80)* _____ (*granular, nongranular*) cells and are the most numerous of all leukocytes, making up 55% to 60% of the total WBC count (Fig. 7-6). Easily recognizable in a peripheral smear, neutrophils or *(81)* _____ _____ are 10 μm to 12 μm in diameter, *(82)* _____ (*smaller, larger*) than an erythrocyte. In its mature form, the PMNL has a nucleus consisting of two to five lobes connected to one another by thin, attenuated strands; hence the term polymorphonuclear. Since the polys or *(83)* _____ are fully differentiated, no nucleoli are evident.

Besides the highly characteristic *(84)* __ ____ ____ _____ lobes, the cytoplasm of the neutrophil has, when stained properly, numerous reddish purplish granules called azurophil granules. These granules, often absent at the cell periphery where fine filaments are evident, contain myeloperoxidase, lysozyme, and acid phosphatase. These enzymes are important in antibacterial activity.

79 *neutrophils*
80 *granular*

81 *polymorphonuclear leukocytes*
82 *larger*

83 *neutrophils*

84 *two to five*

In addition to having lytic granules containing
(85) _____, *(86)* _____, and
(87) _____ _____, PMNL or *(88)* "_____" are avidly phagocytic. By being able to engulf bacteria, the neutrophil can help control infection. [You should finish #90 at this point.]

85 *myeloperoxidase*
86 *lysozyme*
87 *acid phosphatase*
88 *polys*

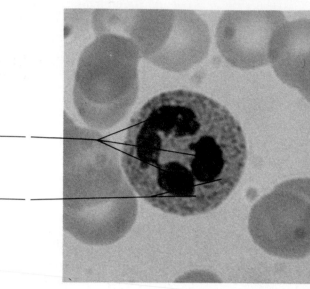

(90) _____
_____

(89) _____
_____

89 *azurophilic granules*
90 *multilobed nucleus*

FIG. 7-6. Polymorphonuclear leukocyte, Wright's stain (original magnification ×225).

Eosinophilic Leukocytes

Constituting 1% to 3% of the total WBC count, eosinophils are found in
(91) _____ *(lesser, greater)* number than the PMNLs, which total
(92) _____ to _____% of the total count (Fig. 7-7). Eosinophils are also 10 μm to 12 μm in diameter *(93)* _____ *(unlike, like)* the neutrophils. While the neutrophils have *(94)* _____ to _____ lobes, eosinophils have only
(95) _____ *(two, four)* lobes connected to one another by a narrow isthmus. Eosinophilic leukocytes *(96)* _____ *(do, do not)* have granules in their cytoplasm
(97) _____ *(unlike, like)* the neutrophils. The granules in the eosinophil stain a brilliant red, making identification of the cell easy. When the eosinophilic granules are isolated they contain *(98)* <u>myelo_____</u>, acid
(99) _____, but no lysozyme. Eosinophils do not have direct antibacterial action like neutrophils nor are they highly phagocytic. Eosinophils are important in hypersensitivity states and allergic reactions. (See Fig. 7-7.)

91 *lesser*
92 *50% to 60%*
93 *like*
94 *two to five*
95 *two*
96 *do*
97 *like*

98 *peroxidase*
99 *phosphatase*

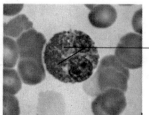

(100) _____
_____

100 *azurophilic granules*

FIG. 7-7. Eosinophilic leukocyte, Wright's stain (original magnification ×250).

Granular Leukocytes

Basophilic Leukocytes

Smallest in number of all granulocytes, basophils range from 0.5% to 0.7% of the total *(101)* __ __ __ count (Fig. 7-8). Like the other granulocytes,

101 WBC

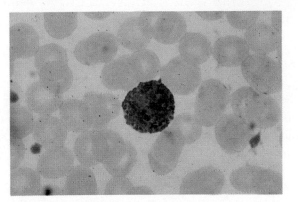

FIG. 7-8. Basophilic leukocyte, Wright's stain (original magnification ×250).

(102) _____ and *(103)* _____, the basophil is *(104)* ____ to ____ μm in diameter, and *(105)* _____ *(contains, is missing)* granules in its cytoplasm. The nucleus of the basophil is "U"-shaped and does not contain two discrete lobes as does the *(106)* _____ or two to five lobes as does the *(107)* _____. The granules in its cytoplasm are rounder and stain a bluish metachromasia. These granules, like the brilliant red granules of the *(108)* _____ *(eosinophil, PMNL)*, are azurophilic granules and obscure the nucleus. Unlike the other azurophilic granules, the granules found in the basophil are missing all three of the antibacterial enzymes, *(109)* _____, *(110)* _____, and *(111)* _____. Found in these granules are two important pharmacologic agents, histamine and heparin.

102 neutrophils
103 eosinophils
104 10 to 12
105 contains
106 eosinophil
107 neutrophil

108 eosinophil

109 lysozyme
110 myeloperoxidase
111 acid phosphatase

Granulopoiesis

The formation of the granulocytes, *(112)* _____ or *(113)* _____, *(114)* _____ and *(115)* _____ is called *(116)* _____ and takes place in the *(117)* _____. Granulopoiesis (granulocyte formation) is virtually identical for all three types of granulocytes. Discussion of granulopoiesis will concern itself with that of neutrophils, *(118)* __ __ __ __, and will be followed by an examination of the distinguishing features of the development of the other granulocytes, *(119)* _____ and *(120)* _____. (See Figs. 7-9 through 7-12, 7-14, and 7-15.)

112 neutrophils
113 polys
114 eosinophils
115 basophils
116 myelopoiesis
117 bone marrow
118 PMNL
119 eosinophils
120 basophils

Neutrophilic Granulopoiesis

MYELOBLAST Like erythropoiesis, granulopoiesis has as its first cell a highly nondistinct cell, the *(121)* _____ _____. With the proper stimulation, this cell will differentiate into the first true cell of the granulocyte cell line, the myeloblast. (See Fig. 7-9.) A relatively

121 pluripotential stem cell

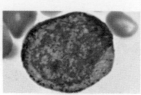

FIG. 7-9. Myeloblast, Wright's stain.

small cell, the **(122)** _____ blast, is 10 μm to 15 μm in diameter. The nucleus is oval, stains a light purple, and has two or three visible nucleoli. The cytoplasm of the myeloblast has a **(123)** _____ philic-staining character and it is devoid of granules.

122 myelo

123 baso

PROMYELOCYTE Upon the appearance of granules in the myeloblast, the cell becomes a promyelocyte. (See Fig. 7-10.) These small metachromatic-staining gran-

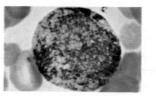

FIG. 7-10. Neutrophilic promyelocyte, Wright's stain.

ules (only at this stage) are the azurophil granules discussed above. The granules, composed of **(124)** _____, **(125)** _____ _____, and lysozyme are important in **(126)** _____ _____ (antibacterial action, immunoglobulin production). As the cell matures, it increases in size to 15 μm to 20 μm; this is in contrast to a decrease in size that occurs in the development from a proerythroblast to a **(127)** _____ _____ in **(128)** _____ poiesis. The nucleus is essentially unchanged and stays a nondistinguishing **(129)** _____ color.

124 myeloperoxidase
125 acid phosphatase
126 antibacterial action

127 basophilic erythroblast
128 erythro
129 purple

MYELOCYTE With further differentiation of the promyelocyte, the myelocyte is formed. (See Fig. 7-11.) It is at this stage that one can first distinguish between all three types of granulocytes. Found in the myelocyte are the secondary or specific granules that distinctly identify the eosinophilic **(130)** _____, the basophilic **(131)** _____, and the **(132)** _____ _____. In addition to the azurophilic granules that are round and dense, the specific or **(133)** _____ granules contain alkaline phosphatase and antibacterial proteins, yet are considerably smaller and less dense. Also, the specific granules do not stain as deep as the azurophilic granules do. In the myelocyte stage, the proportion of the specific granules to azurophilic granules, which contain **(134)** _____ _____, **(135)** _____, and **(136)** _____, is roughly 1:3.

Averaging 12 μm to 18 μm in diameter, the neutrophilic myelocyte is **(137)** _____ (smaller, larger) than the promyelocyte and

130 leukocyte
131 leukocyte
132 polymorphonuclear leukocyte
133 secondary

134 acid phosphatase
135 lysozyme
136 myeloperoxidase
137 smaller

Granulopoiesis

138 larger

139 two to five
140 protein
141 decreased

142 nucleus

(138) _____ _____ (*smaller, larger*) than the myeloblast. For the first time, the nucleus exhibits some slight indentation that will eventually lead to the *(139)* ____ to ____ lobes found in the mature neutrophil. Usually, nucleoli are indistinct, indicating that active *(140)* _____ _____ synthesis has *(141)* _____ _____ (*increased, decreased*). (See Fig. 7-12. You should finish #142 at this point.)

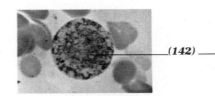

(142) _____

FIG. 7-11.   Neutrophilic myelocyte, Wright's stain.

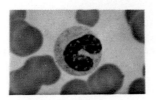

FIG. 7-12.   Neutrophilic metamyelocyte, Wright's stain.

143 indented or lobular

144 purple
145 lighter
146 1:3
147 more
148 azurophilic

149 myelocyte
150 12 to 18

151 myelocyte
152 stab

153 specific
154 azurophilic
155 band

156 10 to 12
157 greater

158 band

METAMYELOCYTE   Further maturation of the myelocyte produces very distinct changes, and in turn the next cell type is called the metamyelocyte. The nucleus is visibly more *(143)* _____ in shape, and attentuation of nuclear material becomes more evident. Often kidney-bean shaped, the nucleus of the metamyelocyte stage stains *(144)* _____ yet *(145)* _____ (*deeper, lighter*) than in previous stages. In the myelocyte stage, the ratio of specific granules to azurophilic granules is *(146)* ___:___; yet in the metamyelocyte stage, there is a total reversal: *(147)* _____ (*more, less*) specific granules than *(148)* _____ granules. Finally, the cell size of the metamyelocyte is equivalent to its precursor, the *(149)* _____ : *(150)* _____ to _____ μm in diameter.

BAND OR STAB GRANULOCYTE   Subsequent maturation of the *(151)* meta_____ produces the band or stab granulocyte. The most distinguishing feature of the band or *(152)* _____ granulocyte is the sausage shape of the nucleus. While the identification of the lobes of the nucleus becomes evident, the final degree of lobulation is still not achieved at this stage. The nucleus is highly visible and is not obscured by the *(153)* _____ and *(154)* _____ granules (Fig. 7-13).

In addition to the nuclear changes in the stab or *(155)* _____ granulocyte, there is a diminution of the cell size to virtually the mature cell size, *(156)* _____ μm to _____ μm in diameter. While the number of specific granules is *(157)* _____ (*greater, less*) than the number of azurophilic granules, it is the azurophilic granules that are most easily visible in a light micrograph.

At this point, in the bone marrow the stab or *(158)* _____ neutrophil undergoes final maturation. (You should be able to identify most of these forms in a normal adult's bone marrow; they are usually clustered near one another.) The mature neutrophil has *(159)* _____ to _____ lobes and an *(160)* _____ (*easy, difficult*)-to-see nucleus; it is *(161)* _____ (*highly, rarely*) phagocytic and is found in roughly *(162)* ___%__ to ___%__ of the total *(163)* __ __ __ count. This whole maturation process takes 10 days to 14 days, while the mature cell lasts only 10 hr to 12 hr in the bloodstream.

159 *two to five*
160 *easy*
161 *highly*
162 *50% to 60%*
163 *WBC*

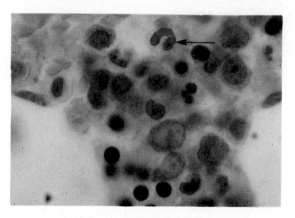

FIG. 7-13. Arrow points to a *(164)* _____ of a neutrophilic band cell, Wright's stain.

Eosinophilic Granulopoiesis

164 *nucleus*

Like neutrophilic granulopoiesis, eosinophilic granulopoiesis starts with the *(165)* _____ _____ _____ that matures into the *(166)* _____. The myeloblast, *(167)* _____ (*smaller, larger*) than its immediate progeny, will mature into a still nondistinguishable granulocyte, the *(168)* _____. From this cell, further maturation produces the *(169)* _____, and this cell can then be identified as to the specific granulocyte cell line.

165 *pluripotential stem cell*
166 *myeloblast*
167 *smaller*
168 *promyelocyte*
169 *myelocyte*

MYELOCYTE The eosinophilic myelocyte first starts to have an indentation of the nucleus *(170)* _____ (*unlike, like*) that of the neutrophilic myelocyte, but its nucleus is *(171)* _____ (*less, more*) visible because of its *(172)* _____ and *(173)* _____ granules. (See Fig. 7-14.) Unlike the neutrophil at this stage, the eosinophils have almost equal numbers of both types of granules.

170 *like*
171 *less*
172 *azurophilic*
173 *specific*

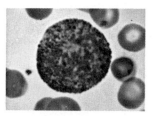

FIG. 7-14. Eosinophilic myelocyte, Wright's stain.

Granulopoiesis

METAMYELOCYTE Maturation of the myelocyte produces the
(174) _____, and this has a slightly *(175)* _____
(*more, less*) indented nucleus. (See Fig. 7-15.) The specific and

174 *metamyelocyte*
175 *more*

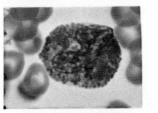

FIG. 7-15. Eosinophilic
metamyelocyte, Wright's
stain.

(176) _____ granules obscure the nuclear outline
(177) _____ (*unlike, as*) in the neutrophilic metamyelocyte.
    In the maturation of the metamyelocyte to the *(178)* _____ or stab
granulocyte, there is little change histologically except that further indentation of
the nucleus occurs. The bright *(179)* _____ (*red, purple*) granules that so char-
acterize the mature eosinophil obscure the *(180)* _____ (*one, two, three*)-lobed
nucleus.
    Finally, the mature eosinophil, with *(181)* _____ lobes and bright
(182) _____ granules, is released into the blood stream through the
(183) _____. Only *(184)* ___% to ___% of the total WBC count, the
eosinophils are identifiable in the bone marrow by their highly characteristic
granules.

176 *azurophilic*
177 *unlike*
178 *band*

179 *red*
180 *two*

181 *two*
182 *red*
183 *sinusoids*
184 *1% to 3%*

Basophilic Granulopoiesis
In the formation of a mature basophilic leukocyte, the sequence is identical to
that of the other leukocytes: pluripotential *(185)* _____ _____,
(186) _____, *(187)* _____,
(188) _____, *(189)* _____, band or
(190) _____ cell, and, finally, the mature basophil that is released through
the *(191)* _____ of the *(192)* _____ _____.
    There are no important morphologic differences discernable in basophilic
granulopoiesis except that the granules stain a deep *(193)* _____ (*red,
purple*) and *(194)* _____ (*always, rarely*) obscure the nuclear outline.
These granules are *(195)* _____ (*dissimilar, similar*) pharmacologically to those found in eosinophils and neutrophils. Finally, the nucleus of
the basophil will slowly assume a *(196)* ___ shape unlike the *(197)* _____ to
_____ lobes of the neutrophil or *(198)* _____ lobes of the eosinophil.

185 *stem cell*
186 *myeloblast*
187 *promyelocyte*
188 *myelocyte*
189 *metamyelocyte*
190 *stab*
191 *sinusoids*
192 *bone marrow*
193 *purple*
194 *always*
195 *dissimilar*
196 *U*
197 *two to five*
198 *two*

Nongranular Cells
    The two other types of leukocytes are the nongranular cells:
(199) _____ and *(200)* _____. The most
abundant of these two are the lymphocytes. Constituting 25% to 35% of the total
(201) ___ ___ ___ count, lymphocytes are the *(202)* _____ (*secondmost, most*) abundant white cell. Lymphocytes can be divided into two
groups by their size: small and large lymphocytes.

199 *monocytes*
200 *lymphocytes*
201 *WBC*
202 *secondmost*

Blood

203 *equivalent in size to*

204 *baso*
205 *cytoplasm*

Lymphocytes

SMALL LYMPHOCYTES In a normal peripheral smear, the small lymphocyte is 7 μm to 8 μm in diameter and is therefore *(203)* _____ _____ (*considerably smaller than, equivalent in size to*) an erythrocyte. These cells have a nucleus of 5 μm in diameter that stains deeply *(204)* _____philic and is slightly indented. Surrounding the nucleus is a thin rim of blue *(205)* _____ with a normal complement of organelles. (See Fig. 7-16.)

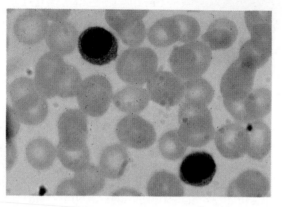

FIG. 7-16. Small lymphocyte, Wright's stain (original magnification ×225).

203 *equivalent in size to*

204 *baso*
205 *cytoplasm*

LARGER LYMPHOCYTES Larger lymphocytes are 12 μm in diameter and therefore of similar size to *(206)* _____ (*neutrophils, erythrocytes*). The nucleus of larger lymphocytes is 7 μm in diameter and stains the same as do the small lymphocytes, *(207)* _____philic. Also, the nucleus of the larger lymphocytes is *(208)* _____ (*slightly, greatly*) indented. The cytoplasm-to-nucleus ratio is greater in larger lymphocytes and serves as a means of differentiating between the small and large lymphocytes. The cytoplasm of the larger lymphocytes also stains *(209)* _____ but contains more organelles than that of the smaller cell.

Infrequently, in both sizes of lymphocytes, azurophilic granules typical of *(210)* _____, *(211)* _____, and *(212)* _____ are evident.

Both sizes of lymphocytes are involved in some way in the immunologic defense of the body. Small lymphocytes are subdivided by cytochemical techniques and physiological actions into T and B lymphocytes. T and B lymphocytes, both *(213)* _____ (*small, large*) lymphocytes, are identical histologically. They are *(214)* __ μm to _____ μm in diameter, and have a thin *(215)* _____ rim of cytoplasm and a deep-staining *(216)* _____philic nucleus. The differences between T and B *(217)* _____ must be understood in order to properly comprehend the histology of the immune system and other organ systems. (For a complete discussion of T and B lymphocytes, please consult a histology textbook.)

B LYMPHOCYTES B lymphocytes are most likely formed in the bone marrow and circulate in the blood. For immunologic protection, an antigen (a foreign substance) must come into contact with the B *(218)* _____. Specific antigens cause specific B lymphocytes to undergo a reaction called the primary response, whereupon they develop into B memory cells and plasma cells.

206 *neutrophils*

207 *baso*
208 *slightly*

209 *blue*

210 *neutrophils*
211 *basophils*
212 *eosinophils*

213 *small*
214 *7 to 8*
215 *blue*
216 *baso*
217 *lymphocytes*

218 *lymphocyte*

Nongranular Cells

The B memory cell is that cell, nondistinct histologically from B lymphocytes, that will differentiate into plasma cells upon repeated contact with the same antigen; this is called the secondary response. B memory cells enable the body to be "ready" when it comes into contact with the same antigen, and therefore to mount a more rapid and effective immune response.

The plasma cell, a differentiated (219) ___ (B, T) (220) _____, is responsible for most of the immunoglobulin or antibody produced. These cells have a(n) (221) _____ (central, eccentric) cartwheel-shaped nucleus and a (222) _____philic-staining cytoplasm. In order to produce the protein, immunoglobulin, or (223) _____, rough (224) _____ _____ is necessary in abundant amounts in the plasma cell's (225) _____ (cytoplasm, nucleus). The cytoplasm stains a rich (226) _____philia because of this large amount of (227) ___ ___ ___. Mature plasma cells sometimes accumulate eosinophilic droplets in their (228) _____philic cytoplasm. These (229) _____philic droplets are termed Russell bodies.

219 B
220 lymphocyte
221 eccentric
222 baso

223 antibody
224 endoplasmic reticulum
225 cytoplasm
226 baso
227 rER

228 baso
229 eosino

T LYMPHOCYTES T lymphocytes originate in the thymus and not the (230) _____ _____ like B lymphocytes. Identical histologically to B lymphocytes, T (231) _____ do not manufacture antibodies and therefore do not possess a highly extensive (232) ___ ___ ___. Upon the initial activation of the T lymphocyte by an antigen, the (233) _____ response, there will be differentiation into several subtypes, one of which is a T memory cell. As with B memory (234) _____, the subtypes of T lymphocytes equip the body with a ready defense system if a second contact with the same antigen occurs—the (235) _____ (primary, secondary) response. (Discussion of the T lymphocyte subtypes is beyond the scope of this text.)

230 bone marrow
231 lymphocytes
232 rER
233 primary

234 cell

235 secondary

Lymphopoiesis
Myelopoiesis, the development of (236) _____, is called lymphopoiesis when lymphocyte formation is meant. (237) ___ (B, T) lymphocytes are formed in the bone marrow and go through various stages of development. Identification of the specific cell stages has not been fully understood and will not be discussed here.

236 leukocytes
237 B

Monocytes
The other nongranular white blood cells are the (238) _____ (Figs. 7-17 and 7-18). Constituting 2% to 8% of the total (239) ___ ___ ___ count, monocytes are (240) _____ (less, more) abundant than lymphocytes. Monocytes are 12 μm to 15 μm in diameter, and therefore are generally (241) _____ (smaller, larger) than mature lymphocytes. (The large size of the monocyte aids in the initial separation from all other WBCs.)

238 monocytes
239 WBC
240 less

241 larger

Blood

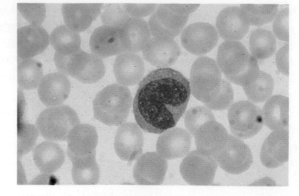

FIG. 7-17. Identify the type of cell: **(242)** _____. Wright's stain.

242 monocyte

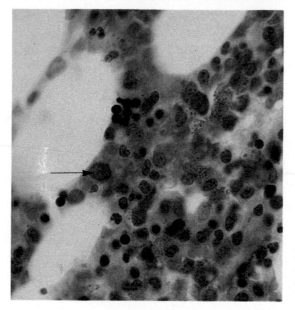

FIG. 7-18. Identify the type of cell indicated by arrow: **(243)** _____. Wright's stain.

243 lymphocyte

244 baso

245 blue

246 does not

247 baso

248 nongranular

249 larger

250 baso

251 irregular

252 azurophilic

The nucleus of the monocyte varies in shape—from ovoid to indented. Staining a paler blue or **(244)** _____philic, the nucleus of the monocyte is more euchromatic than the lymphocyte yet does not stain a **(245)** _____ (color) like the lymphocyte nucleus.

The cytoplasm of the monocyte contains the usual organelles with very small amounts of rER. One notices that the cytoplasm **(246)** _____ (does, does not) stain as deeply **(247)** _____philic as does the cytoplasm of the lymphocytes. While called a **(248)** _____ (granular, nongranular) cell, monocytes do have azurophilic granules that function as lysosomes and are not infrequently seen in a routine light micrograph.

To properly identify the monocyte, one must examine it for a **(249)** _____ (smaller, larger) size than other WBCs, a deeply **(250)** _____philic, **(251)** _____ (regular, irregular)-shaped nucleus, and occasional sparse **(252)** _____ granules.

The monocytes function as the immediate precursors of the mononuclear phagocytic system (MPS). The MPS includes all of the macrophages of the body, including the osteoclasts. Although having a similar function, the phagocytic PMNL is not considered part of the MPS because it is not mononuclear.

Nongranular Cells

253 phago
254 monocytes
255 connective tissue
256 macrophage

257 T

258 bone marrow

259 platelets

260 smaller

261 Wright's

262 ovoid

263 hyalo

Macrophages are highly *(253)* _____ ^cytic^ and so are their blood precursors, the *(254)* _____. The monocyte will stay in the blood circulatory system anywhere from 1 day to 3 days, and then migrate into *(255)* _____ _____ to form the *(256)* _____.

Monopoiesis

Like all other WBC development, except that of *(257)* ___ (B, T) lymphocytes, myelopoiesis (called monopoiesis when describing monocyte formation) takes place in the *(258)* _____ _____. The stages of development and identification of each cell line has not been fully distinguished, nor are they sufficiently clear cut to warrant any histologic discussion.

Thrombocytes

Thrombocytes or *(259)* _____ circulate in the blood and are neither a component of RBCs nor WBCs. In an ordinary peripheral smear, thrombocytes are identifiable as flattened, sometimes irregular in shape but usually ovoid, small clumps of cytoplasm (Fig. 7-19). Much

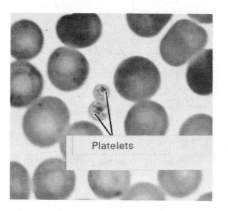

Platelets

FIG. 7-19. Thrombocyte.

(260) _____ (smaller, larger) than RBCs, platelets can be seen to be composed of two distinct areas (best seen under oil immersion), outer and inner zones.

Outer Zones

The outer zone stains a clear pale blue with a *(261)* _____ stain that is normally used for a peripheral smear. This zone is called the hyalomere. The hyalomere consists of microtubules, which are only visible with electron microscopy (EM), and filaments. The tubules are important in maintaining cell shape, usually *(262)* _____, and are also important in transporting intracellular agents outside the cell. The tubules that transport are appropriately called the surface canalicular system. If seen in cross section, they appear to be membrane-bound vesicles in the *(263)* _____ ^mere^ (Fig. 7-20).

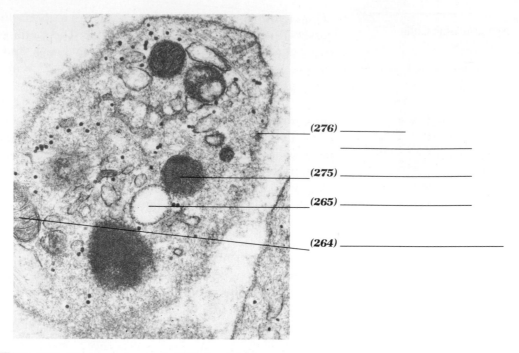

264 mitochondria
265 vesicles

FIG. 7-20 Electron micrograph (EM) of a platelet.

Another and not so readily identifiable tubular system in addition to the surface (266) _____ _____, is the dense tubular system. Its function is as yet unknown. Rarely are any organelles found in the outer zone or (267) _____ mere.

266 canalicular system

Inner Zone

267 hyalo

The inner area is an electron-dense area and is called the granulomere. (268) Granulo _____ area is so named because of the numerous granules found on EM. The granules are either alpha or very dense granules. An alpha granule is an electron-dense membrane-bound area containing a plethora of pharmacologically active agents necessary for aiding coagulation. These sub-

268 mere

stances will be released outside the cell by the (269) _____ _____ system.

The very dense (270) _____ is more electron dense than the (271) _____ granule. Similar in position to the alpha granules, the very dense granules can be found in the (272) _____ mere. The very

269 surface canalicular

(273) _____ granule also contains pharmacologically active agents impor-

270 granule
271 alpha
272 granulo
273 dense
274 coagulation
275 glycogen
276 cell membrane

tant in (274) _____. (You should finish #276 at this point.)

Thrombopoiesis

As in hematopoiesis (the development of (277) _____), thrombopoiesis, which is the maturation of (278) _____ or thrombocytes, occurs in the (279) _____ _____. The sequence of events leading up to the release of a mature thrombocyte consists of a series of cells called the megakaryocytic series. The first cell in this cell line is the megakaryoblast.

277 erythrocytes
278 platelets
279 bone marrow

Thrombopoiesis

280 megakaryoblast
281 larger
282 bone marrow

283 two
284 baso

285 large
286 baso
287 azurophilic
288 increases

289 largest
290 bone marrow

291 promegakaryocyte

292 megakaryocytes
293 megakaryocytes

294 azurophilic

295 megakaryocytes
296 megakaryocytes
297 platelet
298 megakaryocyte

Megakaryoblast

The first recognizable member of the megakaryocytic series is the
(280) _____. Ranging from 15 μm to 25 μm in
diameter and therefore *(281)* _____ (*larger, smaller*) than most other
cell line precursors, the megakaryoblast is found in the *(282)* _____
_____ (*bone marrow, circulating in the blood*). This cell has a light-
staining basophilic cytoplasm with two nuclei, both purple. In addition to the
(283) _____ (*one, two*) nucleus (nuclei) there are numerous mitochondria and
Golgi apparatuses in the *(284)* _____philic cytoplasm. At the cell periphery,
the cytoplasm, usually stippled with azurophilic granules, is devoid of both the
granules and the organelles.

The megakaryoblast's nuclei will fuse and then undergo replication without
concomitant cytokinesis. These nuclear divisions result in a nuclear center of
abundant nuclear material (two to eight times the normal chromatin material).
The cell at this point is termed the promegakaryocyte. (Do not expect to identify
this *specific* stage of the megakaryocytic series in the bone marrow.)

Reserve Megakaryocyte

Subsequent differentiation of the promegakaryocyte, defined by a
(285) _____ (*small, large*) nuclear center, involves a marked increase in
cytoplasmic volume with the disappearance of the lightly *(286)* _____philic-
staining nature of the cytoplasm. The *(287)* _____ granules
are dispersed as the cytoplasm *(288)* _____ (*increases, decreases*) in volume. Although not active in platelet formation, the reserve megakaryocyte is fully formed. (The terminology is confusing, and one might often see
the term *promegakaryocyte* used in place of *reserve megakaryocyte*.)

The reserve megakaryocyte is a very large cell, 50 μm to 70 μm in diameter,
and therefore is the *(289)* _____ (*smallest, largest*) blood cell precursor found in the *(290)* _____ _____. The nucleus is very lobulated,
and fine granules are widely dispersed throughout the cytoplasm. Unlike its
precursor, the *(291)* _____, this cell has gran-
ules at the periphery. (This cell is readily identifiable in the bone marrow; even
under low-power magnification it can be identified by its enormous size.)

Platelet-Forming Megakaryocytes

The differentiation of the reserve *(292)* _____ from
the active platelet-forming *(293)* _____ is not easy
using any routine light micrograph; EM is needed. Clustering of the
(294) _____ granules into distinct areas separated from
one another by agranular areas enables one to identify platelet-forming
(295) _____ from reserve
(296) _____. The active
(297) _____-forming *(298)* _____ then
forms vesicular plates that elongate and form a three-dimensional network of
clefts called platelet-demarcation membranes (Fig. 7-21). The platelet-demarcation

299 *vesicular plates*

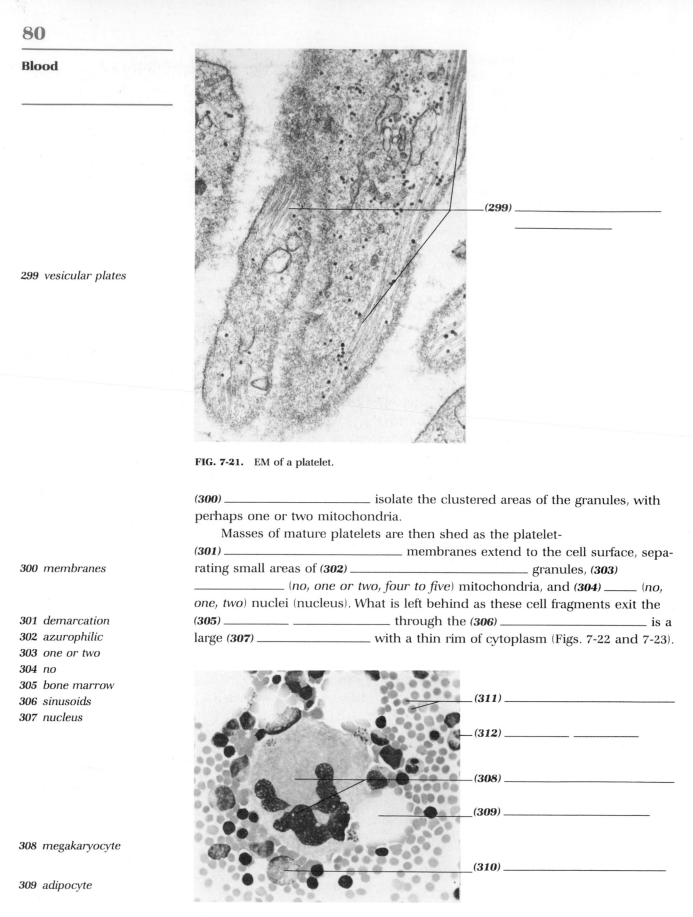

FIG. 7-21. EM of a platelet.

(299) _____

_____

(300) _____ isolate the clustered areas of the granules, with perhaps one or two mitochondria.

Masses of mature platelets are then shed as the platelet-
(301) _____ membranes extend to the cell surface, separating small areas of *(302)* _____ granules, *(303)* _____ *(no, one or two, four to five)* mitochondria, and *(304)* _____ *(no, one, two)* nuclei (nucleus). What is left behind as these cell fragments exit the *(305)* _____ _____ through the *(306)* _____ is a large *(307)* _____ with a thin rim of cytoplasm (Figs. 7-22 and 7-23).

300 *membranes*

301 *demarcation*
302 *azurophilic*
303 *one or two*
304 *no*
305 *bone marrow*
306 *sinusoids*
307 *nucleus*

308 *megakaryocyte*

309 *adipocyte*

(311) _____

(312) _____ _____

(308) _____

(309) _____

(310) _____

FIG. 7-22. EM of a megakaryocyte.

310 *eosinophil*
311 *erythrocytes*
312 *band (stab) cell*

Thrombopoiesis

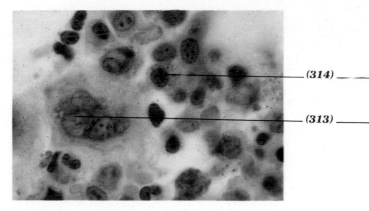

(314) _____

(313) _____

313 megakaryocyte
314 eosinophil

FIG. 7-23. Bone marrow, Wright's stain (original magnification ×400).

8 Muscle

After completing this chapter, you should be able to identify the following:

1 Skeletal muscle
2 Bands, zones, and lines of striated muscle

3 Cardiac muscle
4 Intercalated disks
5 Smooth muscle

Also, after completing this chapter, you should understand the following:

1 The histologic differences between all three types of muscle
2 The histologic changes with muscular contraction
3 The importance of sarcoplasmic reticulum

4 Actin and myosin
5 The importance of intercalated disks.

Muscle consists primarily of specialized contractile cells. Muscle cells contract upon appropriate stimulation owing to the unique, orderly arrangement of various filamentous protein. There are three types of muscle: cardiac, smooth, and skeletal muscle, which can be differentiated by their histologic appearance.

Skeletal muscle cells exhibit regularly spaced transverse bands through their entire length, called cross striations. The cells are syncytial in nature and are under voluntary control. Because the skeletal muscle cell is long and threadlike, the term "fiber" can be used interchangeably with the term "muscle cell." Cardiac muscle cells also exhibit the cross striations, but each cell is a separate cellular unit that has an inherent rhythmic contraction.

Smooth muscle differs from both (1) _____ and (2) _____ muscle by its lack of visible cross (3) _____. Smooth muscle cells are threadlike in appearance, and therefore can be called (4) _____. Like that of cardiac muscle, the contraction of smooth muscle is (5) _____ (*voluntary, involuntary*).

1 *cardiac*
2 *skeletal*
3 *striations*
4 *fibers*
5 *involuntary*

Skeletal Muscle

Often called striated or voluntary muscle, skeletal muscle makes up much of the somatic musculature. Individual skeletal muscles are enclosed by a sheath of dense irregular connective tissue called the epimysium. Bundles of muscle fibers within the muscle are separated by fibrous partitions collectively called the perimysium. This partition serves to conduct blood vessels, nerves, and lymphatics to and from muscle bundles. A more delicate sheath of connective tissue extending between and investing each muscle fiber is the endomysium. The endomysium is rich in capillaries and contains nerves innervating a specific

6 *dense irregular*
connective tissue

7 *more*

8 *bundles of fibers*

9 *endo*

10 *sarcolemma*

muscle fiber. The epimysium, composed of *(6)* _____

_____ _____ _____, has

(7) _____ (*more, fewer*) collagenous fibers than the delicate endomysium does; the perimysium, a partition around

(8) _____ (*separate fibers, bundles of fibers*), conducts blood vessels.

The striated skeletal muscle fiber is long (1 μm to 40 μm long) and cylindrical in shape (Fig. 8-1). Surrounding each muscle fiber is the *(9)* _____<u>mysium</u> and directly beneath that is the muscle fiber's plasma membrane, the sarcolemma. Skeletal muscle fibers are multinucleate, with the nucleus lying just beneath the cell's plasma membrane, the *(10)* _____. Ovoid in shape, each nucleus contains more than one nucleolus. (You should finish #12 at this point.)

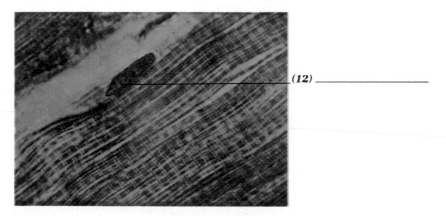

(12) _____

FIG. 8-1. Identify the type of muscle:
(11) _____ _____.
Hematoxylin-eosin (H and E) stain (original magnification × 150).

11 *skeletal muscle*
12 *nucleus*

13 *sarco*

14 *cross*

The cytoplasm of any muscle cell is termed the sarcoplasm. Organelles such as mitochondria and Golgi, small amount of glycogen, plus small amounts of myoglobin are found within the *(13)* _____<u>plasm</u>. The most prominent structures in the sarcoplasm are the myofibrils. The myofibrils are protein filaments and produce the characteristic *(14)* _____ striations. Surrounding the myofibrils is a lacelike network of tubules (discussed later in this chapter) that play an important role in the stimulation of contraction.

Microscopically, in each skeletal muscle cell, one finds various "bands," "zones," or "lines" that represent different components of the myofibrils, the contractile apparatus of the muscle fibers. (It is important to remember the names and associated functions of the zones, bands, and lines in order to understand the basic mechanism of muscular contraction.) In this high-power light micrograph, one can easily see alternating light and dark bands. The dark bands are called A or anisotropic, and the light-staining bands are called the I or isotropic bands (Fig. 8-2). An electron micrograph (EM) enables us to delineate

Skeletal Muscle

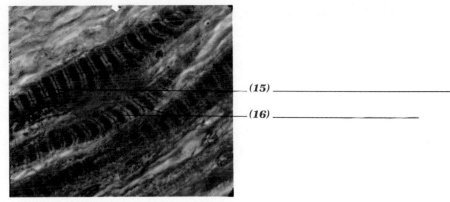

(15) _____

(16) _____

15 anisotropic

16 isotropic

FIG. 8-2. Skeletal muscle, silver stain (original magnification ×180).

subtle detail in the A and I bands. Within the A band or *(17)* _____ band is a noticeably lighter area called the H zone. Traversing the H zone, which is within the *(18)* __ band, is a thin, dark line, the M line. The I band, or *(19)* _____ band, is bisected by a very electron-dense band called the Z band. From one Z band to a successive Z band is a complete functional contractile unit. The unit that stretches from one *(20)* __ to another *(21)* __ band is called a sarcomere and is the definitive contractile apparatus of each muscle fiber (Fig. 8-3). Repeating sarcomeres make up a complete muscle fiber.

17 anisotropic
18 A
19 isotropic

20 Z
21 Z

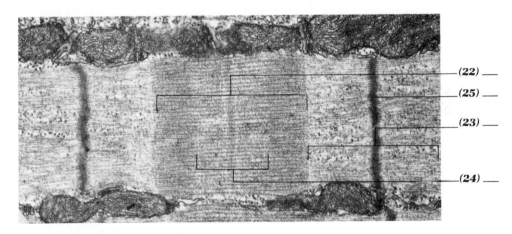

(22) __

(25) __

(23) __

(24) __

FIG. 8-3. Electron micrograph (EM) of skeletal muscle.

22 A
23 I
24 H
25 Z

Further EM and cytochemical analysis has made it possible to identify the specific filaments that make up the *(26)* __, *(27)* __, and *(28)* __ bands, the *(29)* __ zone, and *(30)* __ line. The I band, or *(31)* _____ (*light, dark*) band, is bisected by a *(32)* __ band; the A band consists of a *(33)* __ zone with a bisecting *(34)* __ line.

The light band is composed of a thin protein (500 μm in diameter) called actin. Actin filaments are attached to the Z band and have a free end that terminates in the darker A band. The depth to which the actin—*(35)* _____ (*thin, thick*)—filaments penetrate the darker *(36)* __ band depends upon the degree of contraction.

Thick filaments composed only of the protein myosin are found only in the A band *(37)* _____ (*lighter, darker*) region and are unattached at either end. Myosin is 100 nm in diameter and is *(38)* _____ times thicker than the

26 A
27 I
28 Z
29 H
30 M
31 light
32 Z
33 H
34 M
35 thin
36 A
37 darker
38 two

39 actin
40 I
41 not attached
42 M
43 H
44 H
45 thick

thin, (39) _____ filaments of the (40) __ band. The thick filaments have tapered ends with a slightly thickened middle section. Thick filaments, (41) _____ (attached, not attached) at either end, are held in register to one another by delicate cross connections, giving rise to the dark (42) __ line within the (43) __ zone. The lighter area of the A band, the (44) __ zone, is lighter because it only consists of thick filaments in the relaxed state, and not both thick and thin filaments (Fig. 8-4). The myosin—(45) _____—

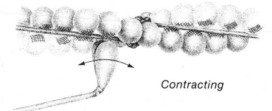

thin filament

Relaxed

Myosin head
(attached to thick
filament)

Active site
of actin
(exposed)

Contracting

FIG. 8-4. Diagram of actin and myosin interaction.

46 I

47 thinner

48 thin or actin
49 globular
50 thick (myosin)

51 thin
52 Z
53 I
54 stretched
55 contracted
56 A
57 remaining constant

58 Z
59 H

filaments of the (46) __ band are composed of subunits that make it possible for contraction. On each thick filament, there are numerous globular heads jutting out. These globular heads are responsible for direct interdigitation with the (47) _____ (thicker, thinner) actin filaments. The myosin globular head is flexible enough to be able to oscillate back and forth, permitting the sliding of actin filaments, and hence contraction.

The process of contraction involves the sliding of (48) _____ filaments over the (49) _____ head of the (50) _____ filaments. This process is called the sliding filament mechanism and involves the use of energy. When a muscle contracts, the sarcomere changes histologically. Since contraction involves the movement of only the (51) _____ (thin, thick) filaments toward each other from their connection to (52) __ bands, the total area of the (53) __ (I, A) band changes. The I band, therefore, is most prominent in (54) _____ (stretched, contracted) muscle, and least prominent in (55) _____ (stretched, contracted) muscle. As the thin filaments penetrate into the (56) __ band, the Z bands are drawn closer together with the A band area always (57) _____ (remaining constant, becoming smaller). Upon contraction, the thin filaments approaching from each (58) __ band get close enough to obliterate the light zone of the A band, the (59) __ zone.

There is an elaborate network of tubules that surrounds the myofibrils and functions in the excitation of the myofibrils, causing them to contract. This threadlike canalicular network around each myofibril is called the sarcoplasmic

60 *endoplasmic*

61 *rough endoplasmic*

62 *darker*

reticulum (SR) and is similar in structure to *(60)* _____
reticulum of other cells. The SR is devoid of ribisomes, unlike the
(61) _____ _____ _____ reticulum (rER). It is important to
realize that the SR is a highly repetitious network that bears a constant relationship with each sarcomere and the specific bands. The SR consists of both a
different morphologic and physiological function for each different band it in-
vests. In skeletal muscle, the part of the SR that overlies the A band, or
(62) _____ (*darker, lighter*) band, is a longitudinal canaliculus that anastomoses greatly in the H zone region. The tubules lying on the A band are called
sarcotubules. At regular intervals, the sarcotubules become confluent and inter-
sect tubules of a much larger caliber. These larger sized, transversely oriented
tubules are called terminal cristae or terminal cisterna and store calcium. Terminal cristae run in parallel pairs along the H band (Fig. 8-5).

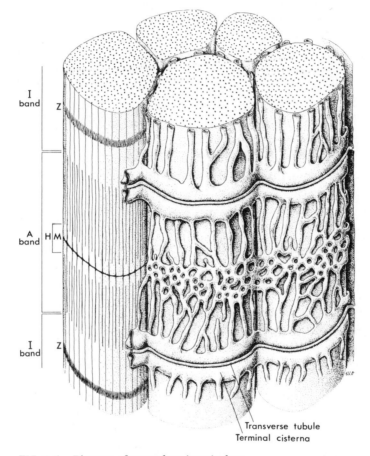

FIG. 8-5. Diagram of sarcoplasmic reticulum.

63 *sarcotubular*

64 *T tubules*

65 *transverse tubule*
66 *reticulum*
67 *plasma membrane*

Between terminal cristae is a closely juxtaposed tubule that is not directly
confluent with the terminal cristae, as the *(63)* _____ _____
are, and is a slender transversing tubule called a T tubule or transverse tubule.
The three together, the terminal cristae, *(64)* ___ _____ _____, and terminal
cristae, constitute the triad of skeletal muscle. The T tubule, or
(65) _____ _____, is not really a part of the sarcoplasmic *(66)* _____, but it is instead continuous with the sarcolemma, the muscle cell's *(67)* _____ _____. The T-tubule
lumen communicates with the extracellular space at the cell surface. Therefore,

Muscle

68 sarco

69 T tubule
70 calcium
71 sarcomere
72 sliding-filament
73 actin (thin)
74 thick
75 myosin
76 I
77 H
78 A
79 voluntary

80 sarcolemma
81 membrane
   (sarcolemma)

82 sliding-filament
83 motor neuron
84 muscle fiber
85 T tubule
86 terminal cristae
87 calcium

88 terminal cristae
89 T tubules
90 terminal cristae
91 H
92 abundant
93 energy (cATP)
94 thin
95 actin
96 SR

97 red
98 white
99 skeletal
100 red

the T tubule is a slender invagination of the (68) _____ lemma that penetrates deep into muscle fibers. T tubules are commonly referred to as the T system.

SR acts in the conduction of the impulse for the myofibrils. Transmitting the impulse from the sarcolemma, the (69) __ _____ causes the SR to release its stored (70) _____. The release of calcium will enable contraction of each individual (71) _____. Contraction, as described by the (72) _____-_____ mechanism, is the movement of (73) _____ filaments over the stationary (74) _____ filaments composed of (75) _____. The muscle in the contracted state makes the (76) __ band smaller and the (77) __ zone disappear while the (78) __ band stays the same.

Skeletal muscle contraction is (79) _____ (voluntary, involuntary), and involves the propagation of an impulse through nerves to specialized arrangements at or directly on the muscle fiber itself. Each muscle fiber is supplied by an efferent motor axon, or a branch of an axon. The motor neuron, or efferent axon, and the muscle fiber(s) it supplies constitute a motor unit. Where these motor neurons synapse on the muscle fiber are highly specialized areas called motor end plates. When the motor neuron synapses with the muscle fiber it may lose its protective myelin sheath. This unmyelinated nerve will then form terminal arborizations within the highly invaginated plasma membrane of the muscle, the (80) _____. The nerves themselves do not come in direct contact with the (81) _____ but are separated by a 40 nm to 60 nm area called a synaptic cleft. Upon stimulation, the nerve releases substances into the synaptic cleft that in turn stimulates the (82) _____-_____ mechanism. What are the two constituents of a motor unit? (83) _____ _____ and (84) _____ _____. The sarcolemma, which is continuous with the (85) __-_____ system, stimulates the tubules, which in turn cause the (86) _____ _____ to release the stored (87) _____; and hence contraction ensues.

Cytochemical and histologic differences among skeletal fibers make it possible to identify three distinct types of skeletal muscle. The three types of fibers, red, white, and intermediate, are identical in most cytologic characteristics. Red fibers are distinctly smaller in diameter than most muscle fibers, highly vascular, and very rich in myoglobin and mitochondria. Fine microscopy reveals thicker Z bands and a much more complex SR, which consists of (88) _____ _____, (89) __ _____, and (90) _____ _____, and anastomoses at the (91) __ zone. The very (92) _____ (abundant, sparse) mitochondria with increased numbers of cristae indicate a high production of (93) _____. White fibers are larger in diameter than red, contain less myoglobin and mitochondria, and have thinner Z bands, attachments to (94) _____ (thin, thick) (95) _____ (actin, myosin) filaments. The surrounding canalicular network about the myofibrils, the (96) __ __, is expectedly less complex in white fibers.

Intermediate fibers are so named because their cytologic characteristics fall between those of (97) _____ and (98) _____ fibers. A more precise means of identifying these typical (99) _____ muscle fibers is by the production of an enzyme by mitochondria, succinodehydrogenase. Since (100) _____ (red, white) fibers have more mitochondria, the amount of the enzyme *(101)* _____ dehydrogenase present will be *(102)* _____ *(little, very evident)* and stain *(103)* _____ *(lighter, darker)*.

101 *succino*
102 *very evident*
103 *darker*

Cardiac Muscle

Cardiac muscle, like skeletal muscle, is *(104)* _____ muscle owing to its *(105)* _____. While skeletal muscle fibers are a syncytium, cardiac muscle is composed of individual cells joined by a specialized cell junction (Fig. 8-6). Control of skeletal muscle function is voluntary while

104 *striated*
105 *cross striation*

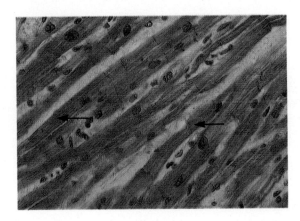

FIG. 8-6. Cardiac muscle. Arrows indicate intercalated discs. H and E stain (original magnification ×150).

cardiac muscle cells possess an inherent rhythm and therefore contraction is *(106)* _____. Within the cardiac *(107)* _____ plasm are myofibrils that are arranged almost identically to those of *(108)* _____ muscle. *(109)* __, *(110)* __, and *(111)* __ bands, *(112)* __ zone, and *(113)* __ line can be easily identified in cardiac muscle. The individual cardiac muscle cell has a(n) *(114)* _____ *(centrally, eccentrically)* placed nucleus within the sarcoplasm, and causes the myofibrils to diverge around it. Skeletal muscle has a nucleus that lies just beneath the *(115)* _____, and therefore the nucleus assumes a(n) *(116)* _____ *(central, eccentric)* position.

At the nuclear poles of cardiac muscle are prominent Golgi apparatuses and other organelles. Mitochondria are found not just around the centrally placed *(117)* _____, but are abundant throughout the cell (Fig. 8-7). Cardiac

106 *involuntary*
107 *sarco*
108 *skeletal*
109 *A*
110 *I*
111 *Z*
112 *H*
113 *M*
114 *centrally*
115 *sarcolemma*
116 *eccentric*

117 *nucleus*

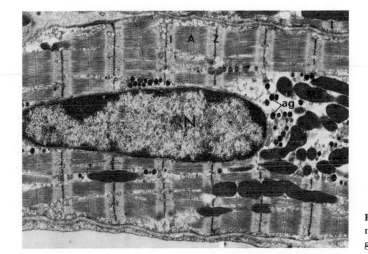

FIG. 8-7. EM of a cardiac muscle cell. ag = aging granules.

muscle cells have more mitochondria, each with an increased number of cristae, than do skeletal muscle cells. Mitochondria, which are necessary for *(118)* _____ production, use the numerous glycogen and lipid droplets found within the *(119)* _____ plasm. A yellow brown pigment is deposited in cardiac muscle *(120)* _____ plasm as one ages. Often called an aging pigment, lipofuscin can indicate the general age of the tissue.

There are repeating dark-staining lines that adjoin individual cardiac muscle *(121)* _____ *(fibers, cells)*. These dark lines represent a specific surface modification that provides extensive interdigitation between cardiac muscle cells and are called intercalated discs (Fig. 8-8). Skeletal muscle

118 energy
119 sarco
120 sarco

121 cells

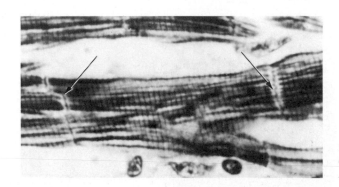

FIG. 8-8. Photomicrograph of *(122)* _____ _____.

(123) _____ *(does, does not)* have intercalated discs adjoining individual fibers. The intercalated disc cuts transversely across the cardiac muscle cell, and is composed of specific cell attachments similar to those found adjoining epithelial cells. One part of the intercalated *(124)* _____ is the macula adherens, or *(125)* _____. As in epithelia, the macula adherens provides for powerful cell-to-cell adhesion. The term for this expanded desmosome or *(126)* _____ _____ in cardiac muscle is fascia adherens. Not as easily recognizable as the desmosomes are small discontinuations of the adjoining cell membranes called gap junctions, or *(127)* _____. Gap junctions serve to transmit impulses across a small space, enabling rapid conduction from cell to cell.

In addition to the *(128)* _____ portion, there is another portion of the intercalated disc that runs longitudinally. The longitudinal portion of the *(129)* _____ disc is composed of larger *(130)* _____ junctions or *(131)* _____, and therefore plays a *(132)* _____ *(lesser, greater)* role in impulse conduction.

Like skeletal muscle, cardiac muscle has an SR surrounding it, but one that is considerably less well developed. There is in cardiac muscle no comparable transverse element like the terminal cristae. In place of the terminal cristae are small expansions juxtaposed to the outer *(133)* _____ tubule. The classic triad, which is composed of a *(134)* _____, *(135)* _____, and *(136)* _____ _____, is not evident in *(137)* _____ muscle because of the small nature of the terminal ends of the *(138)* _____ _____. The intimate anastomoses of the sarcotubules found in skeletal muscle are also less complex in cardiac muscle.

T tubules, an extension of the *(139)* _____, along with the terminal cisternae, is found at the *(140)* ___ band in skeletal *(141)* _____. The reticulum system of cardiac muscle has the end ves-

122 cardiac muscle

123 does not

124 disc
125 desmosome

126 macula adherens

127 nexus

128 horizontal

129 intercalated
130 gap
131 nexus
132 greater

133 T terminal
134 cristae
135 T tubule
136 terminal cristae
137 cardiac
138 terminal cristae

139 sarcolemma
140 H
141 muscle

Cardiac Muscle

142 SR

143 cardiac and skeletal

144 basal lamina

145 cross striation

146 nucleus

scls of the **(142)** __ __ over the Z band. T tubules of cardiac muscle are also twice as large as in skeletal muscle and arc lined with a basal lamina that is external to the sarcolemma. In both types of striated muscle, **(143)** _____ and _____, T tubules are important in impulse transmission. Since the T tubules of cardiac muscle are lined with a **(144)** _____ _____, they also provide additional surface area for exchange of metabolites between the extracellular space and the cardiac muscle cell. Specialized cardiac muscle cells of the heart will be discussed in Chapter 10.

Smooth Muscle

Smooth muscle, as its name implies, lacks the identifying **(145)** _____ _____ of striated muscle (Fig. 8-9). Like skeletal muscle fibers,

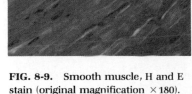

(146) _____

FIG. 8-9. Smooth muscle, H and E stain (original magnification ×180).

smooth muscle cells are arranged in a long, spindle shape, and therefore the terms "cell" and "fiber" are interchangeable. Closer examination reveals the fibers arranged in bundles or sheaths (Fig. 8-10). These bundles or sheaths of fibers

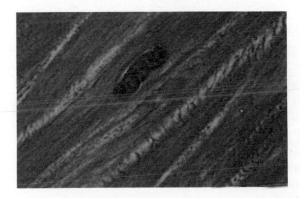

FIG. 8-10. Identify the type of muscle: **(147)** _____ _____. H and E stain (original magnification ×275).

147 smooth muscle

148 *involuntary*

149 *extra*

150 *smooth muscle*

151 *fibroblasts*

152 *fiber*

153 *cardiac*
154 *acidophilic*

155 *middle*
156 *end*

157 *end*

158 *longitudinal and
smooth muscle*
159 *cross section of
smooth muscle*

160 *centrally*

freely interdigitate, forming a single functional unit. These bundles play important roles in the gastrointestinal and respiratory tracts and also in blood vessel walls and the walls of the viscera. Control of smooth muscle is like that of cardiac muscle—*(148)* _____ (*voluntary, involuntary*).

Fine examination of the smooth muscle fiber informs us that each individual fiber is encased in an extracellular matrix of collagen, elastic fibers, and an amorphous component. The *(149)* _____cellular material surrounding the fibers is synthesized by the muscle cell itself. The matrix between each fiber is 40 nm to 60 nm thick, and is similar in function to the basal lamina of epithelial cells and the external lamina of other cells. The collagen surrounding each smooth muscle fiber merges with the collagen of the connective tissue that surrounds a bundle of the fibers. Whereas the collagen around each muscle fiber is, for the most part, produced by the *(150)* _____ _____ fiber, the collagen of connective tissue origin is synthesized by *(151)* _____. Both the collagen meshwork between the individual fibers and the connective tissue surrounding the muscle *(152)* _____ help to maintain fiber relationship in the alternating cycles of stretching and contraction. Each individual smooth muscle cell is a spindle-shaped fiber and can be as small as 10 μm, as in small blood vessels, or as long as 0.2 mm, as in the uterus. The nucleus of the smooth muscle fiber is centrally located, as in *(153)* _____ muscle. The center of the *(154)* _____ (*basophilic, acidophilic*) fiber bulges slightly to accommodate the nucleus. Smooth muscle fibers are juxtaposed in a way so the bulging *(155)* _____ (*end, middle*) of one fiber is adjacent to the thin tapered *(156)* _____ (*end, middle*) of another cell. This arrangement in sheets of fibers produces, on cross section, fibers that are round and polygonal. The absence of the nucleus in some fibers indicates that the section of the fiber is at its *(157)* _____ (*end, middle*), and not where the nucleus is (Fig. 8-11).

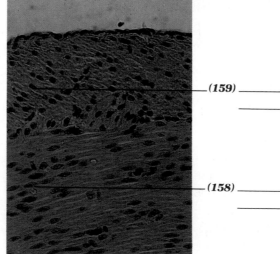

(159) _____ _____ _____

_____ _____

(158) _____ _____

_____ _____

FIG. 8-11. Identify the section and the type of muscle. H and E stain (original magnification ×125).

The sarcoplasm of smooth muscle contains organelles and glycogen granules that are primarily confined to the sarcoplasm around the *(160)* _____ (*centrally, eccentrically*) located nucleus. The highly

Smooth Muscle

visible *(161)* ___ fibrils ___ of *(162)* ___ and
(163) ___ muscle are not evident in smooth muscle; there are
filaments in the fiber involved in contraction. Throughout the sarcoplasm of a
smooth muscle fiber are randomly arranged thick, thin, and intermediate filaments (Fig. 8-12). The thin filaments, measuring 7 μm in diameter, are composed

161 myo
162 skeletal
163 cardiac

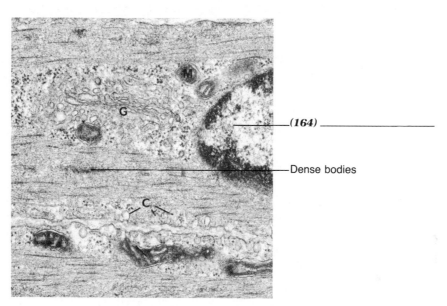

(164) ___

Dense bodies

164 nucleus

FIG. 8-12. EM of smooth muscle. M = mitochondria; G = Golgi; C = caveolae.

of actin whereas the thick filaments are composed of *(165)* ___
(*actin, myosin*) and are 17 μm in diameter. These filaments do not form
(166) ___ ___ like striated muscle, because they
do not overlap and are not organized into the contractile unit like the
(167) ___ mere.

165 myosin

166 cross striations

167 sarco

Intermediate fibers have only recently been studied; they may play a crucial
role in smooth muscle contraction. Measuring 10 μm in diameter, intermediate
fibers represent a continuous system that pulls on the cell membrane from its
attachment to randomly dispersed areas of the smooth muscle cell called dense
bodies. Dense bodies, as their name describes and Figure 8-12 shows, are electron *(168)* ___ and serve as points of attachment for
(169) ___ filaments. The exact function of the dense
bodies is unknown, but evidence leads to a Z-band counterpart in that they serve
as an area for attachment for the basic contractile mechanism. The mechanism
of contraction is believed to be very much like that of striated muscle contraction, the *(170)* ___-___ mechanism.

168 dense
169 intermediate

Smooth muscle fibers have an SR and a T tubule system, but it is considerably less well developed than that of *(171)* ___ or ___
muscle. In skeletal muscle, *(172)* __ tubules anastomose in the *(173)* __ band,
while in cardiac muscle anastomosis is at the *(174)* __ band.

170 sliding-filament

Smooth muscle's SR does not invest the filaments, *(175)* ___ or
myosin, *(176)* ___ or *(177)* ___, and intermediate filaments that
are directly associated with contraction. Instead, the SR is associated with narrow, longitudinal rows of subsurface vesicles called caveolae. Caveolae are invaginations of the plasma membrane, the *(178)* ___, and trans-
mit the impulse down into the cell. Carrying the impulses into the cell, the
caveolae assume a role similar to the *(179)* __ ___ system of striated
muscle.

171 cardiac or skeletal
172 T
173 H
174 Z
175 thick
176 thin
177 actin

178 sarcolemma
179 T tubule

9 Nervous Tissue

After completing this chapter, you should be able to identify the following:

1 Neuron: cell body, axon, dendrite   5 Neuroglia
2 Schwann's cells   6 Oligodendrocytes
3 Gray matter   7 Astrocytes
4 White matter

Also, after completing this chapter, you should understand the following:

1 The function of myelin   3 The components of the motor
2 The histologic differences be-   unit
   tween the spinal cord, cerebellar   4 Motor spindles
   cortex, and cerebral cortex

The structural and functional unit of nervous tissue is the nerve cell, or neuron. There are over 10 billion of these *(1)* _____ in the human nervous system. Most neurons have processes called nerve fibers, which are thin extensions of cytoplasm covered by a *(2)* _____ _____.

Neurons can be classified by the number of processes (Fig. 9-1). Unipolar neurons, found in the retina, have one *(3)* _____ _____ extending out from the cell body, or soma. Neurons with two nerve fibers, such as in structures associated with hearing and balance, are classified as *(4)* bi_____. Pseudo-unipolar neurons, found in sensory ganglia, have two nerve fibers branching off a single process of the cell body. Most neurons of the body have numerous nerve *(5)* _____ and are classified as multipolar neurons. The processes can be of two types.

1 neurons

2 plasma (cell)
* membrane*

3 nerve fiber

4 polar

5 fibers

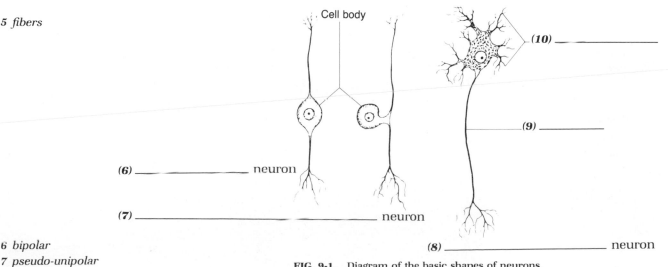

FIG. 9-1. Diagram of the basic shapes of neurons.

6 bipolar
7 pseudo-unipolar
8 multipolar
9 axon
10 dendrites

11 axon

12 unipolar
13 axon

14 soma

Each neuron can have one, and only one, axon, which tends to be very straight. Axons usually carry the electrical impulse away from the soma to the other neurons. The longer the length of the *(11)* _____, the larger the soma will be. Dendrites are branchlike structures and are usually very numerous. These processes usually receive the electrical impulse and carry it to the cell body. In a *(12)* pseudo-_____ neuron, one of the branch fibers serves as the dendrite, while the other serves as the *(13)* _____.

Cell Body

The cell body, or *(14)* _____, is usually very large (up to 135 μm in diameter), although some are small (about 4 μm). The shape is generally round, although certain specialized neurons have cell bodies with different shapes (Fig. 9-2). The

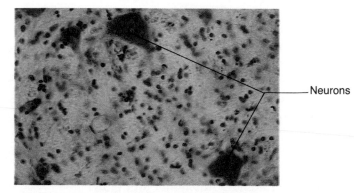

—Neurons

FIG. 9-2. Photomicrograph of nervous tissue, hematoxylin-eosin (H and E) stain (original magnification ×200).

15 centrally

16 nucleolus

17 euchromatin

18 basophilic
19 Nissl

20 ribosomes

21 dendrites

large nucleus is located *(15)* _____ (*centrally, peripherally*), and is also rounded. The most prominent feature of the nucleus is the large central *(16)* _____, which gives the neuron what has been called an "owl's eye" appearance. The chromatin of the nucleus is usually in the extended form, called *(17)* _____, and chromatin granules cannot be seen.

The most prominent feature of the cytoplasm of large neurons are the clumps of *(18)* _____ (*eosinophilic, basophilic*) material called Nissl bodies. Also found in large dendrites, *(19)* _____ bodies are areas of cytoplasm containing increased amounts of flattened cisternae of rough endoplasmic reticulum (rER) with numerous free and attached *(20)* _____. These function to synthesize proteins and enzymes to be carried by the continuous flow of cytoplasm into both axons and *(21)* _____ (Fig. 9-3).

Cell Body

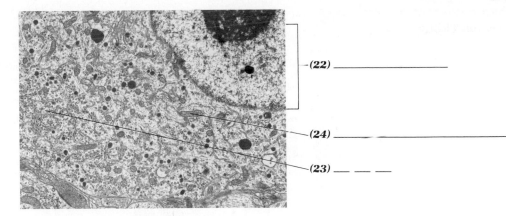

(22) _____

(24) _____

(23) __ __ __

FIG. 9-3. Electron micrograph (EM) of a part of the cell body of a neuron (original magnification ×15,000).

22 *nucleus*
23 *rER*
24 *mitochondria*

Neurofilaments (also called intermediate filaments) are filaments 10 nm in diameter found clumped into fibrils called neurofibrils. Their exact composition and function are generally unknown. Neurotubules, which are typical microtubules *(25)* _____ μm in diameter, function to maintain the *(26)* _____ of the neuron and aid in the *(27)* _____ of materials through the cytoplasm and into the processes. Golgi complexes and mitochondria can also be found.

25 *25*
26 *shape*
27 *movement*

Axon

The axon, of which there is usually *(28)* _____ (*one, more than one*) per neuron, is the most prominent process. Its length can vary from 1 mm to 1 m, and its diameter, from 1 μm to 15 μm. The part of the soma that protrudes outward and continues as the axon is called the axon hillock. There is no rER in the initial portion, or axon *(29)* _____, but neurofilaments and *(30)* _____ tubules are numerous.

28 *one*

The plasma membrane of the axon is referred to as the axolemma, and the cytoplasm as *(31)* _____ plasm (Fig. 9-4). Numerous mitochondria are present and oriented parallel to the long axis of the neuron. Portions of smooth endoplasmic reticulum (sER) are visible, and are referred to as oxoplasmic vesicles.

29 *hillock*
30 *neuro*

31 *axo*

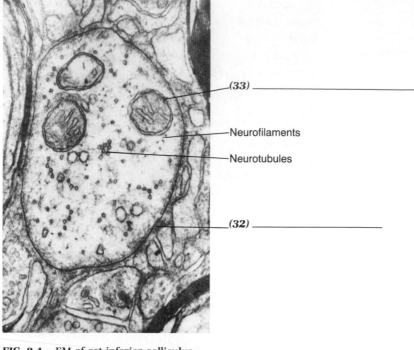

(33) _____

—Neurofilaments

—Neurotubules

(32) _____

32 axolemma
33 mitochondria

FIG. 9-4. EM of cat inferior colliculus (original magnification ×40,000). (Courtesy of Dr. Edward G. Jones, Washington University School of Medicine, St. Louis, Missouri)

Ribosomes are scarce, and two organelles are noticeably absent in the axoplasm. What are they? *(34)* __ __ __ and *(35)* _____. Because of this absence, the axon is totally dependent upon the cell body, or *(36)* _____, to synthesize its protein. Transport through the axoplasm occurs with the aid of *(37)* _____. Thus, the longer the axon, the *(38)* _____ *(larger, smaller)* the cell body must be to support it.

34 rER
35 Golgi
36 soma
37 neurotubules
38 larger

Axons may be covered with myelin, which greatly increases the speed of conduction of the electrical impulse. Myelin is composed of the same elements as the cell membrane, protein and *(39)* <u>phospo   </u>, and is produced by specialized cells in both the central (CNS) and peripheral nervous system (PNS). This process of myelinization will be discussed later.

39 lipid

Dendrites

Dendrites, which usually carry the electrical impulse *(40)* _____ *(away, toward)* the cell body, are shorter and *(41)* _____ *(more, less)* numerous than axons (usually 5 to 15 dendrites per cell). Large dendrites have clumps of rER in the cytoplasm called *(42)* _____ _____, which decrease in number the farther the dendrites are from the cell body. Most dendrites contain multiple small protrusions called dendritic spines, which function in the communication process. These spines increase in number the farther they are from the soma. Each dendritic *(43)* _____ is a pedunculated structure with an expanded tip on a narrow stalk 0.5 μm to 1.0 μm long. To help maintain its shape, the stalk usually contains *(44)* _____.

40 toward
41 more

42 Nissl bodies

43 spine

44 neurotubules

Synapse

The synapse is the site of communication between neurons. It is an area where the electrical impulse is delivered from the end of one nerve fiber, called the presynaptic terminal, and received by another nerve fiber, called the postsynaptic terminal. The presynaptic terminal is usually part of the fiber that carries impulses away from the cell body, the **(45)** _____. The postsynaptic terminal is usually part of the highly branched nerve fiber, the **(46)** _____.
This type of synapse, where an axon comes in contact with a dendrite, is called axodendritic. It is common for the axon to synapse on the protrusion of the dendrite, the **(47)** _____ _____. There are also axosomatic synapses, in which the axon comes in contact with the **(48)** _____ _____ of another neuron, or axo-axonal synapses in which the presynaptic terminal contacts an unmyelinated portion of another **(49)** _____. The synaptic cleft is the small space between the presynaptic and postsynaptic **(50)** _____ and is usually 20 nm to 30 nm wide (Fig. 9-5).

The presynaptic terminal has numerous mitochondria and many synaptic vesicles, which resemble **(51)** _____ vesicles found in glandular cells. The synaptic vesicles are usually 40 nm to 50 nm in diameter, and generally are spherical. Attached to the cytoplasmic face of the plasma membrane of the **(52)** pre_____ terminal is a hexagonal array of electron-dense particles (60 nm in diameter) that are joined by filaments. This whole structure is called the presynaptic vesicular grid and allows the **(53)** ____ _____ vesicles to pass through and reach the plasma membrane.

The postsynaptic terminal, like the presynaptic terminal, has an area of electron-dense particles beneath its plasma membrane. However, the area is more electron dense on the postsynaptic side. (You should finish #54 to 57 at this point.)

45 axon
46 dendrite

47 dendritic spine
48 cell body

49 axon

50 terminals

51 secretory

52 synaptic

53 synaptic

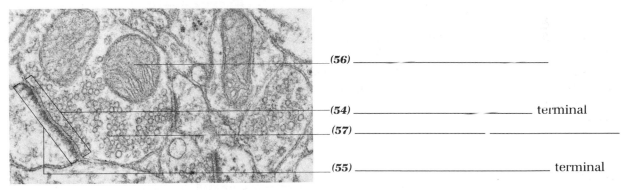

(56) _____ _____

(54) _____ _____ terminal

(57) _____ _____

(55) _____ terminal

FIG. 9-5. EM of synapses in the brain (original magnification ×41,000).

54 presynaptic
55 postsynaptic
56 mitochondria
57 synaptic vesicles
58 20
59 30

The synaptic cleft, usually **(58)** ____ nm to **(59)** ____ nm wide, contains an electron-dense area composed of fine threadlike extensions of the plasma membrane from both the presynaptic and postsynaptic membranes that intertwine and function to hold the two terminals together. Which type of intercellular junction do these modifications on the presynaptic and postsynaptic membrane and the synaptic cleft resemble in structure and function? **(60)** _____ _____

The release of the neurotransmitter (NT) contained within the synaptic vesicle occurs when the electrical impulse travels down the axon and reaches the **(61)** _____synaptic terminal. The NT is released through the same process

60 macula adherens

61 pre

62 *exocytosis*
63 *axolemma*

64 *outer*

65 *coated vesicle*

66 *synaptic vesicle*

67 *synaptic*
68 *exocytosis*
69 *coated*
70 *basket*

by which secretions are released from secretory vesicles, **(62)** _____; this involves fusion of the membrane of the vesicle with the membrane of the axon, called the **(63)** _____ (Fig. 9-6). The membranes of the synaptic vesicles are recycled between the axolemma and the rER from which they originate. Certain areas of the inner membrane of the axolemma have a bristled appearance and are destined to be pinched off into the cytoplasm. Because a whole section of membrane pinches off into the cytoplasm, the bristled border will appear on the **(64)** _____ (*inner, outer*) layer of the newly formed "coated vesicle." The coating, referred to as a basket, is of unknown composition and falls off before the vesicle reaches the rER, where the vesicular membrane fuses with the membrane of the rER.

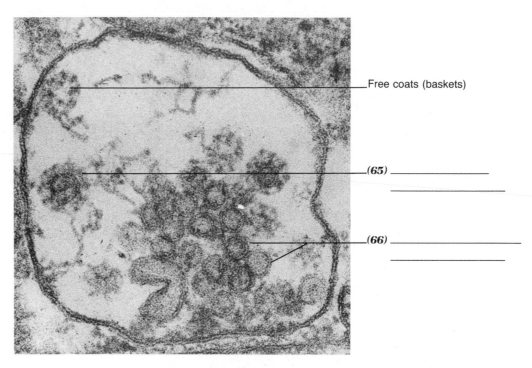

Free coats (baskets)

(65) _____

(66) _____

FIG. 9-6. EM of a synapse in the cerebral cortex.

Thus, the recycling mechanism is composed of the formation by the rER of the **(67)** _____ vesicle, the release of its contents by the process of **(68)** _____, the formation from bristled axolemma of **(69)** _____ vesicles, and its eventual fusion, once the **(70)** _____ falls off, with the rER.

Peripheral Nervous System

The PNS is composed of ganglia, nerves, nerve endings, and organs of special sense. Ganglia are little nodules containing the cell bodies of neurons. They are either central (or spinal) ganglia, which contain the cell bodies of sensory (afferent) neurons; or peripheral (or autonomic) ganglia, which contain the cell bodies of effector (efferent) neurons of the autonomic nervous system. Nerves exist as cordlike structures containing a great number of nerve fibers. Effector nerve endings usually terminate in glands or muscles. Sensory nerve endings and their related organs of special sense will not be discussed here.

Peripheral Nervous
System

Peripheral Nerves

The most obvious feature of a peripheral nerve is the extensive connective tissue component, which can be divided into three layers (Fig. 9-7). The epineurium is the outer tubelike layer of dense irregular connective tissue that encases the whole nerve. The epineurium is not as thick or as resistant to stretch as the inner tube of (71) _____ _____ connective tissue, the (72) peri-_____. Each tube of perineurium encases a fascicle (or bundle) of nerve fibers. Each nerve fiber is enclosed by a tube of connective

71 dense irregular
72 neurium

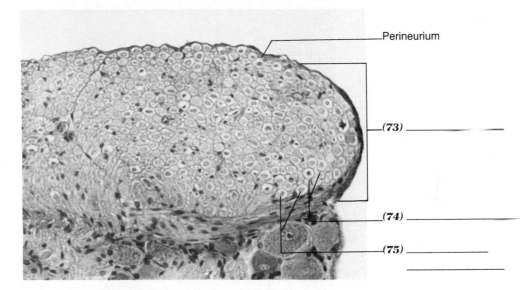

Perineurium

(73) _____

73 fascicle (bundle)

(74) _____

(75) _____

74 endoneurium

FIG. 9-7. Photomicrograph of a cross section of a peripheral nerve (original magnification × 125).

75 nerve fibers

tissue called the endoneurium. Some of the thinner nerve fibers may not have an (76) endo_____. A nerve fiber with its covering, the (77) _____, may penetrate the perineurium and pass from one (78) _____ to another. The majority of nerve fibers in a peripheral nerve are usually the longest of the nerve fibers, the (79) _____.

The neurolemma (or sheath of Schwann) is a thin cytoplasmic covering, directly over the nerve fiber, produced by specialized cells of the PNS called Schwann's cells. Myelinated fibers have an extensive myelin covering between the nerve fiber and the overlying (80) _____, or (81) _____ of Schwann. The myelin is produced by the same cells whose cytoplasm forms the neurolemma, the (82) _____ cells. Unmyelinated fibers have the cytoplasm of the (83) _____ cell directly apposed to the nerve fiber. Covering both the neurolemma and the myelin sheath, if it exists, is the innermost connective tissue covering, the (84) _____.

A peripheral nerve will appear differently depending on the type of stain used in the preparation. A hematoxylin-eosin (H and E) stain will dissolve most (85) _____-soluble substances and the myelin will be washed out. Consequently, all that is observed is the nerve fiber with a surrounding empty space where the (86) _____ should be; the covering (87) _____ of the Schwann's cells remains. The nucleus of the Schwann's cell is visible, as is the cell that produces the endoneurium, the (88) _____.

76 neurium
77 endoneurium
78 fascicle (bundle)

79 axons

80 neurolemma
81 sheath
82 Schwann's
83 Schwann's

84 endoneurium

85 lipid

86 myelin
87 neurolemma

88 fibroblast

In longitudinal or oblique views, the nerve shows a wavy, snakelike appearance representing the fibers, with nuclei of Schwann's cells and fibroblasts observable (Fig. 9-8).

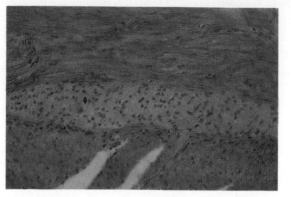

FIG. 9-8. Photomicrograph of a longitudinal section of a peripheral nerve, H and E stain (original magnification ×125).

Osmic acid, which specifically stains myelin, will produce a different view of a peripheral nerve (Fig. 9-9). The dark-staining ring of myelin surrounds an empty space where the *(89)* _____ _____ should be.

89 nerve fiber

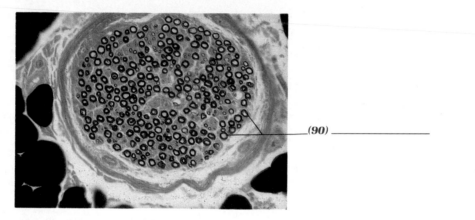

_(90) _____

90 myelin

FIG. 9-9. Photomicrograph of a cross section of a peripheral nerve, osmic acid stain (original magnification ×125).

Schwann's Cells

The myelin is not continuous over the whole length of the axon, but is interrupted at regular intervals called nodes of Ranvier. At these sites, cytoplasmic processes of two neighboring Schwann's cells may interdigitate to cover the axon, but do not totally seal it off from the intercellular space. There is one Schwann's cell between two nodes of *(91)* _____, and the distance between nodes varies from 0.3 mm to 1.5 mm. Nodes are necessary for rapid conduction of the electrical impulse. If the nerve fibers branch, they do so at the *(92)* _____ of Ranvier (Fig. 9-10).

91 Ranvier

92 nodes

Peripheral Nervous System

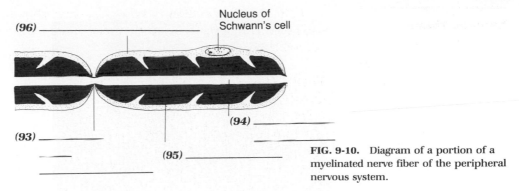

(96) _____

Nucleus of Schwann's cell

(94) _____

(93) _____

_____   *(95)* _____

_____

FIG. 9-10. Diagram of a portion of a myelinated nerve fiber of the peripheral nervous system.

93 node of Ranvier
94 nerve fiber
95 myelin
96 neurolemma
97 one
98 peripheral

Each Schwann's cell can myelinate a portion of only one fiber, and there is *(97)* _____ *(one, more than one)* Schwann's cell located between adjacent pairs of nodes. Schwann's cells are located in the *(98)* _____ *(central, peripheral)* nervous system; oligodendrocytes perform a similar function, the production of *(99)* _____, in the CNS. While Schwann's cells can myelinate *(100)* _____ *(one, more than one)* fiber, oligodendrocytes can myelinate numerous fibers by sending out numerous cytoplasmic processes.

99 myelin

100 one

Unmyelinated fibers of the PNS fit into grooves in the Schwann's cell cytoplasm and are thus protected. Between 5 and 20 fibers can be protected by a single Schwann's cell. The periaxonal space (10 nm–15 nm) is the space between the nerve fiber and the *(101)* _____ _____ cell membrane around it.

101 Schwann's

Central and Peripheral Ganglia

Ganglia are little nodules composed of the *(102)* _____ _____ of neurons (Fig. 9-11). The neurons found within ganglia are referred to as ganglia cells. Central ganglia, also called *(103)* _____ ganglia, contain the cell bodies of *(104)* _____ *(sensory, motor)* neurons. These neurons are of the *(105)* _____ _____ *(pseudo-unipolar, multipolar)* variety. The cell bodies are usually *(106)* _____ *(round, columnar)* and very large (up to 120 μm). The nucleus is *(107)* _____ *(peripherally, centrally)* located and pale staining except for the prominent *(108)* _____. In the cytoplasm, basophilic clumps called *(109)* _____ _____ can be seen. Capsule cells, also called amphicytes, form a single flattened layer of cells around each ganglion cell. The connective tissue framework of the ganglion is similar to that of a peripheral nerve, consisting of a peripheral *(110)* _____neurium___, an inner *(111)* _____, and an *(112)* _____ around each nerve fiber.

102 cell bodies

103 spinal
104 sensory

105 pseudo-unipolar

106 round

107 centrally

108 nucleolus
109 Nissl bodies

110 epi
111 perineurium
112 endoneurium

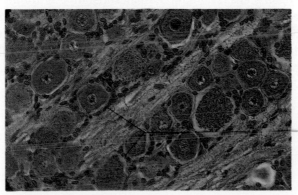

(113) _____

FIG. 9-11. Photomicrograph of a central ganglion, H and E stain (original magnification ×200).

113 amphicytes (capsule cells)

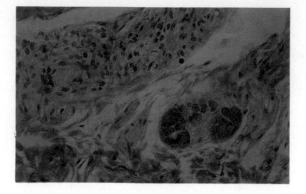

FIG. 9-12. Photomicrograph of a peripheral ganglion, H and E stain (original magnification ×200).

Peripheral ganglia contain the cell bodies of *(114)* _____ *(afferent, effector)* neurons of the autonomic nervous system (Fig. 9-12). These ganglia are also called *(115)* _____ ganglia. They are similar to central ganglia, with a connective tissue framework and a surrounding layer of *(116)* _____ cells around the cell bodies. The ganglion cells are multipolar and the numerous *(117)* _____ *(axons, dendrites)* are responsible for the more irregular shape of the cell body. The capsule cells, or *(118)* _____, are less uniform and not all cell bodies are surrounded by them. The cell bodies themselves are smaller than central ganglion cell bodies, and the nucleus is located *(119)* _____ *(centrally, eccentrically)*.

Central Nervous System

The CNS is composed of the brain and spinal cord with its associated central, or *(120)* _____, ganglia. The billions of neurons of the CNS are not supported by the usual connective tissue, but by cells of neural origin called neuroglial cells. There are three types of *(121)* _____glial cells: astrocytes, microglia, and the cells responsible for the production of myelin in the CNS, *(122)* _____.

Gray Matter

The brain and spinal cord can be divided into gray and white matter, which can be differentiated both grossly and microscopically. The gray matter contains the cell bodies of the neurons and the supporting *(123)* _____ cells. The neuropil, which is seen as background material, is composed of a mass entanglement of fibers, mostly unmyelinated dendrites, and the processes of neuroglial cells. The intercellular substance of the neuropil, referred to as fine intercellular spaces, constitutes 10% to 20% of the brain volume; it is composed of glyosaminoglycans. Extracellular fibers such as *(124)* _____ are lacking. The supporting function normally provided for by such fibers is accomplished in the CNS by the *(125)* _____ cells.

114 effector

115 autonomic

116 capsule
117 dendrites

118 amphicytes

119 eccentrically

120 spinal

121 neuro

122 oligodendrocytes

123 neuroglial

124 collagen

125 neuroglial

Central Nervous System

White Matter

The white (126) _____ is composed almost entirely of myelinated fibers, which provide the gross white coloring. Cell bodies of neurons are lacking, although neuroglial cells such as the myelin-producing (127) _____ are present. The fibers in the white matter originate from cell bodies in (128) _____ matter and from spinal ganglia.

126 matter

Spinal Cord

The spinal cord is organized into a central gray matter covered by the white matter (Fig. 9-13). In an osmic-acid stain the myelin appears (129) _____. Therefore, the (130) _____ matter located (131) _____ (*inside, outside*), which is virtually all myelinated fibers, will appear black; and the gray

127 oligodendrocytes
128 gray

129 black
130 white
131 outside

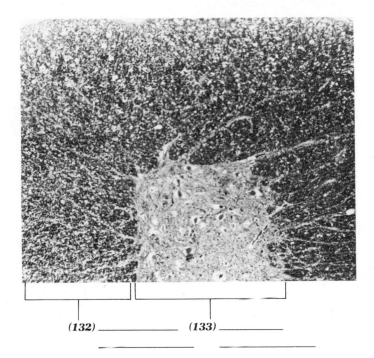

(132) _____ (133) _____

FIG. 9-13. Photomicrograph of a part of the spinal cord, osmic acid stain (original magnification × 125).

matter, which is lacking in myelin, stains white. The cerebrum and cerebellum are organized in an opposite manner, with the gray matter located (134) _____ (*inside, outside*) the white matter.

132 white matter
133 gray matter

134 outside

Cerebral Cortex

The gray matter of the cerebral cortex varies in thickness from 1.5 mm to 5 mm and is found **(135)** _____ (*superficial to, beneath*) the white matter (Fig. 9-14). It is organized into a specific pattern, which varies slightly in relation to specialized functions. Generally, there are six layers of cell bodies of neurons. The most superficial layer is the molecular layer, and contains few cell bodies but numerous fibers from cell bodies of deeper layers. The second layer is the outer granular layer, which appears very **(136)** _____ (*cellular, acellular*), thus producing the granular appearance. The third layer is the pyramidal-cell layer containing large neurons with a pyramidal shape. The inner granular layer, the fourth layer, contains small neurons and is similar to the **(137)** _____ (*first, second*) layer. The internal pyramidal layer is the fifth layer, and the polymorphic (many shapes) cell layer is the innermost layer or the sixth layer. (You should finish #143 at this point.)

135 superficial to

136 cellular

137 second

(138) _____ _____

(139) _____ _____
_____

(140) _____ _____
_____

(141) _____ _____
_____

(142) _____ _____
_____

(143) _____ _____ ____
_____

White matter

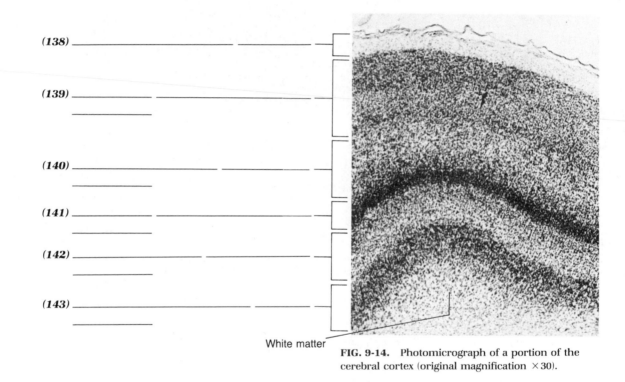

FIG. 9-14. Photomicrograph of a portion of the cerebral cortex (original magnification ×30).

138 molecular layer
139 outer granular layer
140 pyramidal-cell layer
141 inner granular layer
142 internal pyramidal layer
143 polymorphic cell layer
144 molecular

145 neurons

Cerebellar Cortex

The gray matter of the cerebellar cortex is divided into three layers (Fig. 9-15). The outer layer is similar to the outer layer of the cerebral cortex, the **(144)** _____ layer. The middle layer is the Purkinje's cell layer and contains large, flask-shaped cells. The innermost layer is the innergranular layer, which contains numerous small **(145)** _____ (*neurons, fibers*).

Central Nervous System

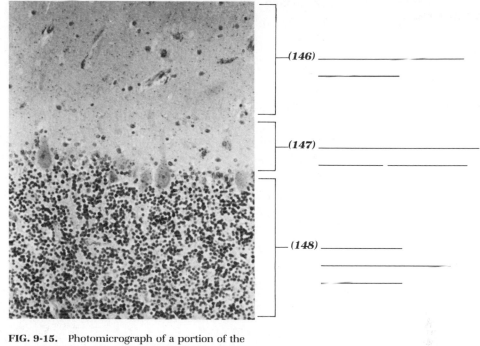

_(146)_ _____

_(147)_ _____

_(148)_ _____

146 _molecular layer_

147 _Purkinje's cell layer_

148 _inner granular layer_

FIG. 9-15. Photomicrograph of a portion of the cerebellar cortex (original magnification ×125).

Neuroglia

The three types of neuroglia are _(149)_ _____,
_(150)_ _____, and
_(151)_ _____. What is the general function of
neuroglia? _(152)_ _____.

   Oligodendrocytes vary in size and have fine nonbranching cell processes (Fig. 9-16). Ribosomes and microtubules are very abundant. As

149 _microglia_
150 _astrocytes_
151 _oligodendrocytes_
152 _support the neurons, produce myelin_

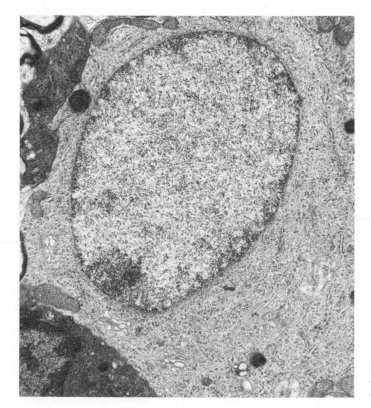

FIG. 9-16. EM of an oligo-dendrocyte (original magnification ×15,000).

153 dendrocytes

154 myelin
155 more than one

156 Schwann's

157 no
158 astrocyte

159 astrocyte foot

(153) <u>oligo_____</u> mature, they decrease in size and become more electron dense. The least mature cells are the predominant functioning cells, and are responsible for the production of *(154)* _____, which covers the fibers of the neurons. One oligodendrocyte can myelinate *(155)* _____ *(one, more than one)* nerve fiber, unlike the *(156)* _____ cells of the PNS. More mature oligodendrocytes function to maintain the myelin sheaths.

    Astrocytes appear as dark stars against a yellow background when stained with Cajal's gold-chloride sublimate method. The processes of the astrocytes may or may not be branched. Are the processes of oligodendrocytes branched? *(157)* _____. When an astrocyte process contacts a blood vessel it widens to form an astrocyte foot. The *(158)* _____ foot spreads over the surface of the capillary and interdigitates with other astrocyte feet in contact with the capillary. The cytoplasm of the astrocyte contains numerous dark-staining lysosomes and bundles of filaments (Fig. 9-17). Each filament of the bundle is 8 nm to 9 nm in diameter and is of unknown composition, but it functions in maintaining the rigidity of the process and expanded portions, the *(159)* _____ _____. Astrocytes have a large, light-staining nucleus, and ribosomes and rER are uncommon.

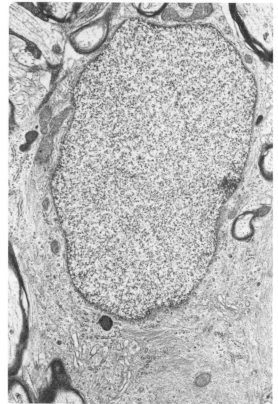

FIG. 9-17. EM of an astrocyte (original magnification × 13,800).

    Microglia can be visualized by using the weak silver carbonate method of Hortega. The presence of numerous lysosomes in these small cells suggests a possible *(160)* _____ *(phagocytic, hormone-producing)* function. Unlike the other two neuroglial cells, the *(161)* _____ and *(162)* _____, microglia are not of neural-cell origin. These cells are probably a form of migratory macrophage.

160 phagocytic
161 astrocyte
162 oligodendrocyte

Motor Unit

Motor Unit

The motor unit is a specialized structure made of an efferent motor axon and the skeletal muscle fibers it supplies (Fig. 9-18). Every skeletal muscle fiber is sup-

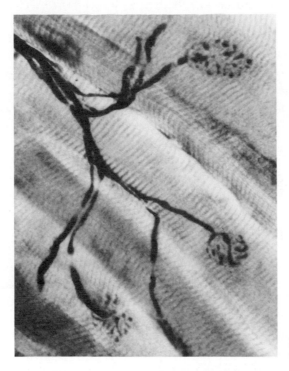

FIG. 9-18. Photomicrograph of a motor unit (original magnification ×250).

plied by an axon or a branch of an axon. The synapse between the axon and the plasma membrane, or *(163)* _____, of the muscle fiber occurs on a little mound called the motor end plate. At the mound, or *(164)* _____ _____ plate, the myelin produced by the *(165)* _____ cells is absent, but the cytoplasm of these cells forms a protective covering over the exposed area of the axon. The axon is highly branched at its terminal, each branch synapsing with a part of the highly folded sarcolemma. Separating the axon branches from the sarcolemma is a gap called the *(166)* _____ _____. Release of the synaptic vesicles, approximately 40 nm to 50 nm in diameter, occurs by the same process that all synaptic vesicles are released, *(167)* _____.

163 sarcolemma

164 motor end

165 Schwann's

166 synaptic cleft

167 exocytosis

Muscle Spindles

Muscle spindles, which are specialized structures found within most skeletal muscle bundles, function to regulate the tension of the muscle (Fig. 9-19). The

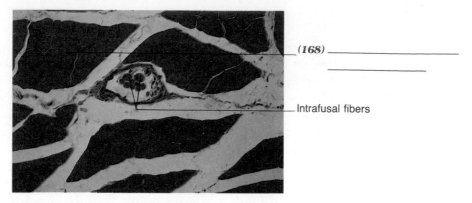

(168) _____

_____

Intrafusal fibers

FIG. 9-19. Photomicrograph of a muscle spindle, H and E stain (original magnification ×125).

168 *skeletal muscle*

specialized fibers found within the spindle are called intrafusal fibers, and are *(169)* _____ (*larger, smaller*) than normal skeletal muscle fibers. Sensory nerve fibers pierce the connective tissue capsule and lose their protective *(170)* _____ covering as they approach the intrafusal fiber bundles. The synapse involves the interdigitation of the axon branches with the highly folded plasma membrane of the muscle fiber, the *(171)* _____. The synapse is similar to the one involving regular skeletal muscle fibers, referred to as the motor *(172)* _____ _____.

169 *smaller*

170 *myelin*

171 *sarcolemma*

172 *end plate*

10 Cardiovascular System

After completing this chapter, you should be able to identify the following:

1 Epicardium, endocardium, and myocardium
2 Cardiac valves
3 Nodal cells
4 Purkinje's fibers

5 Arteries (all sizes)
6 Capillaries
7 Veins (all sizes)
8 Lymphatics

Also, after completing this chapter, you should understand the following:

1 The histologic differences of cardiac muscle and nodal cells
2 The histologic differences of artery sizes

3 The histologic differences between veins and arteries

In humans, the blood vascular system consists of a muscular pump, two circuits, and two continuous systems of tubular vessels. The two circuits are the pulmonary and systemic circuits or circulations. Transport of blood to and from the lungs involves the pulmonary circulation and the heart. Systemic circulation is the transport to and the collection of blood from all other tissues and organs of the body. The vessels that carry the blood from the heart, in both circulations, *(1)* _____ and *(2)* _____, are called arteries, and blood travels back to the *(3)* _____ through veins. Arteries, which conduct blood *(4)* _____ (*to, from*) the *(5)* _____, constitute a continuous system beginning with large elastic arteries, to muscular arteries, large arterioles, arterioles, and finally capillaries. The venous system, also a *(6)* _____ (*discontinuous, continuous*) system, includes the capillaries, and their smallest vessels, the venules; small veins; medium-sized veins; and the great vessels that lead to the heart.

Another vascular system, the lymphatic system, serves as a drainage system and is composed of vessels of various calibers. The principal function of the lymphatic system is to return to the blood vascular system the fluid, plasma proteins, and lymphocytes that "escape" from the circulation.

Heart

The functional and anatomic differences of the heart must be examined briefly in order to best understand the histologic aspect of the organ. Functionally, the heart is divided into two separate pumps. The left pump or left side of the heart receives highly oxygenated blood from the lungs. It then pumps this blood to all parts of the body; the *(7)* _____ circulation. The right pump or right side of the heart receives blood from the *(8)* _____ (*veins, arteries*) of the systemic circulation and then delivers this blood to the lungs for oxygenation.

1 pulmonary
2 systemic
3 heart
4 from
5 heart
6 continuous

7 systemic
8 veins

111

Anatomically, the heart consists of four chambers, the right and left atria and the right and left ventricles. The atria form the upper part of the heart and serve as reservoirs of the incoming blood. The right atrium contains specialized arrangements of cardiac cells that are responsible for the synchronous beating of the heart.

Blood flows from the atrium into the ventricle through valves that separate the two chambers. The ventricles are the major pumping apparatus of the heart. The left ventricle wall is considerably thicker than the right owing to the greater pressure it must pump against.

The histologic discussion of the heart focuses on the three layers of the heart chambers, the cardiac fibrous skeleton, the cardiac valves, the sinoatrial (SA) nodal and atrioventricular (AV) nodal cells, and the Purkinje's fibers.

The wall of the heart in both atria and ventricles consists of three layers. The layers include an external layer or epicardium, an internal layer or endocardium, and a middle muscular layer, the myocardium.

Epicardium

Essentially a fibroblastic membrane, the epicardium, the *(9)* _____ (*external*, *internal*) layer also consists of three defined layers, which are not easily defined. The superficial layer of the epicardium consists of flattened mesothelial cells or *(10)* _____ _____ epithelium. Immediately beneath the simple *(11)* _____ epithelium or *(12)* _____ cells is a thin plane of connective tissue rich in elastic fibers, small blood vessels, lymphatics, and nerves. The deepest section of the epicardium consists of loose connective tissue with a considerable amount of adipose tissue. The loose connective tissue is directly juxtaposed to the endomysium that surrounds *(13)* _____ (*muscle bundles, individual muscle cells*) of the muscular *(14)* _____ (*middle, outer*) myocardium.

Myocardium

The middle layer of the heart, the *(15)* _____ is composed of *(16)* _____ muscle (Fig. 10-1). Intercalated discs, which are composed of *(17)* _____ and *(18)* _____ _____, connect the highly anastomosing muscle cells. The *(19)* _____ allows electrical transmission and therefore carries depolarization from cell to cell. Most myocardial cells of the atria do not differ from the ventricular cells. (You should finish #20 at this point.)

9 external

10 simple squamous
11 squamous
12 mesothelial

13 individual muscle cells
14 middle

15 myocardium
16 cardiac
17 nexus
18 macula (fascia) adherens
19 nexus or gap junction

Heart

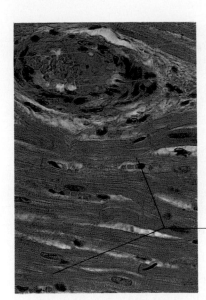

(20) _____ _____

20 *intercalated disc*

FIG. 10-1. Myocardium, hematoxylin-eosin (H and E) stain (original
magnification ×200).

Atrial myocardial cells, sandwiched between the
(21) _____ and *(22)* _____ layers, are
smaller in diameter than the ventricular myocardial cells, and T tubules are few
or absent. Found at the poles of the nucleus and only in atrial cells are membrane-bound spherical granules that cannot be seen in a routine light micrograph. These granules, detectable only on electron microscopy (EM), are called
specific atrial granules, and their function has yet to be determined. The atrial
myocardial cells *(23)* _____ (*smaller, larger*) than ventricular myocardial cells, are also invested by a network of fibers far richer in elastic fibers than
the ventricular myocardial cells. These elastic fibers are composed mainly of the
protein *(24)* _____ and intermingle with the outermost segment of
the *(25)* _____ cardium.

21 *epicardium*
22 *endocardium*

23 *smaller*

Endocardium

The innermost layer of the heart wall, the *(26)* _____, like
the *(27)* _____ (*myocardium, epicardium*), is composed of
three indistinct sublayers. The innermost sublayer consists of an endothelium
supported by a delicate connective tissue network. The endothelium is continuous with the vessels leaving or entering the heart and also covers the valves and
its surrounding attachments. The middle sublayer is the thickest, and is composed of dense connective tissue rich in elastic fibers, like the
(28) _____ (*first, second, third*) layer of the epicardium. Bundles of
smooth muscle are evident in the middle sublayer of the *(29)* _____ cardium,
especially in the septum that separates the ventricles (Fig. 10-2).

24 *elastin*
25 *endo*

26 *endocardium*
27 *epicardium*

28 *second*
29 *endo*

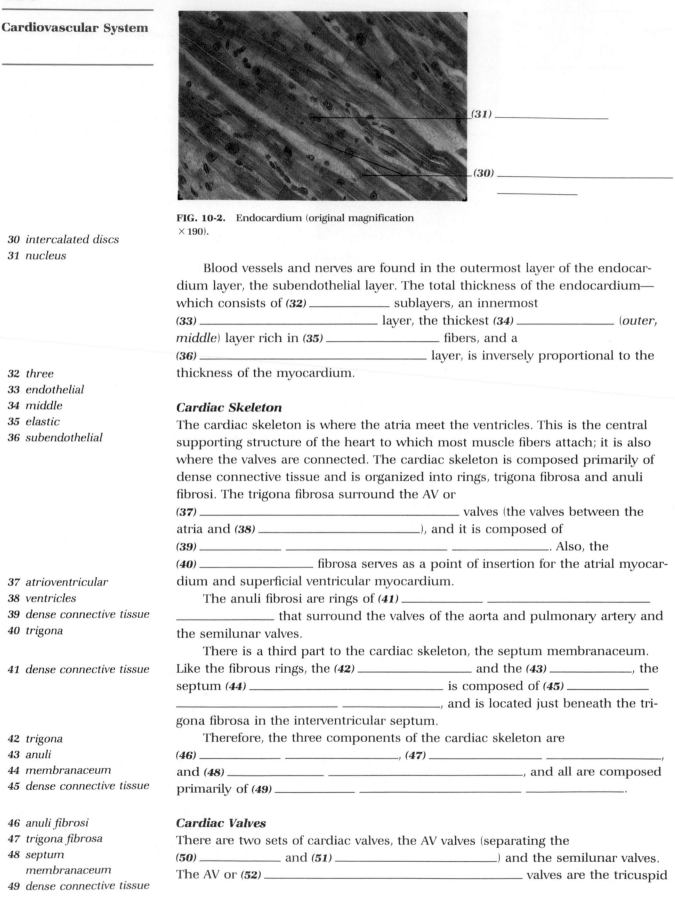

FIG. 10-2. Endocardium (original magnification ×190).

30 *intercalated discs*
31 *nucleus*

Blood vessels and nerves are found in the outermost layer of the endocardium layer, the subendothelial layer. The total thickness of the endocardium—which consists of *(32)* _____ sublayers, an innermost *(33)* _____ layer, the thickest *(34)* _____ (*outer, middle*) layer rich in *(35)* _____ fibers, and a *(36)* _____ layer, is inversely proportional to the thickness of the myocardium.

32 *three*
33 *endothelial*
34 *middle*
35 *elastic*
36 *subendothelial*

Cardiac Skeleton

The cardiac skeleton is where the atria meet the ventricles. This is the central supporting structure of the heart to which most muscle fibers attach; it is also where the valves are connected. The cardiac skeleton is composed primarily of dense connective tissue and is organized into rings, trigona fibrosa and anuli fibrosi. The trigona fibrosa surround the AV or *(37)* _____ valves (the valves between the atria and *(38)* _____), and it is composed of *(39)* _____ _____ _____. Also, the *(40)* _____ fibrosa serves as a point of insertion for the atrial myocardium and superficial ventricular myocardium.

37 *atrioventricular*
38 *ventricles*
39 *dense connective tissue*
40 *trigona*

The anuli fibrosi are rings of *(41)* _____ _____ _____ that surround the valves of the aorta and pulmonary artery and the semilunar valves.

41 *dense connective tissue*

There is a third part to the cardiac skeleton, the septum membranaceum. Like the fibrous rings, the *(42)* _____ and the *(43)* _____, the septum *(44)* _____ is composed of *(45)* _____ _____ _____, and is located just beneath the trigona fibrosa in the interventricular septum.

Therefore, the three components of the cardiac skeleton are *(46)* _____ _____, *(47)* _____ _____, and *(48)* _____ _____, and all are composed primarily of *(49)* _____ _____ _____.

42 *trigona*
43 *anuli*
44 *membranaceum*
45 *dense connective tissue*

46 *anuli fibrosi*
47 *trigona fibrosa*
48 *septum membranaceum*
49 *dense connective tissue*

Cardiac Valves

There are two sets of cardiac valves, the AV valves (separating the *(50)* _____ and *(51)* _____) and the semilunar valves. The AV or *(52)* _____ valves are the tricuspid

50 *atria*
51 *ventricles*
52 *atrioventricular*

Heart

53 ventricle

54 mitral
55 two
56 trigona

57 middle

58 atrium, ventricles

59 endocardium
*60 collagenous middle
   layer*
61 endocardium

62 tricuspid
63 mitral
64 bicuspid
65 dense
66 middle
67 tendineae

68 tendineae
69 papillary
70 ventricular

valves situated between the right atrium and right *(53)* _____ and the bicuspid (more commonly called the mitral valve) on the left side of the heart. These valves are composed of thin leaflets. The tricuspid valve has three leaflets while the bicuspid or *(54)* _____ valve has *(55)* _____ leaflets, as its name implies. Each leaflet is a trilayer tissue arrangement that originates from a part of the cardiac skeleton, the *(56)* _____ fibrosa.

   The three layers of the leaflets of the AV valves are as follows: a thick middle layer of dense connective tissue surrounded on both sides by the endocardium; the collagenous *(57)* _____ (*middle, outer*) layer that lends support to the thin valves; and the endocardium, which is thicker on the atrial side of the valves because of further extension by the atrial myocardium onto the valve (Fig. 10-3). While capillaries may be present at the base of the valve, the valves are essentially avascular. The valves derive oxygen and nutrients from the blood that surrounds them and flows around them in passing from *(58)* _____ to _____. (You should finish #61 at this point.)

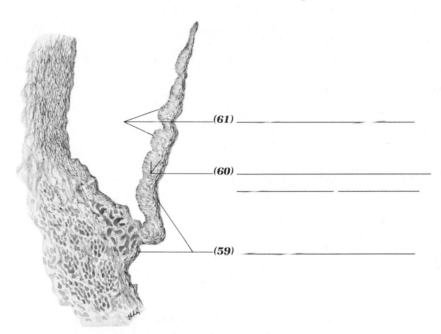

(61) _____

(60) _____

_____ _____

(59) _____

FIG. 10-3. Aortic valve, H and E stain (low-power magnification).

   AV valves, *(62)* _____ and *(63)* _____ or *(64)* _____, are able to withstand the pressures of ventricular contraction because of their *(65)* _____ connective tissue *(66)* _____ (*middle, outer*) layer and specialized support cords. These cords, chordae tendineae, are long tendinous cords composed of dense connective tissue. Chordae *(67)* _____ extend from specialized muscular extensions of the heart wall, the papillary muscles (discussed below). Found only in the ventricles, the chordae *(68)* _____ from their attachment to *(69)* _____ muscles insert onto the *(70)* _____ (*ventricular, atrial*) side of the leaflet and merge with the middle layer. Upon contraction of the papillary muscles at ventricular contraction, the chordae tendineae hold the valve tight and prevent it from blowing out into the atrium.

71 semi

72 three

73 dense collagenous layer

74 AV

75 mitral

76 bicuspid

77 ventricle

78 avascular

79 diffusion

80 tendineae

81 lunar

82 lunar

83 myocardium

84 intercalated discs

85 sinoatrial

86 generation

87 fewer

88 SA

Pulmonary and aortic valves or *(71)* _____ lunar valves are also composed of *(72)* _____ (*one, two, three, four*) layers: endocardium, middle *(73)* _____ _____ _____, and endocardium. Semilunar valves are not cuspid in shape like the *(74)* ___ valves but crescent in shape. These valves are thinner than the tricuspid and *(75)* _____ or *(76)* _____ valves. The endothelium of the vessel (aorta or pulmonary) forms one layer of endothelium covering the valve, while endothelium continuous from the *(77)* _____ (*ventricle, atrium*) covers the other surface of the valve. Like the AV valves, the semilunar valves are *(78)* _____ (*vascular, avascular*), and therefore get their oxygen and nutrients by *(79)* _____. There are no chordae *(80)* _____ lending support to the *(81)* semi _____ valves, but on the ventricular side of the valves there is a great deal of elastic tissue, which provides the necessary flexibility. Last, the *(82)* semi _____ valves have gross nodular thickenings in the middle of the free edge of the leaflets, which are called the noduli aranti.

Most of the contractile muscle of the heart, the *(83)* _____, is composed of identical muscle cells connected by *(84)* _____ _____. In addition to these cells of the myocardium, there are cells whose primary function is not contraction but generation of the stimulus for the heart beat. There are also muscle cells so modified as to be best able to conduct the impulse most rapidly. These impulse-generating cells and the rapidly conductile fibers make up the conducting system of the heart—the SA and AV nodal cells, AV bundle or bundle of His.

Sinoatrial Node

The SA node is located just beneath the epicardium at the junction of the superior vena cava and right atrium. Often called the pacemaker of the heart, the SA node fires at a set beat in normal people, and therefore sets the heart rate.

Histologically, the SA node or *(85)* _____ cells are specialized cardiac muscle cells embedded in a dense network of dense connective tissue (Fig. 10-4). Since the function of these nodal cells is basically

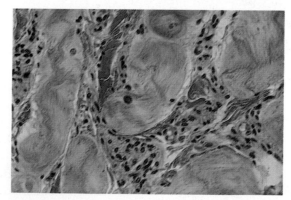

FIG. 10-4. Sinoatrial nodal cells, H and E stain (original magnification ×200).

(86) _____ (*generation, rapid conduction*) of an impulse, the fine structure of the cells is so modified. The cells have considerably less contractile function and therefore in an EM one finds *(87)* _____ (*fewer, more*) myofibrils that *are not* in an orderly arrangement with easily identifiable bands. The nodal artery supplies the *(88)* __ __ nodal cells and aids in identifying the location of these cells in a light micrograph. This area is richly innervated by both sympathetics and parasympathetics (Fig. 10-5). The SA cells are in direct

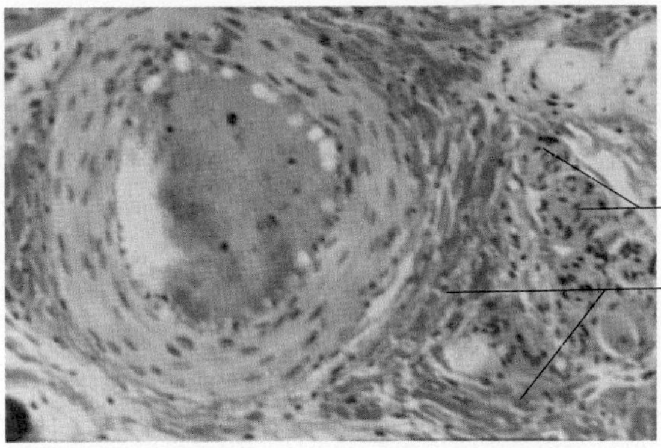

Heart

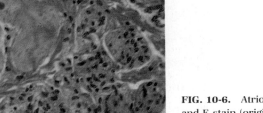

(89) _____

(90) _____

_____

_____

FIG. 10-5. Nodal artery, H and E stain (original magnification ×125).

89 nerves

90 cardiac muscle cells

contact with ordinary cardiac muscle cells, enabling conduction of the impulse to the rest of the heart. Located in the **(91)** _____ (_right, left_) atrium, the SA node sends impulses through both atria and down to the other node, the **(92)** _____.

Atrioventricular Node

91 right

92 AV

The AV node is located beneath the endocardium (not the **(93)** _____ as the SA node is) in the lower part of the interatrial septum next to the tricuspid valve. The AV nodal cells are histologically similar to those of the SA node. AV nodal cells are slender cardiac muscle cells embedded in a network of **(94)** _____ _____

93 epicardium

_____ (Fig. 10-6). Like that of the SA nodal cells, the AV or

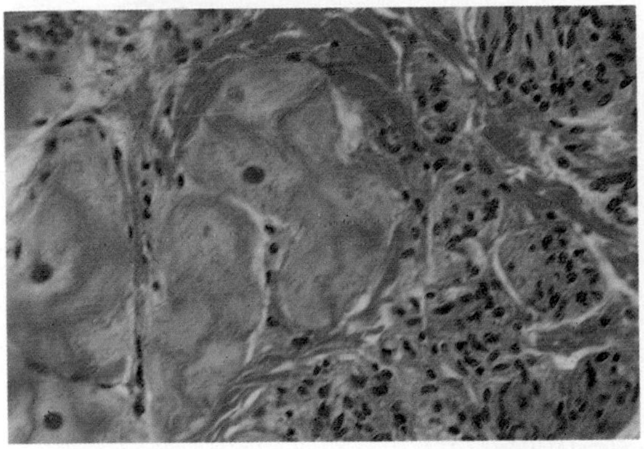

94 dense connective tissue

FIG. 10-6. Atrioventricular nodal cells, H and E stain (original magnification ×200).

(95) _____ nodal cells' primary function _____ (_is, is not_) contraction, and therefore they contain **(97)** _____ (_fewer, more_) myofibrils in **(98)** _____ (_an orderly, a random_) arrangement. Both nodal areas, **(99)** __ __ and **(100)** __ __, are in direct contact with ordinary **(101)** _____ muscle so as to be able to transmit the impulse that leads to cardiac contraction.

95 atrioventricular
96 is not
97 fewer
98 a random
99 AV
100 SA
101 cardiac

An important physiological distinction should be made between the nodes. AV nodal cells do not ordinarily generate an impulse but delay the impulse from the SA node and then conduct it to the ventricles. The _only_ contact between muscle fibers of the atria and ventricles is where the AV node conducts the impulse to the ventricles. The rest of the muscle fibers are separated by a fibrous dense connective tisse, the cardiac **(102)** _____.

102 skeleton

Cardiovascular System

---

103 *SA*
104 *both*
105 *AV*
106 *the only*
107 *ventricles*
108 *bundle*

109 *His*
110 *cardiac muscle cells*

111 *ventricle*

112 *myocardium*
113 *bundle*

114 *fibers*
115 *reticulum*
116 *unlike*

117 *intercalated*
118 *macula adherens*
119 *adhesion*

120 *Purkinje's fibers*

121 *nexus*
122 *communication*
123 *lack*
124 *lack*
125 *have*
126 *nexus*

Bundle of His

The impulse generated by the *(103)* ___ ___ node passes through *(104)* _____ *(one, both)* atrium (atria) to the *(105)* ___ ___ node. The AV nodal cells contact a specialized bundle of cells of the ventricle, the bundle of His; *(106)* _____ _____ *(the only, one of many)* connection(s) between atria and *(107)* _____. The AV bundle or the *(108)* _____ of His at its origin consists of cardiac muscle cells that assume an intermediate position histologically between nodal cells and ordinary cardiac muscle cells. The bundle of *(109)* _____ lacks the very orderly arrangement found in most *(110)* _____ *(cardiac muscle cells, nodal cells)*. The AV bundle divides into two separate bundles, one for each *(111)* _____ *(atrium, ventricle)*. These bundles then ramify into extensive plexuses from the endocardium into the contractile layer of the heart wall, the *(112)* _____.

The branches of the *(113)* _____ of His consist of distinctive cardiac muscle cells called Purkinje's fibers (Fig. 10-7). The Purkinje's *(114)* _____ consist of one or two centrally located nuclei with randomly arranged myofibrils. The sarcoplasmic *(115)* _____ of the Purkinje's fibers is not well developed and *(116)* _____ *(unlike, like)* cardiac muscle cells, it lacks T tubules. These fibers have various and unusual shapes that send out large processes producing extensive interdigitation with other Purkinje's cells and ordinary myocardial cells. There are no typical *(117)* _____ disks between the rapidly conducting Purkinje's fibers but desmosomes or *(118)* _____ _____ are randomly distributed, increasing cell-to-cell *(119)* _____ *(adhesion,*

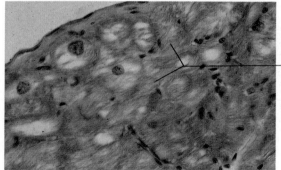

(120) _____ _____

FIG. 10-7. Left ventricle, Purkinje's cell, H and E stain (original magnification × 125).

communication). There is a sufficient number of gap junctions or *(121)* _____ between cells to facilitate cell-to-cell *(122)* _____ *(communication, adhesion)*.

Purkinje's fibers *(123)* _____ *(have, lack)* T tubules, *(124)* _____ *(lack, have)* intercalated disks and, *(125)* _____ *(lack, have)* gap junctions or *(126)* _____, which make it possible for uniform and virtually simultaneous contraction of both ventricles.

Blood Vessels

Blood Vessels

Blood is transported through vessels. Vessels conducting the blood
(127) _____ (*to, from*) the heart are arteries and veins carry the blood
(128) _____ (*from, to*) the heart. Identification of the type of vessel is based on
simple histologic landmarks.

127 *from*
128 *to*

Arteries

Arteries can be subdivided into three major types. These three types are, in
successively smaller sizes, the large elastic arteries, muscular or distributing
arteries, and the smallest arteries, the arterioles. The organization of the vessel
wall is basically the same for all **(129)** _____ (*two, three*) major types of
arteries, elastic, **(130)** _____ or distributing arteries, and
(131) _____. All vessels consist of three concentric layers or
tunics. The innermost layer or tunica intima is the layer in direct contact with
the blood. The tunica intima consists of longitudinally arranged endothelial cells.
An intermediate layer that follows the **(132)** _____ intima consists of
circumferentially arranged smooth muscle cells with elastic fibers; it is termed
the **(133)** _____ _____ media. Last, the outer layer, the tunica adventitia, is
made up of fibroelastic and fibrous elements oriented longitudinally. The
(134) _____ adventitia merges with the loose connective tissue that
accompanies all blood vessels.

129 *three*
130 *muscular*
131 *arterioles*

132 *tunica*

133 *tunica*

134 *tunica*

Separating each tunica are distinct boundaries of elastic tissue. Between the
(135) _____ intima and **(136)** _____ _____ is a scal-
loped-appearing line of elastic tissue, the internal elastic lamina or elastic interna. Separating the **(137)** _____ adventitia and the tunica
(138) _____ is another thinned line of elastic tissue called the external
elastic lamina or elastic externa (Fig. 10-8).

135 *tunica*
136 *tunica media*
137 *tunica*
138 *media*

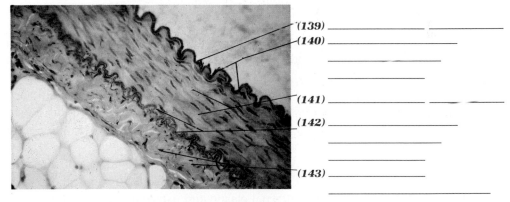

(139) _____ _____
(140) _____
_____
_____
(141) _____ _____ _____
(142) _____
_____
_____
(143) _____

139 *tunica intima*

140 *internal elastic lamina*

141 *tunica media*

FIG. 10-8. Aorta, H and E stain (original magnification
× 100).

142 *external elastic lamina*

143 *tunica adventitia*

The three concentric layers and the lamina differ in size and proportion, and
on the various-sized arteries.

ARTERIOLES The **(144)** _____ are the smallest of all arteries,
and their vessel walls vary more than those of other arteries. Arterioles are
arteries with a diameter of less than 100 μm. Arterioles can be further subdivided
into those whose diameter is between 100 μm and 40 μm and those whose
diameter is less than 40 μm; corresponding, yet difficult to visualize, histologic
differences can be found.

144 *arterioles*

145 *intima*
146 *media*
147 *adventitia*
148 *endothelium*
149 *internal elastic*

150 *smooth*
151 *circumferentially*
152 *smooth muscle*
153 *tunica*
154 *internal elastic*

Arterioles of 100 μm to 40 μm have a cell wall with all three tunicae, *(145)* _____, *(146)* _____, and *(147)* _____. The tunica intima consists of a thin layer of *(148)* _____ with a basal lamina applied to the boundary elastin layer, the *(149)* _____ _____ lamina. The internal elastic lamina in these "large" arterioles is nearly continuous but retains occasional narrow fenestrations. The tunica media in the arterioles varies in the number of *(150)* _____ muscle cells, but usually contains two to three *(151)* _____ *(longitudinally, circumferentially)* arranged *(152)* _____ _____ cell layers. Separating the tunica media and the *(153)* _____ adventitia is a thin *(154)* _____ _____ lamina that is visible only in the largest arterioles (it is often very difficult to distinguish; Fig. 10-9). The tunica

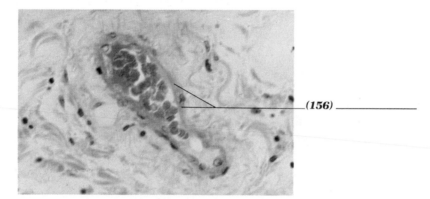

(156) _____

FIG. 10-9. The endothelium of the tunica *(155)* _____ is not visible here, nor are the two laminae. Mesentery, H and E stain (original magnification ×225).

155 *intima*
156 *media*

157 *loose connective*

158 *two to three*
159 *media*

160 *1:1*

161 *unlike*
162 *internal elastic*
163 *external elastic*
164 *smooth*
165 *tunica media*

adventitia has the same thickness as the tunica media and is composed of fibroblasts and collagenous fibers. The tunica adventitia merges with the *(157)* _____ _____ tissue surrounding the blood vessel. The arteriole wall and lumen are almost equal in diameter. By using the wall-to-lumen ratio (1:1) and the number of smooth muscle cell layers *(158)* _____ to _____ in the tunica *(159)* _____, one can differentiate between arterioles and small arteries.

Arterioles less than 40 μm also have all three tunics. The wall-to-lumen size stays a *(160)* ___:_____ ratio as both the wall and lumen decrease proportionately. The internal elastic and external elastic laminae are often absent in the small arteriole, *(161)* _____ *(unlike, as)* in the larger arterioles. The lamina, both *(162)* _____ _____ and *(163)* _____ _____ contain numerous large slitlike fenestrations disrupting the lamina continuity. A very small *(164)* _____ muscle cell layer, the *(165)* _____ _____, is found in those small arterioles. Also, the tunica adventitia is often very thin and consists primarily of collagenous fibers. Both small and large arterioles derive nutrients for the tunicae by diffusion from the blood in the lumen.

Blood Vessels

166 distributing
167 larger
168 three
169 more

170 tunica intima

171 tunica media

172 muscular

173 muscular
174 internal elastic

175 interna
176 media

177 media
178 smooth
179 circular
180 media
181 smooth muscle
182 distributing
183 elastin

184 external elastic lamina

185 tunica media

186 media
187 adventitia

188 connective tissue

189 media
190 tunica
191 smooth muscle

192 adventitia

MUSCULAR ARTERIES   Most numerous in number, the muscular or *(166)* _____ arteries are *(167)* _____ (*larger, smaller*) than arterioles, and therefore all *(168)* _____ (*one, two, three*) tunics are *(169)* _____ (*less, more*) easily identified.

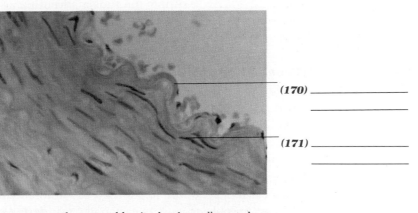

(170) _____
_____

(171) _____
_____

FIG. 10-10.   The external lamina has been disrupted owing to staining techniques. This is a *(172)* _____ artery. H&E stain. (Original magnification ×125.)

     The tunica intima of the distributing or *(173)* _____ arteries consists of an endothelium bound by the *(174)* _____ _____ lamina (Fig. 10-10). Slender endothelial cell processes are found coursing through narrow slitlike fenestrations in the elastica *(175)* _____ and establish contact with the smooth muscle cells of the tunica *(176)* _____. These processes possibly act as a means of transporting nutrients to the avascular tunica *(177)* _____. Consisting almost exclusively of *(178)* _____ muscle cells arranged in *(179)* _____ (*longitudinal, circular*) layers, the tunica *(180)* _____ has an elastin intercellular substance that holds the muscle cells together. More than three *(181)* _____ _____ layers can be found in the tunica media of muscular or *(182)* _____ arteries, and are held together by *(183)* _____ (*elastin, collagen*).

     Separating the tunica media from the tunica adventitia is the *(184)* _____ _____ _____ _____, and this is considerably thicker than the internal elastic lamina that separates the *(185)* _____ _____ from the tunica intima. Like the internal elastic lamina, the external elastica has fenestrations that permit the smooth muscle cells of the tunica *(186)* _____ to bulge through into the tunica *(187)* _____.

     The tunica adventitia, thicker than the tunica media in muscular arteries, consists of bundles of longitudinally arranged elastic and collagen bundles. The collagen bundles merge with the surrounding loose *(188)* _____ _____. Nerves run through the tunica adventitia but do not penetrate the external elastic lamina and enter the tunica *(189)* _____. Since the *(190)* _____ media consists primarily of *(191)* _____ _____ cells, the nerves that will affect contraction must send transmitter substances across the external elastic lamina. In the largest muscular arteries, tiny blood vessels are evident in the tunica *(192)* _____. These blood vessels are called the vasa vasorum—vessels of vessels—and are more abundant in the larger elastic arteries'

193 *adventitia*
194 *avascular*

195 *vasorum*
196 *vessels of vessels*

197 *diffusion*

198 *distributing*
199 *three*

200 *endothelial*
201 *internal elastic lamina*

202 *internal elastic lamina*

203 *lamina*

204 *tunica media*

205 *tunica adventitia*
206 *internal elastic lamina*

tunica *(193)* _____. Since the tunica media is *(194)* _____ (*avascular, vascular*), oxygen and nutrients are supplied by diffusion in the small muscular arteries and arterioles. In the larger arteries, the vasa *(195)* _____ or *(196)* _____ of _____ supply the tunica adventitia and the outer two thirds of the tunica media with the rest of the wall supplied by simple *(197)* _____.

ELASTIC ARTERIES   The elastic arteries are the largest of all arteries and consist of the aorta and its major branches. Like the arterioles and muscular or *(198)* _____ arteries, the large elastic arteries have all *(199)* _____ (*one, two, three*) tunics. The tunica intima is quite thick in elastic arteries, and it consists of a number of sublayers. Lining the vessel lumen are the *(200)* _____ cells. They are *not* adjacent to the *(201)* _____ _____ _____ as found in smaller arteries, but are juxtaposed to a thin subadjacent layer of collagen bundles, fibroblasts, and, occasionally, wandering cells and various undifferentiated cells. The next sublayer of the tunica intima is a thin layer of elastic fibers, some collagenous fibrils, and small but not evident smooth muscle cells. Do not expect to see all these sublayers in a routine light micrograph.

The bundle of smooth muscle cells and elastic fibrils of the tunica intima join a fenestrated lamina, the *(202)* _____ _____ _____. It is difficult to outline clearly the internal elastic *(203)* _____ because of the abundance of fenestrating elastic laminae in the adjacent tunica media (Fig. 10-11).

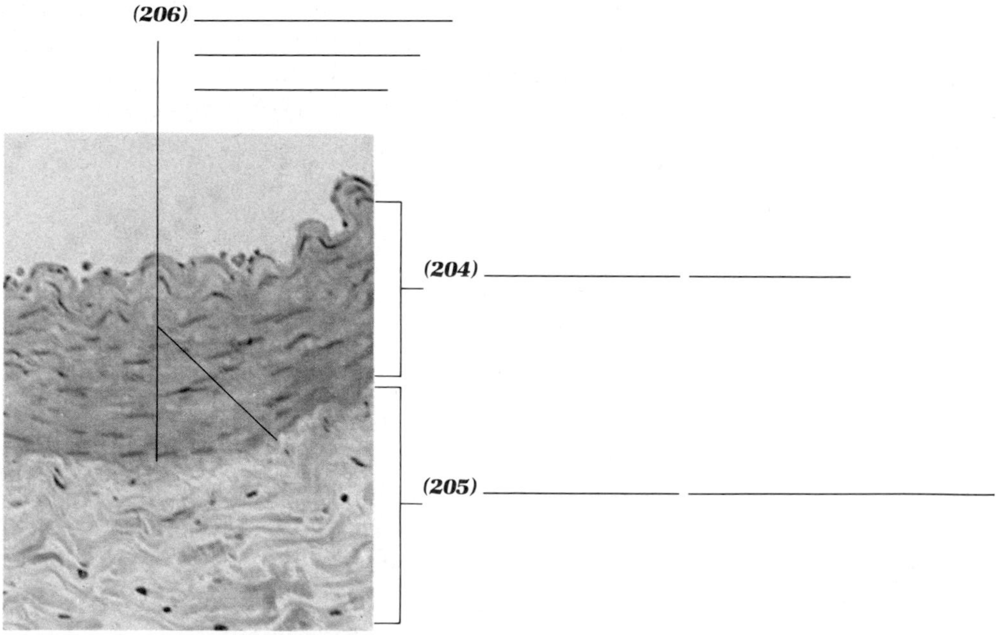

(206) _____
_____
_____

(204) _____ _____

(205) _____ _____

FIG. 10-11.   Medium-sized elastic artery, H and E stain (original magnification ×125).

Blood Vessels

Under the microscope, one can see that the tunica media consists of regularly repeating, concentrically arranged, fenestrated laminae (10 in the smallest elastic artery to 75 in the aorta). Between these dark-staining wavy lines are thin layers of connective tissue, collagenous and elastic fibers, and **(207)** _____ _____ muscle cells with metachromatic-staining intercellular cement. The smooth muscle cells are circumferentially arranged and flattened, and have characteristically elongate nuclei. Clearly, the tunica media constitutes the major part of the wall.

The tunica adventitia, separated by the **(208)** _____ _____ from the tunica **(209)** _____, is a thin layer of connective tissue and collagenous fibrils. The tunica adventitia has nerves, lymphatics, and blood vessels—**(210)** _____ _____ _____—coursing through it. Both the nerves and blood vessels in the tunica **(211)** _____ supply the tunica **(212)** _____ and the tunica **(213)** _____ but **(214)** _____ _____ (do, do not) penetrate the lamina.

CAPILLARIES Arterioles, the **(215)** _____ _____ (largest, smallest) of arteries, lead to capillaries. Capillaries are the thinnest vessels of the blood vascular system and are the greatest in number. Found in vastly anastomosing networks called capillary beds, capillaries allow the movement of oxygen and nutrients across their wall into the tissues and receive the tissues' waste products.

The capillary wall is one cell thick, and it is an endothelial cell wall. Most capillaries consist of two to three endothelial cells in a circle; the smallest capillaries have a cell wall of only one endothelial cell. Underlying this **(216)** _____ cell thick wall is a very thin basal lamina similar in all aspects to the basal lamina underlying epithelia. The lumen varies in diameter but it is usually 8 μm and therefore slightly **(217)** _____ (smaller, larger) than the diameter of a red blood corpuscle or RBC (Fig. 10-12). Detailed analysis of the capillaries has revealed two similar but very distinct types of capillaries, continuous and fenestrated.

207 smooth

208 elastic external
209 media

210 vasa vasorum
211 adventitial
212 adventitia
213 media
214 do not

215 smallest

216 endothelial

217 smaller

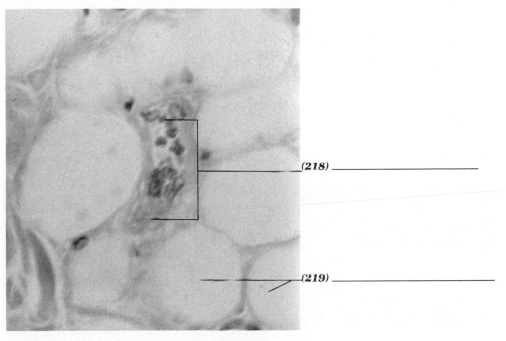

(218) _____

(219) _____

218 capillary

219 adipocytes

FIG. 10-12. Connective tissue, H and E stain (original magnification ×300).

Continuous capillaries are found throughout the body's muscles, connective tissue, and central nervous system (CNS). The fine structure of the capillary indicates a(n) **(220)** _____ cell wall in which the cells are thickened at the nucleus and often very attenuated at the periphery. The bulging nucleus can often assume one fourth the capillary's lumen, which is roughly **(221)** _____ in diameter. The plasma membrane of the continuous capillary endothelium resembles a typical unit membrane, a **(222)** _____ laminar _____ membrane composed of lipids and **(223)** _____. Closer examination of the membrane under an electron microscope reveals conspicuous vesicular invaginations or caveolae (Fig. 10-13). These "pits," 80 nm in diameter, are essentially pinocytotic vesicles. The vesicles traverse the capillary membrane, transporting material back and forth. Partial overlapping of contiguous endothelial cells often occurs, producing a flap projecting into the lumen. The purpose of this flap or marginal fold has yet to be determined.

220 endothelial

221 8 μm
222 tri
223 protein

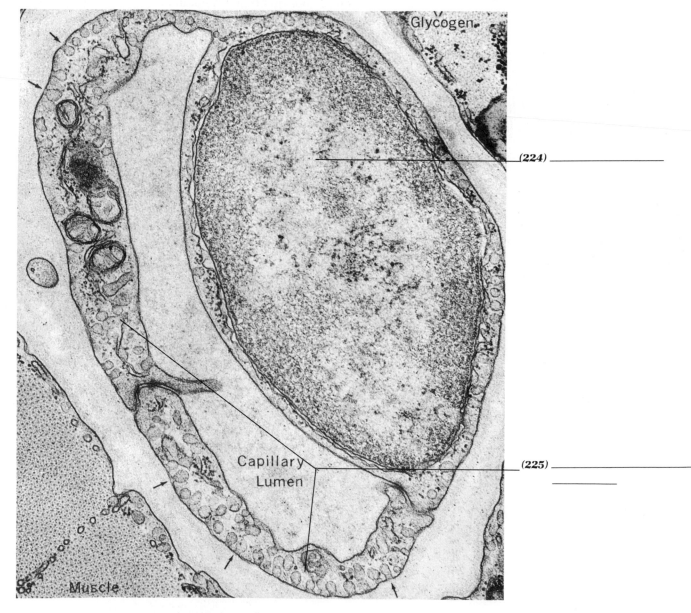

FIG. 10-13. Electron micrograph (EM) of a capillary.

224 nucleus
225 endothelial cell

Blood Vessels

226 endothelial
227 plasma membrane
228 desmosome
229 adherens

230 tight

231 endothelial cells

232 adherens

233 as is

234 continuous
235 fenestrated

236 postcapillary
237 endothelium
238 basement

239 does not
240 possible
241 protein

242 muscle

243 collecting venules

244 arterioles
245 endothelial
246 membrane

While the vesicular invaginations traverse the (226) _____ cell's (227) _____ _____, the boundary between adjacent endothelial cells is joined by tight junctions of the fascia adherens type. This is a sort of expanded (228) ___ _____ or macula (229) _____ _____, and therefore the junction does not occupy the entire margins of the continuous cells. The areas of the cells not joined by (230) _____ junctions enable tissue fluid to seep out of the capillary. One exception concerning the continuous capillaries is found in the CNS. In the CNS, tight junctions between adjacent (231) _____ _____ are continuous and of the zonula occludens type (not the macula (232) _____ type), and therefore encircle the whole cell. The tight junction and the underlying basal lamina make a secure blood–brain barrier.

Fenestrated capillaries, on the other hand, do not have an uninterrupted endothelium. The fenestrated capillaries are found in the renal glomeruli, endocrine glands, lamina propria of the intestine, and elsewhere. This type of capillary is characterized by extremely attenuated areas of the endothelium that have circular fenestrae or perforations. These pores are 80 nm to 100 nm wide but are not true holes. Covering the pore area is a thin single-membrane diaphragm that is not derived from the cell membrane itself. Immediately beneath the endothelium there is a basal lamina (233) _____ (as is, not) found in continuous capillaries. As will be shown, the renal glomerulus capillaries do not even have a diaphragm over the fenestrae and therefore fluid passes out of the vessel at a far greater rate than it does in either of the two types of capillaries, (234) _____ and (235) _____.

Capillaries coursing through capillary beds lose oxygen to surrounding tissue and receive carbon dioxide and waste. This deoxygenated blood is returned to the heart by a system of veins. Blood flow through the venous system starts from the postcapillary venule to the collecting venules, which merge into muscular venules. The muscular venules then empty into collecting veins, which form larger veins until the blood reaches the heart.

Veins

Several capillaries merge into the smallest of the venules, the (236) _____ venule. Like all other blood vessels, the postcapillary venule is lined with (237) _____, surrounded by longitudinally oriented reticular fibers. Immediately beneath the fibers is a thin (238) _____ membrane. The postcapillary venules are permeable. The tight junction adjoining the cells is of the fascia adherens type, and therefore it (239) _____ (does, does not) encircle the cell, making it (240) _____ (possible, impossible) for fluids to leak out. Also, the endothelial cells are rich in actin, a (241) _____ (protein, lipid) that with proper hormonal stimulation enables the cells to alter their shape, as (242) _____ cells do, and alter capillary permeability.

Collecting Venules

Postcapillary venules empty into the larger (243) _____ _____, which are 30 μm to 50 μm and equivalent in size to (244) _____ _____ (small arteries, arterioles). These vessels have an (245) _____ ___ cell lining and a basement (246) _____ surrounding them too. There is also a noticeable adventitia that is composed of fibroblasts and collagenous fibers. Collecting venules, **(247)** _____ (*larger, smaller*) than postcapillary venules but **(248)** _____ (*much smaller, equivalent in size*) to arterioles, have a unique cell outside the endothelium called the pericyte. A pericyte lacks the contractile apparatus and filaments necessary for contraction, but can differentiate into smooth muscle cells with all the contractile machinery.

The exact nature of the pericytes is not fully known.

Muscular Venules

Collecting venules will become confluent with larger **(249)** _____ venules, which, as the name implies, have a tunica media replete with **(250)** _____ _____ cells (Fig. 10-14). All three tunics are found here.

247 *larger*
248 *equivalent in size*

249 *muscular*

250 *smooth muscle*

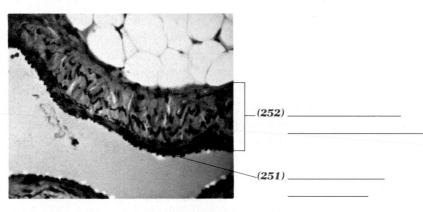

(252) _____

_____

(251) _____

_____

FIG. 10-14. Medium-sized vein, H and E stain (original magnification ×200).

251 *tunica media*
252 *tunica adventitia*

The tunica media, which has one or two **(253)** _____ _____ cell layers, is separated from the endothelium of the tunica **(254)** _____ by an **(255)** _____ _____ lamina. This lamina is thin and *not always* present in the muscular venule (Fig. 10-15).

253 *smooth muscle*
254 *intima*
255 *internal elastic*

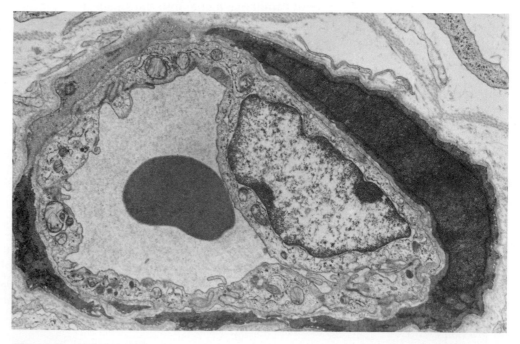

FIG. 10-15. EM of a venule.

Veins

Collecting Vein

The next type of vessel after the muscular venule is a collecting vein, which has a diameter of 100 μm to 300 μm. Collecting veins are small veins whose histology is very similar to that of medium veins. Both small and medium veins, like small and medium arteries, have all three tunicae.

In small, medium, and even large veins, the tunica intima is the least developed layer. Consisting of endothelium, highly irregular in outline, the tunica **(256)** _____ often rests on a visible connective tissue layer, similar to that of muscular arteries. This layer is quite common in large veins. Fine elastic fibers separate the tunica **(257)** _____ from the **(258)** _____, but *do not necessarily* form an internal elastic lamina. The tunica media is considerably thinner than that of arteries of comparable size and consists mainly of **(259)** _____ _____ fibers **(260)** _____ (*longitudinally, circumferentially*) arranged and separated by **(261)** _____ (*longitudinally, circumferentially*) arranged collagenous fibers. There is considerably less elastic tissue in the **(262)** _____ (*veins, arteries*) (Fig. 10-16).

256 intima

257 intima
258 media

259 smooth muscle
260 circumferentially

261 circumferentially

262 veins

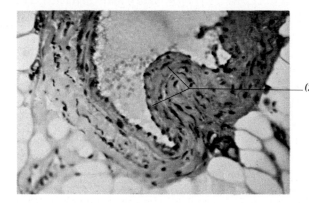
—**(263)** _____ _____

263 tunica media

FIG. 10-16. Identify the type of vessel: **(264)** _____. H and E stain (original magnification × 125).

Veins that travel through muscle need less muscle for support, and therefore their tunica **(265)** _____ is remarkably **(266)** _____ (*thinner, thicker*). Those veins that lack any such supportive tissue (e.g., superficial leg veins) have a great deal **(267)** _____ (*more, less*) **(268)** _____ (*smooth, striated*) muscle in their tunica **(269)** _____, and therefore are considerably **(270)** _____ (*thicker, thinner*).

The tunica adventitia of all medium and small veins consists of loose connective tissue replete with thick longitudinal collagenous fibers and elastic networks, and no **(271)** ^{vaso}_____ or separation from the tunica **(272)** _____ by an **(273)** _____ _____ _____ is evident.

264 vein

265 media
266 thinner
267 more
268 smooth
269 media
270 thicker

271 vasorum
272 media
273 external elastic lamina

Large Veins

Large veins have as the thickest tunic, the tunica adventitia, **(274)** _____ (*similar to, unlike*) large arteries. The tunica adventitia is many times thicker than the tunica media and is loose

274 similar to

275 *connective tissue*

276 *vasorum*
277 *poorly*

278 *vasa vasorum*

279 *adventitia*
280 *vasorum*
281 *adventitia*

282 *endothelial*

283 *small and medium*
    veins
284 *elastic arteries*

285 *internal elastic*
286 *media*
287 *smooth muscle*

288 *tunica intima*

289 *low*

290 *closed*

291 *lymph*

292 *endothelial*

(275) _____ _____ rich in elastic and collagen bundles. In many, but not all, of the largest veins, bundles of longitudinally arranged muscle fibers can be found in the inner part of the tunica adventitia. Large veins (more so than large arteries) are supplied by an abundant (276) vaso_____ and lymphatic vessels. Since the large veins carry (277) _____ (*poorly, richly*) oxygenated blood, the vein wall does not derive enough nutrients from diffusion. The rich blood supply of blood vessels of the (278) _____ _____ in the tunica adventitia supplies the necessary oxygen and nutrients. Also, because of the low pressure that is found in the veins, the vessels in the tunica (279) _____ can approach the tunica intima without collapsing. The (280) vaso_____ of arteries is found only in the tunica (281) _____ because of the high-pressure system.

The tunica intima of large veins is a poorly developed (282) _____ lining that is highly irregular in outline. Immediately beneath the endothelium is a subendothelial layer of connective tissue found also in (283) _____ (*collecting venules, small and medium veins*) and (284) _____ _____ (*arterioles, elastic arteries*). This connective tissue layer is prevalent in all large veins and is thick.

There is no (285) _____ _____ lamina between the tunica intima and tunica (286) _____. Often absent in many large veins is the tunica media, and, if found, it is very thin with few (287) _____ _____ cells.

There are valves in many medium-caliber veins, especially in the extremities. The valves usually consist of two leaflets (there can be one) that are outpocketings of the innermost tunica, the (288) _____ _____. Central reinforcement by connective tissue and elastic fibers gives the valves resiliency. Valves function to prevent blood backflow in this (289) _____ (*low, high*)-pressure system.

Lymphatic Vessels

Blood vessels form a(n) (290) _____ (*closed, open*) circulatory system. The lymphatic system, found in virtually all organs except the CNS, cartilage, bone, bone marrow, thymus, teeth, and placenta, constitutes a drainage system or open circulatory system. Like blood vessels, the smallest lymphatic vessel is a lymphatic capillary. This vessel will carry fluid (lymph) into successively larger vessels that pass through lymph nodes (see Chap. 11), and ultimately converge on lymphatic ducts. The fluid transported, (291) _____, is an ultrafiltrate of blood formed by continual leakage across the capillary (292) _____ (*mesothelial, endothelial*) wall into the surrounding spaces. Collected by lymphatic vessels, lymph is primarily water, electrolytes, and proteins (Fig. 10-17).

Lymphatic Vessels

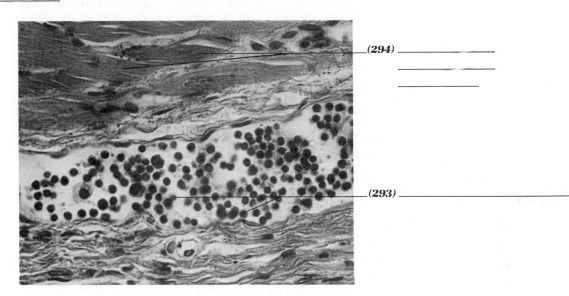

(294) _____

_____

_____

(293) _____

FIG. 10-17. A small lymphatic vessel, H and E stain (original magnification ×312).

293 *lymphocytes*
294 *smooth muscle cells*

Large lymphatic vessels are made up of walls consisting of the three tunics. While the wall is thicker than that of lymphatic capillaries, it is still quite thin. The tunics are not well defined and therefore are hard to differentiate under a microscope. The tunica intima does consist of a lining *(295)* _____. Adjacent to the intima is a thin interlacing layer of elastic fibers. There is no distinct boundary between the tunica intima and the *(296)* _____ _____, the *(297)* _____ _____ _____. The tunica media has one to two layers of

295 *endothelium*

circularly arranged and obliquely arranged smooth *(298)* _____ cells supported by connective tissue fibers.

296 *tunica media*
297 *internal elastic lamina*
298 *muscle*

The outermost tunic, the tunica *(299)* _____ _____, is a well-developed layer composed of elastic fibers, collagen bundles continuous with the surrounding *(300)* _____ _____ _____. In the largest lymphatic vessels, blood vessels (the *(301)* ^vaso-_____) are

299 *adventitia*

found in the tunica *(302)* _____. The best way to differentiate large lymphatic vessels from arteries and veins is by the very large lumen of the lymphatic vessel in relation to the thickness of the vessel wall, a

300 *loose connective tissue*
301 *vasorum*
302 *adventitia*

(303) _____ *(large, small)* lumen-to-wall ratio, and its very irregular shape.

Except in the smallest and occasional large lymphatics, valves are common in these vessels. The valves are folds of the endothelium of the tunica

303 *large*

(304) _____ back to back and supported by a delicate middle connective tissue layer. These valves are far more numerous than those of the *(305)* _____ *(arteries, veins)* and often run close together. The flow of lymph, dependent on the contraction of the surrounding muscles, will have unidirectional flow ensured by the valves.

304 *intima*

The final convergence of the lymphatics is at the base of the neck, where they drain into either the right lymphatic duct or the thoracic duct. Histologically, the lymphatic duct wall is composed of the three tunics. The lumen is

305 *veins*

lined by an endothelial cell with elastic fibers forming a boundary similar to the internal elastic lamina at the junction of the tunica *(306)* _____ and *(307)* _____. The media has more muscle bundles than the great veins, and the tunica adventitia also has smooth muscle bundles surrounded by loose connective tissue.

306 intima
307 media

11

Immunologic System

After completing this chapter, you should be able to identify the following:

1 Lymphocytes	5 Lymph nodes
2 Plasma cells	6 Spleen
3 Thymus	7 Red and white pulp
4 Hassall's bodies	8 Periarterial lymphatic sheaths

Also, after completing this chapter, you should understand the following:

1 The difference between primary and secondary lymphoid organs
2 The parenchymal tissue versus stromal tissue
3 The blood barrier in the thymus
4 The difference between primary and secondary lymph nodules

5 The physiological and histologic differences between red and white pulp
6 The blood supply throughout the spleen

The immune system is a vastly complex system that is composed of different organs and tissues. Throughout the body, this system encompasses the lymphoid organs: thymus, lymph nodes, and spleen; all aggregates of lymphoid tissue in nonlymphoid organs, for example, gastrointestinal (GI), respiratory, and the urinary tracts; lymphocytes of the blood and lymph; and the total population of lymphocytes and plasma cells dispersed throughout the connective tissues and epithelial tissues of the body. The function of the immune system is to protect the body from harmful exogenous and endogenous agents. Discussion in this chapter will center on the lymphoid organs, the lymph *(1)* _____, thymus, and *(2)* _____.

The lymphoid organs are the *(3)* _____ _____, *(4)* _____ and the *(5)* _____, each differing in histologic organization; yet histologic identification of the specific organ can be difficult. A cursory examination of the histophysiology of lymphocytes is necessary in order to understand the histology of the lymphoid organs.

There are two types of lymphocytes, *(6)* __ and *(7)* __. Differentiation of these cells in an ordinary light micrograph is *(8)* _____ (*simple, not possible*). *(9)* __ and *(10)* __ lymphocytes express immunologic specificity, which means that they are programmed to respond to an antigen (foreign substance) specific for each T and B cell. The *(11)* __ lymphocyte reacts to antigens by manufacturing immunoglobulins, whereas *(12)* __-lymphocytes cannot. After contact with the specific antigen, the B-lymphocyte eventually differentiates into two types of cells, plasma cells, which produce and secrete immunoglobulins, and B-memory cells (Fig. 11-1). Plasma cells, as discussed before, have

1 *node*
2 *spleen*
3 *lymph node*
4 *spleen*
5 *thymus*

6 *T*
7 *B*
8 *not possible*
9 *T*
10 *B*
11 *B*
12 *T*

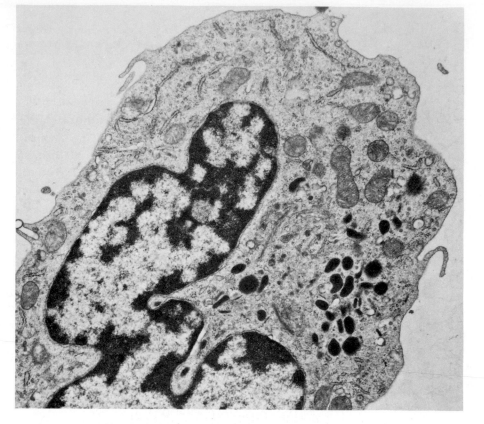

FIG. 11-1. Identify the type of cell: *(13)* _____ _____. Oil immersion.

13 *plasma cell*

a(n) *(14)* _____ (*eccentric cartwheel, central cartwheel*) nucleus in a cytoplasm rich in *(15)* _____ (*sER, rER*) aiding in the manufacture of the protein *(16)* _____.
Antibody will accumulate in the plasma cell in large vacuoles called Russell bodies. These chiefly *(17)* _____philic bodies give a distinct appearance to the cell, and the plasma cell is then called a Russell body cell.

14 *eccentric cartwheel*
15 *rER*
16 *immunoglobulins*

17 *eosino*

18 *B-memory*

    The other cell produced from B-cell differentiation is the *(18)* __-_____ cell. Small B-memory cells are small lymphocytes that upon a second contact with the same antigen will mature into large lymphocytes that rapidly divide into great numbers of plasma cells and other B-memory cells. The production of more plasma cells makes it possible for more
(19) _____ or antibody to be produced.
    T-lymphocytes *(20)* _____ (*do, do not*) produce
(21) _____ and also do not differentiate into
(22) _____ cells and memory cells. Yet T-lymphocytes and macrophages are needed for the proper and full response to occur. Knowing this small amount of histophysiology of the T- and B-*(23)* _____ makes it possible to better understand why the lymphoid organs, the
(24) _____, *(25)* _____, and *(26)* _____ _____ are organized the way they are.

19 *immunoglobulins*
20 *do not*
21 *antibodies*
   (immunoglobulins)
22 *plasma*

23 *lymphocytes*

24 *thymus*
25 *spleen*
26 *lymph node*

Thymus

Thymus

The thymus is a lymphoid organ located anteriorly to the great vessels where they enter and exit the heart, and immediately beneath the sternum. The thymus is the only primary lymphoid organ in humans. Primary describes the development of a subpopulation of hematopoietic stem cells free from antigen into lymphocytic antigen-reactive cells. The thymus produces a subpopulation of lymphocytes called (27) ___-lymphocytes. The bone marrow is thought to serve as the primary site of development of (28) ___-lymphocytes.

Secondary lymphoid organs, the (29) _____ and (30) _____ _____ are areas where the antigen-reactive cells come into contact with the antigen but there is no primary production of lymphocytes. Besides being a (31) _____ (secondary, primary) lymphoid organ, the thymus also differs from the other lymphoid organs in that it attains its greatest size at puberty and then begins a progressive involution in which cells are largely replaced by adipocytes, or (32) _____ _____.

Grossly, the thymus is a bilobed organ in which there is continuity between parenchymal cells of one lobule with parenchymal cells of another. Parenchymal cells indicate the distinguishing cells of a gland or organ supported by a connective tissue stroma. The thymic lobe can be subdivided into three gross areas: a connective tissue capsule that surrounds and subdivides the lobes; a dark-staining peripheral margin called the cortex; and a lighter staining central area—the medulla (Fig. 11-2).

27 T
28 B
29 spleen
30 lymph nodes

31 primary

32 fat cells

33 cortex
34 medulla

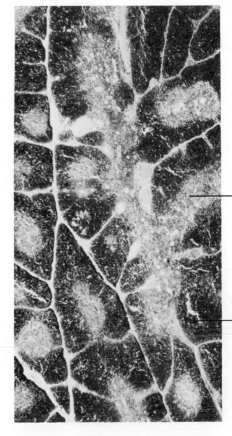

(34) _____

(33) _____

FIG. 11-2. Thymus, hematoxylin-eosin (H and E) stain (low-power magnification).

35 connective tissue

36 two
37 lymphatic

38 darker
39 peripheral

40 stromal

41 stroma
42 spot junctions
43 light
44 reticular

45 T
46 T-lymphocytes

47 lymphocytes

48 dark
49 thymocytes

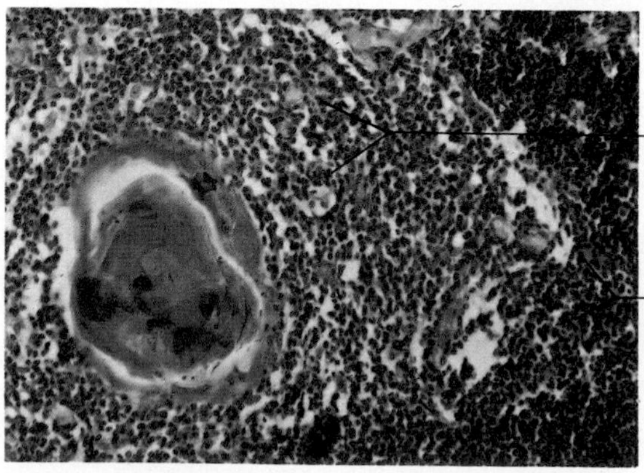

50 cortex
51 medulla

Capsule

Each lobe is invested by a capsule consisting of loose
(35) _____ _____. The capsule contains small
blood vessels that supply the cortex, but no lymphatic vessels enter or drain
from the organ. The capsule then subdivides into connective tissue septa that
incompletely divide each of the **(36)** _____ (*one, two, three, four*) lobes into
lobules. These septa carry blood vessels but no **(37)** _____ vessels, and do not penetrate further than the border between the cortex and
medulla—the corticomedullary border.

Cortex

The cortex, the **(38)** _____ (*lighter, darker*) staining
(39) _____ (*peripheral, central*) area of the thymic lobe, is
made up of three types of cells: stromal cells, lymphocytes, and macrophages.
Stellate epithelial reticular cells constitute the supportive or
(40) _____ cells of the thymus. Arranged in a three-dimensional
spongelike network, the epithelial reticular cells are often obscured by the lymphocytes packed into this network (difficult to visualize with the light microscope). Consisting of light-staining eosinophilic cytoplasm, epithelial cells that
form the **(41)** _____ (*stroma, parenchyma*) of the thymus are joined to
one another by desmosomes or **(42)** _____ _____. Along
the border between the cortex and capsule, attenuated cell processes of the
(43) _____ (*light, dark*)-staining epithelial **(44)** _____ cells
form a continuous sheath that separates the thymic lymphocytes from the
connective tissue capsule.

Lymphocytes—or, as they are often called when found in the thymus, thymocytes—or immature **(45)** ___ (*T, B*)-lymphocytes, are packed tightly in the cortex. The thymocytes or immature **(46)** ___-_____ range in
size from small to large. The large thymocytes constitute a small percentage of
the total population of **(47)** _____ (*lymphocytes, reticular
cells*), and are at the greatest concentration at the periphery of the cortex. These
large thymocytes have a highly basophilic cytoplasm. Inward from the outer
edges of the **(48)** _____ (*light, dark*)-staining cortex, the lymphocytes or immature **(49)** _____ become smaller, and more dying lympho-
cytes are found (Fig. 11-3). The smallest thymocytes are less than one half the

(51) _____

(50) _____

FIG. 11-3. Thymus, H and E stain (original magnification ×170).

Thymus

---

52 baso

53 epithelial reticular
54 spot junction
55 desmosomes

56 reticular cells

57 thymocytes
58 macrophages
59 epithelial reticular cells

60 stromal

61 endothelial
62 basement membrane

63 phagocytize
64 epithelial reticular
65 T-lymphocytes
66 thymocytes
67 T-lymphocytes

68 lymphocytes
69 macrophages
70 lighter
71 decreased
72 epithelial reticular
73 reticular
74 stromal
75 eosinophilic

76 Hassall's
77 thymic
78 bodies
79 thymus
80 medulla

---

size of the largest; they have a thin rim of cytoplasm with few polyribosomes and stain less (52) _____philic_____.

Macrophages are scattered throughout the cortex and are a minor part of the cell population. They increase in number the closer they are to the cortico-medullary junction, and they are difficult to distinguish. Macrophages are quite similar in appearance to the stromal cells, (53) _____ cells, but are not attached to one another by (54) _____ _____ or (55) _____ as are the stromal cells. Other cells found with even less frequency than macrophages are plasma and mast cells. Do not expect to visualize the macrophages or epithelial (56) _____ _____ very well, if at all, under routine photomicroscopy. The tremendous numbers of immature (57) _____ often obliterate the highly phagocytic (58) _____ and the (59) _____ _____ that make up the stroma.

At the corticomedullary junction, the cortex is supplied by arterioles that send out highly anastomosing capillaries into the cortex. These capillaries course through narrow channels formed by the epithelial reticular cells or (60) _____ cells. A blood barrier is formed by the capillary, thereby preventing antigen from passing through. This barrier consists of three parts: the first part of the barrier to antigen passage is the capillary wall, (61) _____ cells and their associated (62) _____ _____. If the antigen successfully passes out of the lumen, macrophages lying between the capillaries would (63) _____ (phagocytize, produce antibodies against) it. Last, the antigen must pass through the (64) _____ _____ cells before contact with the forming (65) ___-_____ or immature (66) _____. This barrier is essential for the proper maturation of (67) ___-_____.

Medulla
Containing the same cells as the cortex (i.e., epithelial reticular cells, (68) _____, and (69) _____), the medulla differs, however, in the proportions of these cells. The medulla is a (70) _____ (darker, lighter) staining area because of the (71) _____ (increased, decreased) proportion of lymphocytes to (72) _____ _____ cells.

The epithelial (73) _____ cells or (74) _____ cells are extremely pleiomorphic in the medulla. Their light-staining (75) _____ (eosinophilic, basophilic) cytoplasm contributes to the "lightness" of the medulla. These stromal cells often wrap themselves around each other forming concentric arrays of epithelial cells called Hassall's bodies or thymic corpuscles. The formation of the (76) _____ bodies or (77) _____ corpuscles is characteristic of only the medulla of the thymus, and no other organ. The Hassall's (78) _____ are an extremely useful clue in identifying the (79) _____ and the specific area of that organ, the (80) _____ (Fig. 11-4).

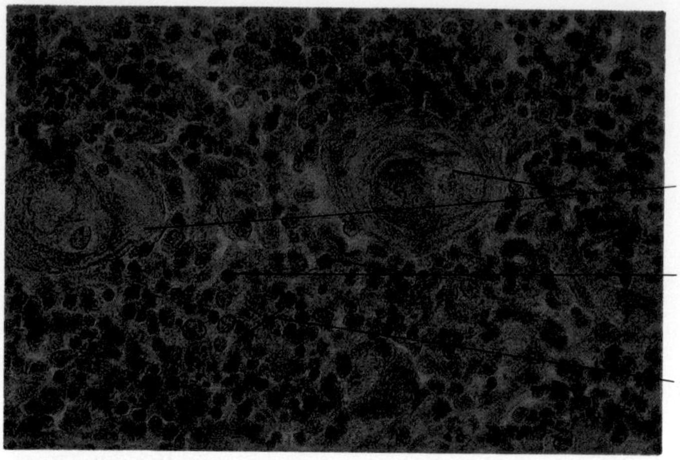

136

pening**Immunologic System**

81 Hassall's bodies

82 epithelial reticular

83 medulla
84 lymphocyte

85 thymus

86 decreased

87 eosinophilic
88 pleiomorphic
89 reticular cells

90 small
91 smaller

92 corticomedullary
93 venules
94 permeable
95 possible
96 medulla
97 endothelial
98 basement membrane
99 epithelial reticular

(81) _____

_____

made up of

(82) _____

_____

cells

(84) _____

(cell type)

(83) _____

FIG. 11-4. Identify this organ:
(85) _____. H and E stain (original magnification ×170).

The (86) _____ (decreased, increased) number of lympho-
cytes in the medullary area of the thymus makes it slightly easier to examine the
(87) _____ (eosinophilic, basophilic)
(88) _____ (regular, pleiomorphic)-shaped epithelial
(89) _____ _____. The lymphocytes here are smaller
than those of the core.

Macrophages, which appear in (90) _____ (large, small) numbers in
the cortex, and plasma cells, which are found in even (91) _____
(greater, smaller) numbers in the cortex, are virtually absent in the medullary
area of the thymus.

The blood supply for the medulla of the thymus is from the arterioles at the
(92) _____ junction. Since the postcapillary
(93) _____ are highly (94) _____ (impermeable,
permeable), they make it (95) _____ (possible, impossible) for mi-
grating T-lymphocytes to enter the bloodstream in the (96) _____
(cortex, medulla) through a barrier: the capillary
(97) _____ barrier with its associated
(98) _____ _____, the macrophage barrier, and the
(99) _____ _____ cell barrier (Fig. 11-5).

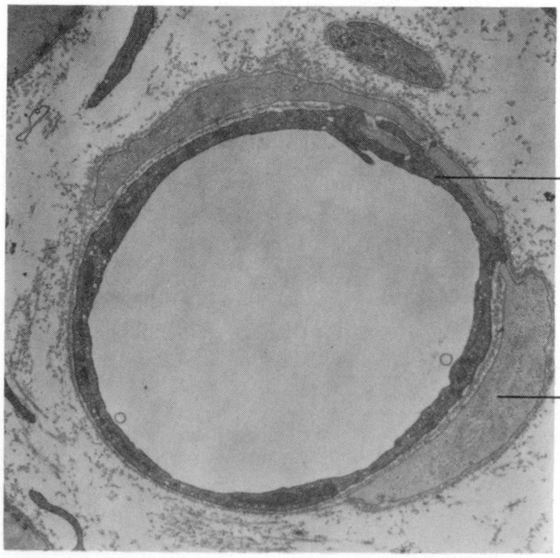

Endothelial
cell

Pericyte

FIG. 11-5. Electron micrograph of a capillary.
(Courtesy of Dr. Rosemary Mazanet)

Lymph Nodes

Lymph nodes are lymphoid organs 1 mm to 25 mm in diameter; they are located along the course of lymphatic vessels. These small organs are flattened and ovoid with a slight indentation on one side. At this indentation, or hilus, blood vessels enter and exit while lymphatic vessels exit only. Lymph is transported to the node by way of afferent lymphatic vessels. The afferent vessels approach the node and give rise to a number of branches that enter the node at various sites along its convex surface, opposite to the hilus. Efferent lymphatic vessels leave the node at the *(100)* _____ and carry lymph away from the node. Lymphatic vessels have valves that ensure *(101)* _____ (bi, uni) *directional* flow of lymph from the *(102)* _____ lymphatic vessel through the *(103)* _____ node and out at the *(104)* _____ by the *(105)* _____ _____ vessels.

The histologic organization of the node consists basically of lymphoid tissue in a recticular stroma, surrounded by a capsule and traversed by specialized lymphatic vessels called sinuses.

100 hilus
101 uni
102 afferent
103 lymph
104 hilus
105 efferent lymphatic

Capsule

Like the thymus, the node is invested by connective *(106)* _____ *(107)* _____. This covering consists of dense collagenous fibers and a few fibroblasts. Muscle fibers can be found in the capsule at the exit and entry points of the *(108)* _____ and *(109)* _____ lymphatic vessels respectively. Thickened at the hilus, the capsule also sends out a number of branching connective tissue trabeculae (Fig. 11-6). These trabeculae are not complete septa but flattened rods of dense *(110)* _____ _____ that carry blood vessels into the node and lend support. The capsule also merges with the surrounding loose connective tissue and adipose tissue. (You should finish #112 at this point.)

106 tissue
107 stroma

108 efferent
109 afferent

110 connective tissue

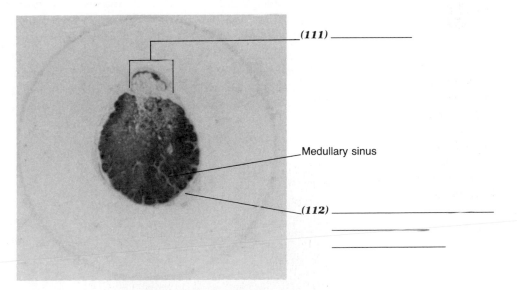

(111) _____

Medullary sinus

(112) _____

_____

FIG. 11-6. Lymph node (low-power magnification).

111 hilus

112 connective tissue
*   capsule*

Stroma

The lymph node has a stroma that holds the free cells in place. This nodal stroma is a reticular net composed of two different types of reticular cells. The first type is called a dendritic reticular cell because of its long nervelike cyto-

plasmic processes. Joined by spot junctions or *(113)* _____,
like the *(114)* _____ _____ _____
that compose the stroma of the thymus, these cells predominate in the outermost and middle areas of the cortex. The second type of stromal cell, stromal
cell type II, has thin interdigitating processes. These stromal cells type II are
found in the medullary region of the nodes—the inner zones. Essentially the
stromal cells, their associated basement *(115)* _____, collagenous
fibers of the capsule, and trabeculae form intertwining reticular nets extending
from the capsule through the cortex and terminating in the medullary area. It is
extremely difficult to visualize the stroma as well as the individual stromal cells
in a routine light micrograph unless a specific reticular stain is applied and the
slide examined under great magnification.

Sinuses

Surrounding and traversing the lymphoid tissue and stroma are specialized
lymphatic vessels called sinuses. These sinuses act as channels to transport the
lymph through the node. Piercing the capsule at its convex side,
(116) _____ lymphatic *(117)* _____ open into a sinus
just beneath the covering capsule. This sinus is called the marginal or subcapsular sinus. The marginal or *(118)* _____ sinus encircles the
node and communicates directly with the efferent lymphatic vessels at the nodal
indentation or the *(119)* _____. The marginal sinus also gives off branches
that follow the course of the *(120)* _____ _____
trabeculae, and they are called intermediate or cortical sinuses. These narrow
sinuses, the cortical or *(121)* _____ sinuses, penetrate
the parenchymal tissue all the way to the medullary area.

In the central area of the node, the *(122)* _____ *(lighter, darker)*
staining *(123)* _____ *(medullary, cortical)* region, the intermediate or *(124)* _____ sinuses are confluent with the larger medullary
sinuses (Fig. 11-7). The medullary sinuses are highly tortuous, wide, branching
channels that are confluent with the encircling marginal or
(125) _____ sinuses at the *(126)* _____ where they
both lead into the *(127)* _____ lymphatic vessel. The branching
and anastomosing of the medullary sinus fragment the medullary parenchymal
tissue into medullary cords (discussed below). (You should finish #129 at this
point.)

116 afferent
117 vessels
118 subcapsular

119 hilus
120 connective tissue

121 intermediate

122 lighter
123 medullary
124 cortical

125 subcapsular
126 hilus
127 efferent

128 medulla
129 cortex

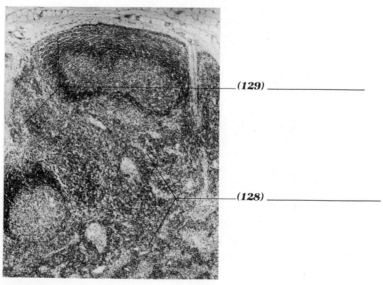

(129) _____

(128) _____

FIG. 11-7. Lymph node, H and E stain
(original magnification ×50).

In summary, the flow of lymph is from the *(130)* _____ lymphatic vessels penetrating the *(131)* _____ (*convex, concave*) side of the node, to the *(132)* _____ or *(133)* _____ sinus, which either runs around the whole node or branches into *(134)* _____ or *(135)* _____ sinuses. The cortical or *(136)* _____ sinuses are then confluent with the highly tortuous *(137)* _____, which in turn are confluent with both the *(138)* _____ or *(139)* _____ sinus and the *(140)* _____ _____ vessel.

All sinuses of the lymph node have the same histology, yet, unlike splenic sinuses, have fibers in them. The adluminal side of the sinuses is lined by a lymphatic endothelium, not unlike the *(141)* _____ lining of blood and lymphatic vessels. Only the endothelium lining the *capsular* side of the subcapsular sinus is continuous. All the sinuses, *(142)* _____ or cortical, *(143)* _____, and the sinus side of the subcapsular or *(144)* _____ sinus have endothelium that is discontinuous. Beyond the endothelium, there is also no definitive basement membrane to further impede the flow of lymphocytes and other cells out of the vessels. Lymphocytes, macrophages (often found attached to the sinus endothelium), fluid, and, possibly, antigens are said to percolate throughout the whole node with some direction provided by the *(145)* _____. This leakage out of all the sinuses maximizes the contact of antigen with lymphocytes and macrophages. The node acts as a filter that eliminates harmful antigens and alerts defense mechanisms.

The lymph node has a cortical and *(146)* _____ area *(147)* _____ (*like, unlike*) the thymus. Yet unlike the thymus, *(148)* _____-lymphocytes constitute an important part of nodal histology.

Cortex

Under low power, the outer cortex of the node appears as a *(149)* _____ (*dark, light*)-staining area that stains progressively *(150)* _____ (*lighter, darker*) as one moves inward (Fig. 11-8). The cortex can be subdivided

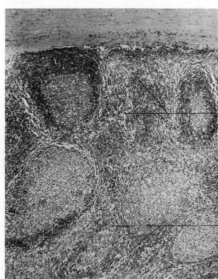

(151) _____

(152) _____

FIG. 11-8. Lymph node, H and E stain (original magnification ×50).

histologically into two areas, the outer cortex and the inner (deep) cortex, more commonly called the paracortex.

The outer cortex consists of primary and secondary nodes, stromal cells, and scattered lymphocytes. Primary nodules, uniform populations of neatly packed small B-lymphocytes, stain considerably darker than surrounding tissue. There are other such nodules throughout the outer cortex, but they have a dark-staining rim and a light-staining central area. These nodules are called secondary nodules and the *(153)* _____ (*dark, light*) central area surrounded by a mantle of densely packed lymphocytes is called the germinal center (Fig. 11-9).

153 light

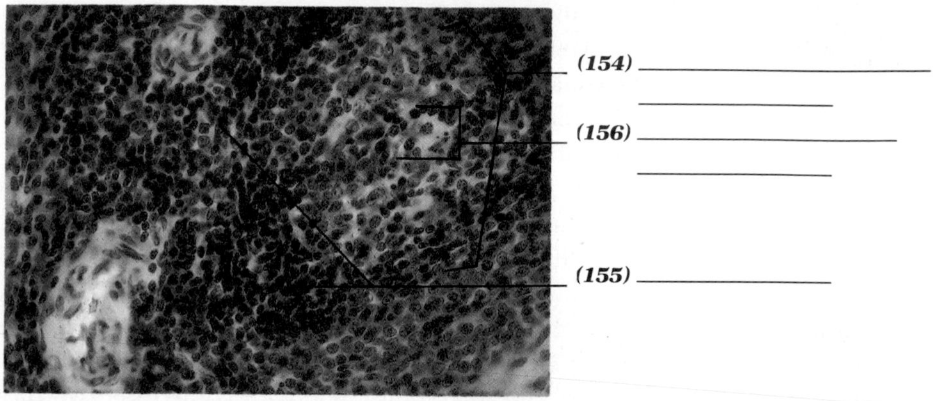

(154) _____

(156) _____

(155) _____

FIG. 11-9.   Lymph node, H and E stain (original magnification × 170).

154 secondary nodule
155 mantle
156 germinal center

The dense-staining mantle contains mainly small lymphocytes. The *(157)* _____ center is a *(158)* _____ (*lighter, darker*) staining area consisting of actively dividing medium and large lymphocytes with some macrophages and a few plasma cells. Because of the predominance of B-lymphocytes, the outer cortex of the node is called the B-dependent area.

The stromal cells of the outer cortex are *(159)* _____ _____ cells, so named because of their long cytoplasmic processes.

157 germinal
158 lighter

Rarely will a primary or secondary nodule be found in the inner cortex or *(160)* _____ cortex. The thymus provides *(161)* ___-lymphocytes and is a *(162)* _____ (*primary, secondary*) lymphoid organ *(163)* _____ (*with, without*) B-lymphocytes. It was found that if the thymus is removed in an infant, the paracortex or *(164)* _____ _____ is depleted of lymphocyte population. The primary lymphocytes in the paracortex are scattered *(165)* ___-lymphocytes, unlike in the B-dependent area or the *(166)* _____ cortex. By ascertaining the type of lymphocytes that predominate, we can call the paracortex area T dependent and the outer cortex *(167)* ___ _____. Dispersed throughout the loosely packed T-lymphocytes of the paracortex are scavenger cells of the body, *(168)* _____ and some plasma cells.

159 dendritic reticular

160 para
161 T
162 primary
163 without
164 inner cortex

165 T
166 outer

167 B-dependent

168 macrophages

Medulla

The medulla of the lymph node is remarkably different from the cortex. The medulla consists mainly of medullary cord and sinuses and scattered cells. The cords are a divergent anastomosing network that separates the sinuses. Rich in reticular fibers, the medullary cords have supporting stromal cells, type *(169)* _____ (*I, II*) that terminate on them. Found within the cords are a few lymphocytes, large numbers of plasma cells, and scattered macrophages. The

169 II

141

medullary area of the node, therefore, contains **(170)** _____ *(more, fewer)* plasma cells than the cortex.

Major blood vessels enter and exit the node at the **(171)** _____ where the **(172)** _____ lymphatic **(173)** _____ **(174)** _____ *(exits, enters)*. Blood vessels reach the cortex and divide into capillary plexuses around the nodules. Arising from the plexuses and traveling deep into the paracortex are postcapillary venules. Like the postcapillary venules of the **(175)** _____ - _____ area of the thymus, those of the node are highly **(176)** _____ *(perme-able, impermeable)*, and therefore passage into and out of the vessels is **(177)** _____ *(difficult, easy)*. Eventually, the postcapillary venule becomes con-fluent with wide but small **(178)** _____ *(veins, arteries)*. These vessels then merge to form larger vessels that exit at the lymph node's **(179)** _____.

Spleen

The spleen is a lymphoid organ that functions as a filter for the blood system. Like the thymus and lymph node, the spleen is important in the immune response, but it also acts to sequester and destroy blood cells. These two physiological actions account for the two widely different histologic areas in the spleen.

The spleen, a highly vascular organ, does not have cortical and medullary divisions like the other immune organs, the **(180)** _____ and **(181)** _____ _____. Instead, the spleen is an encapsulated organ con-sisting of white pulp areas scattered throughout red pulp tissue. Surrounding the parenchymal tissue of the spleen is a highy collagenous **(182)** _____, similar to that of the lymph node. Besides collagen bundles, the capsule also consists of an elastic network and sparse muscle cells. Covering the outside of the capsule is a flattened mesothelium or **(183)** _____ _____ epithelium. The capsule produces inward extensions called trabeculae that penetrate deep into the organ. Since these extensions travel in various directions, a section of the spleen reveals trabeculae that seem detached from the capsule. Like the capsule, the trabeculae function in carrying arteries and veins into and out of the spleen.

The stroma of the spleen, difficult to visualize under most preparations, consists of fine reticular fibers and cells. Attached to the capsule and trabeculae, the stroma forms a meshwork supportive of both red and white pulp areas.

White Pulp

White pulp is not white or lighter than the red pulp under any light micrograph. Instead, white pulp appears as dark grayish blue areas scattered throughout the red-staining red pulp areas (Fig. 11-10). White pulp is lymphatic tissue consisting

Lymph Nodes

170 more
171 hilus
172 efferent
173 vessel
174 exits
175 corticomedullary junction
176 permeable
177 easy
178 veins
179 hilus
180 thymus
181 lymph node
182 capsule
183 simple squamous
184 white pulp
185 red pulp

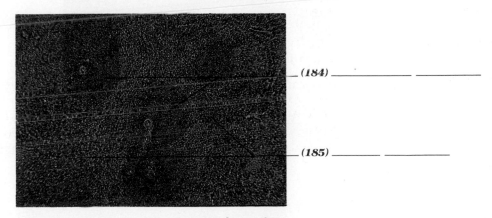

(184) _____ _____

(185) _____ _____

FIG. 11-10. Spleen, H and E stain (original magnifica-tion ×50).

of lymphocytes, plasma cells, macrophages, and reticular cells all surrounding a major blood vessel. White pulp can be subdivided into a periarterial lymphatic sheath (PALS) and lymphatic nodules.

PALS surround an artery in a cylindrical manner. The artery often assumes a central position in the *(186)* _____ lymphatic sheath, and is therefore called a central artery (Fig. 11-11). The sheaths consist of a loose

186 periarterial

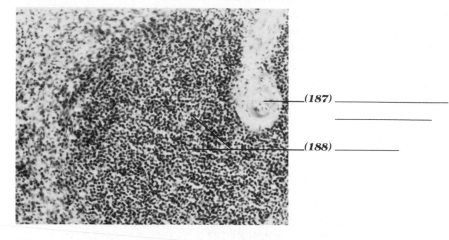

(187) _____
_____

(188) _____

187 central artery

188 PALS

FIG. 11-11. Spleen, H and E stain (original magnification ×125).

framework in which reticular cells are packed with small and medium T-lymphocytes. A small number of marophages and plasma cells are found and increase in number the closer they are to the periphery of the *(189)* _____ _____ sheath.

Lymphatic nodule and *(190)* _____ lymphatic sheath borders are often difficult to delineate. To identify the parts of the white pulp, one must find the central artery. The area closely circumscribing it will be the sheath. Farther away from the artery, easily identifiable lymphatic nodules can be seen (Fig. 11-12). The nodules, like those of the lymph nodes, consist

189 periarterial lymphatic
190 periarterial

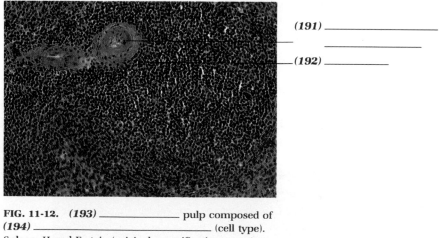

(191) _____
_____

(192) _____

191 central artery
192 PALS

FIG. 11-12. *(193)* _____ pulp composed of *(194)* _____ (cell type). Spleen, H and E stain (original magnification ×135).

193 white
194 lymphocytes

Spleen

195 B
196 germinal centers
197 center
198 secondary nodules
199 centers
200 primary nodules
201 periarterial lymphatic

202 PALS

203 capillaries

204 white pulp
205 secondary
206 central artery
207 red pulp
208 red
209 lymphatic
210 lymph node

211 reticular

212 splenic
213 Billroth's

214 Macrophages

primarily of *(195)* ___-lymphocytes and can contain pale-staining areas, *(196)* _____ _____. Those nodules with a germinal *(197)* _____ are called *(198)* _____ _____, and those without the germinal *(199)* _____ are *(200)* _____ _____. Lymphatic nodules often push the central artery of the *(201)* _____ _____ sheath to a more eccentric position but still within the sheath.

Blood travels to the white pulp through branches of arteries that travel in the trabeculae. These branches give rise to the central artery, which is supported by reticular sheaths as they run through the *(202)* __ __ __ __. Supplying each lymphatic nodule is a branch of the central artery, the lymphatic follicular artery. The follicular artery branches into the smallest of blood vessels, *(203)* _____, in the red pulp.

Red Pulp

Red pulp consists of branching, anastomosing networks of sinuses separated from each other by a reticular meshwork. The reticular meshwork is often called the splenic cords or Billroth's cords. Often called the nonlymphatic area of the

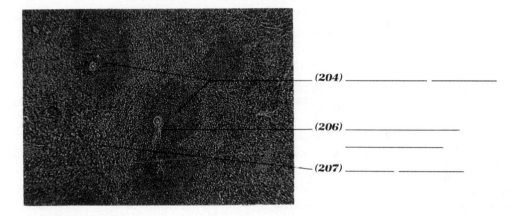

(204) _____ _____

(206) _____ _____

_____

(207) _____ _____

FIG. 11-13. *(205)* _____ (*secondary, primary*) nodule. Spleen, H and E stain (original magnification ×50).

spleen, *(208)* _____ pulp lacks *(209)* _____ nodules and areas of concentrated lymphocytes. Supplied by arteries, the red pulp is drained by vascular sinuses, similar to the *(210)* _____ (*lymph node, thymus*). The color of the red pulp is a reddish brown, and is caused by the abundance of red blood corpuscles (RBCs) in the sinuses (Fig. 11-13).

The splenic cords vary in thickness, and consist of an extensive supportive *(211)* _____ fiber network. Reticular cells and their fibers support the adjacent sinus endothelium as well as the great numbers of free cells. The *(212)* _____ cords or *(213)* _____ cords have large numbers of macrophages. RBCs and a few plasma cells freely float across the cords and into the sinuses. Damaged blood cells can be detained in the cords and it is here that the cells will be phagocytized and removed from circulation. *(214)* _____ (*Plasma cells, Lymphocytes, Macrophages*) are the cells responsible for the phagocytizing of the damaged blood cells.

Immunologic System

BLOOD SUPPLY OF RED PULP The central artery branches after running through the (215) __ __ __ __. These branches become confluent with straight, nonanasto-mosing, slender vessels called penicillar arteries or arteries of the red pulp. (It is very difficult to properly identify the parts of the blood system in the spleen.) Ranging from 25 μm to 50 μm in diameter, these arteries of the red pulp or (216) _____ arteries are histologically identical to arteries of the same size; they are lined by a tall (217) _____ resting on a continuous (218) _____ _____; their tunica media is adjacent to the tunica (219) _____ and (220) _____, one to two (221) _____ _____ cell layers thick, but is not separated on either side by the laminae, (222) _____ _____ and (223) _____ _____. The penicillar arteries or (224) _____ of the (225) _____ _____ either terminate into capillaries called arterial capillaries or, if sheathed, sheathed capillaries. These capillaries will not be confluent with postcapillary (226) _____ but with the vascular sinuses. The sinuses drain into the pulp veins and are there-fore called venous sinuses. Lining the sinusoidal wall are (227) _____ cells that are not attached to one another by desmosomes or other cell junctions.

When the blood from the capillaries, both (228) _____ and (229) _____, pours into the sinuses, (230) __- and (231) __-lymphocytes for the most part are diverted away from the splenic cords, or the (232) _____ _____; the sinuses are then con-centrated in the (233) _____ pulp. The T-lymphocytes will concentrate in the (234) __ __ __ __, and the B-lymphocytes form (235) _____ _____, both primary and (236) _____ with (237) _____ centers. The blood percolating through the sinusoids carries damaged blood cells that are rapidly phagocytized by the abundant (238) _____.

Venous sinusoids empty into the veins. These veins are lined by endothe-lium with a continuous basement (239) _____ and a layer of smooth muscle cells. Supported by the cords, the veins of the pulp become confluent with the veins of the trabeculae. Finally, the veins drain at the hilus of the spleen into splenic veins.

The blood supply of the spleen therefore consists of arteries branching from connective tissue branches. These arteries then give off a central artery that flows through the (240) __ __ __ __ rich in (241) __-lymphocytes and (242) _____ (*always, not always*) central in location. Supplying each lymphatic nodule is a branch of the artery. Another branch of the central artery travels into the red pulp; it is a nonanastomotic (243) _____ artery. This artery in turn is confluent with (244) _____ or sheathed capillaries that empty into the (245) _____ sinuses of the (246) _____ pulp. Blood is eventually drained by the veins that leave the spleen at its (247) _____ as the splenic vein.

Marginal Zone
Separating the white and red pulp areas is a thin, 80 μm to 100 μm in diameter transitional region called the marginal zone. Situated between the (248) _____ pulp and the (249) _____ pulp, the (250) _____ zone is

Spleen

251 red
252 penicillar
253 PALS
254 lymphatic nodules

where the red pulp first receives arterial blood from the arteries of the
(251) _____ pulp or the **(252)** _____ _____ (*central, penicillar*) arteries. This zone is also where circulating T-lymphocytes and B-lymphocytes are diverted from the circulation and can accumulate and form the **(253)** __ __ __ __ and **(254)** _____ _____, respectively (Fig. 11-14).

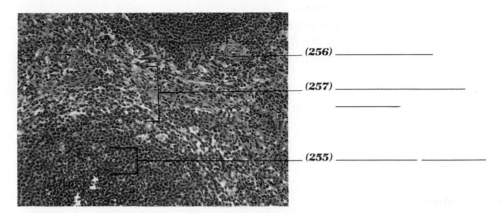

(256) _____

(257) _____

_____

(255) _____ _____

FIG. 11-14. Spleen, H and E stain (original magnification ×50).

255 white pulp
256 artery
257 marginal zone

The lymphocytes can recirculate in the blood system by entering the venous sinuses of the **(258)** _____ pulp. More important, this region—the marginal zone—is where antigen can first contact lymphocytes in the splenic parenchyma and cause an immune response to start in the white pulp, the **(259)** _____ (*nonlymphoid, lymphoid*) area of the spleen. The marginal zone is a border region that contains more lymphocytes than the **(260)** _____ pulp but far less than the **(261)** _____ pulp.

258 red

259 lymphoid

260 red
261 white

Lymph Flow

Lymph flow runs counter to the blood flow. The lymph originates from the red pulp at the venous sinusoids where there is a great deal of seepage across the walls. Lymph flow starts in the **(262)** _____ pulp, crosses the **(263)** _____ zone and the **(264)** _____ pulp, and enters larger lymphatic vessels lying in the trabeculae and surrounding **(265)** _____ _____ capsule. These vessels eventually merge at the hilus to form **(266)** _____ lymphatic vessels that carry the lymph out of the spleen. Unlike the lymph node, the spleen has no **(267)** _____ (*afferent, efferent*) lymphatic vessels, but like the node, it does have **(268)** _____ (*afferent, efferent*) lymphatic vessels that **(269)** _____ (*exit, enter*) at the **(270)** _____ of the organ.

262 red
263 marginal
264 white
265 connective tissue
266 efferent

267 afferent
268 efferent
269 exit
270 hilus

Nonlymphoid Organs with Lymphoid Tissue

Depots of lymphatic tissue scattered throughout the connective tissue are termed nonencapsulated lymphatic tissue. The areas of **(271)** non_____ _____ tissue are usually a solitary nodule, but confluent nodules can be found in the ileum and the oral cavity. Like the nodules in the **(272)** _____ _____ and spleen, these nodules can have pale centers, **(273)** _____ __ _____, and therefore are called **(274)** _____ (*secondary, primary*) lymphatic **(275)** _____. The nonencapsulated

271 encapsulated lymphatic

272 lymph node
273 germinal centers
274 secondary
275 nodules

Immunologic System

276 *lymphatic*

277 *associated lymphatic
tissue*
278 *bronchus*

(276) _____ tissue has the same function as encapsulated tissue.

The major nonlymphoid system associated with lymphatic tissue is the GI tract or *gut associated with lymphoid tissue* (GALT). The bronchus has scattered lymphoid tissue throughout and is called BALT or bronchus-
(277) _____ _____ _____. Last, the urinary tract has lymphoid tissue but it is far less prominent than that found in the GI tract or **(278)** _____.

12

Integumentary System

After completing this chapter, you should be able to identify the following:

1 Layers of the skin
2 All five strata of the epidermis
3 Eccrine sweat glands
4 Hair follicles
5 Sebaceous glands
6 Arrector pili muscles of skin

Also, after completing this chapter, you should understand the following:

1 How skin provides water impermeability
2 Production of pigment

The skin, or integument, is the largest organ in the body. It is composed of an outer layer of *(1)* _____ (*keratinized, nonkeratinized*) *(2)* _____ (*simple, stratified*) squamous epithelium, called the epidermis, and an inner layer of connective tissue called the dermis. The dermis is a highly vascular tissue. The absence of blood vessels in the epidermis aids in the formation of keratin, and forces the epidermis to be totally dependent on the underlying *(3)* _____ for its nutrients through the process of diffusion.

There are two types of skin, determined by the thickness of the covering epithelium, or *(4)* _____, and not by the thickness of the entire skin. The thickness varies from 0.5 mm to 4 mm. Thick skin, found on the palms of the hands and the soles of the feet, has a thick epidermis with a very thick dead, outer layer of *(5)* _____. Thin skin is found covering the rest of the body surface, and has both a thin epidermis and keratin layer.

There are four cell types found in the epidermis: the epithelial cells, referred to as keratinocytes; melanocytes, which produce the pigment melanin; Langerhans' cells, which are probably migratory macrophages (such as the *(6)* _____ cells in the central nervous system); and Merckel's cells, which are specialized sensory cells (Fig. 12-1).

1 keratinized
2 stratified

3 dermis

4 epidermis

5 keratin

6 microglial

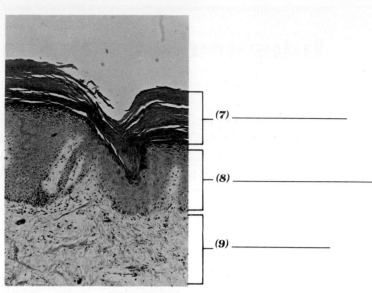

FIG. 12-1. Photomicrograph of the epidermis and dermis of the skin (original magnification ×30).

(7) _____

(8) _____

(9) _____

7 keratin

8 epidermis

9 dermis

The keratinized epithelium acts as a barrier to invading organisms, and is important in regulating fluid loss through its relative **(10)** _____ (*permeability, impermeability*) to water. Protection against the damaging effects of excessive ultraviolet (UV) radiation is provided by melanin contained in **(11)** _____ lying in the basal layers of the epidermis.

The layers of skin rest on a bed of subcutaneous tissue called the hypodermis. The composition of the **(12)** <u>hypo</u>_____ is variable, and may include adipose tissue, loose or dense irregular connective tissue, or a combination. Bundles of collagen fibers attach the dermis to the hypodermis and aid in the anchoring of the skin. These are similar to the collagenous fibers that anchor the periosteum to the underlying bone, called **(13)** _____ fibers. Skin appendages, which may be located in the hypodermis, include sweat and sebaceous glands, hair follicles, and nails.

10 impermeability

11 melanocytes

12 dermis

13 Sharpey's

Thick Skin

Because thick skin has a full complement of layers, it will be discussed first. Where is thick skin found? **(14)** _____ and **(15)** _____. Cell division occurs in the most basal layer, and in thick skin it can take up to 1 month to fully replace all the cell layers. As the basal cells proliferate, the older cells get pushed toward the surface. This places these cells farther from the nutrients supplied by blood vessels in the **(16)** _____. Consequently, degeneration occurs in the most **(17)** _____ (*apical, basal*) cell layers, and these cells are transformed into the protective layer of **(18)** _____.

14 soles
15 palms

Epidermis
The most basal layer of the epidermis is one-cell-layer thick, and is called the stratum germinativum (stratum basale; Fig. 12-2). As with most epithelia, the basal layer of cells rest on a **(19)** _____ _____, composed

16 dermis
17 apical
18 keratin

19 basement membrane

Thick Skin

20 reticular lamina
21 reticular lamina
22 germinativum
23 produce

24 hemidesmosome
25 columnar
26 most

27 round

28 macula adherens

29 tonofilaments
30 germinativum

31 stratum

32 flattened
33 basophilic

34 keratin
35 hyalin
36 membrane-coating
37 spinosum
38 exocytosis

39 aid in total water
   impermeability

of a basal lamina and a **(20)** _____. Which layer is usually thicker? **(21)** _____. The epithelial cells of the stratum **(22)** _____, which **(23)** _____ (*produce, do not produce*) the more superficial layer of the basement membrane, adhere to it by what intercellular junction? **(24)** _____. The cells of the stratum germinativum have a **(25)** _____ shape and are the **(26)** _____ (*most, least*) proliferative of the epidermal cells. There are numerous ribosomes and polysomes essential for proliferation and production of the intermediate (10 nm) tonofilaments, which are a component of keratin (Fig. 12-2).

The stratum spinosum, the second layer, is a few cell layers thick, and the cells are **(27)** _____ (*round, squamous*). This layer is also called the prickle-cell layer because the cell borders are separated from one another by small spaces traversed by spinelike processes. Because of shrinkage artifact, these spines are actually strands of cytoplasm drawn out from the cells as a result of the desmosomes, or **(28)** _____ _____, that join them. What filaments are usually found on the cytoplasmic side of such a junction? **(29)** _____. The intermediate tonofilaments found in the deeper stratum **(30)** _____ are organized into bundles in the stratum spinosum, and are then referred to as tonofibrils. Membrane-coating granules, also called lamellated bodies, are membrane-bound granules found within the cells of this layer. These granules, which contain cell products essential for total water impermeability, are released by the cells as these cells become part of the next superficial layer, the **(31)** _____ granulosum.

The stratum granulosum is two- to four-cell-layers thick and the cells appear **(32)** _____ (*round, flattened*). These cells contain granules that stain deeply **(33)** _____, called keratohyalin granules. They provide an important component of the matrix of the superficial layer of **(34)** _____. These **(35)** kerato _____ granules are not membrane bound, unlike the **(36)** _____-_____ granules found in this layer and the stratum **(37)** _____. These latter granules are released like most granules, through the process of **(38)** _____, and their contents then adhere to the outer layer of the plasma membrane. What is their function? **(39)** _____.

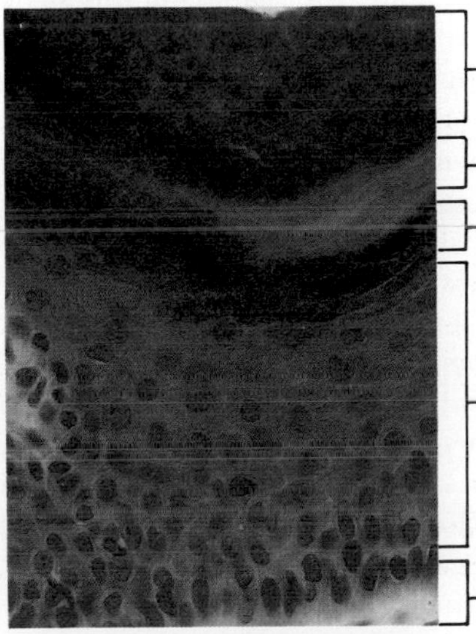

(54) _____
_____
(53) _____
_____
(52) _____
_____
(51) _____
_____
(50) _____
_____

FIG. 12-2. Photomicrograph of the layers of the epidermis, hematoxylin-eosin (H and E) stain (original magnification ×300).

Superficial to the stratum granulosum is the stratum lucidum, a layer not always seen (Figs. 12-2 and 12-3). It consists of a thin, clear, bright, homogeneous line resulting from the production of eleidin. Eleidin is a transformation product of the non-membrane-bound *(40)* _____ granules.

The stratum corneum is the most superficial layer (Fig. 12-2). The cytoskeleton persists, although there is neither a nucleus nor organelles. The cell junc-

40 kerato-hyalin

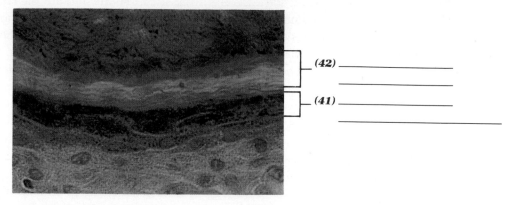

(42) _____

_____

(41) _____

_____

41 stratum granulosum
42 stratum lucidum

FIG. 12-3. Photomicrograph of a part of the epidermis, H and E stain (original magnification ×500).

tions, the *(43)* _____, most evident in the stratum *(44)* _____, are still present. The cells, totally composed of the protein *(45)* _____, are referred to as squames. What two cellular products previously described are important in the production of keratin? *(46)* _____ granules and *(47)* _____. The squames of the stratum *(48)* _____ are stacked with overlapping edges to ensure a watertight seal. What other cell product, although not a part of keratin, is important in water impermeability? *(49)* _____-_____ _____. (You should finish #54 at this point.)

43 desmosomes
44 spinosum
45 keratin
46 keratohyalin
47 eleidin
48 corneum
49 membrane-coating
  granules
50 stratum germinativum
51 stratum spinosum
52 stratum granulosum
53 stratum leucidum
54 stratum corneum
55 germinativum
56 basement membrane
57 reticular

Dermis

The dermis is the layer beneath the stratum *(55)* _____ of the epidermis (Fig. 12-4). What connective tissue structure separates the dermis from the epithelial cells? *(56)* _____ _____. The *(57)* _____ lamina of this structure is produced by the fibroblasts of the dermis. Variations in the thickness of the dermis occur throughout the body, although the difference between thin and thick skin is attributable to differences in the thickness of the *(58)* _____. The dermis is composed of two layers. Beneath the epidermis is the papillary layer, composed of *(59)* _____ _____ connective tissue. This layer makes up the connective tissue papillae that extend up between the ridges of epidermis (called the rete ridges or rete pegs). The thicker layer of the dermis is the reticular layer, and it is composed of *(60)* _____ irregular connective tissue. The two layers, the *(61)* _____ layer and the reticular layer, merge at a level approximately even with the base of the connective tissue papillae. Elastic fibers, in the form of bundles, can be found running through the thicker *(62)* _____ layer. Capillaries are found in greatest abundance in the layer closest to the epidermis, the *(63)* _____ layer. Fat cells, also called *(64)* _____, and macrophages are abundant in the dermis. (You should finish #67 at this point.)

58 epidermis

59 loose irregular

60 dense
61 papillary

62 reticular
63 papillary
64 adipocytes

Thick Skin

65 *rete ridges*

66 *papillary layer*

67 *reticular layer*

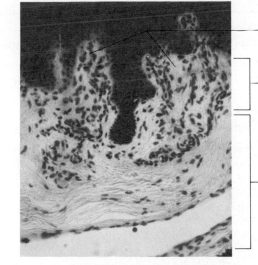

(65) _____ _____

(66) _____

_____

(67) _____

_____

FIG. 12-4. Photomicrograph of the dermis of the skin (original magnification ×125).

Thin Skin

Thin skin is differentiated from thick skin by having a thinner **(68)** _____, and a thinner dead layer of **(69)** _____ (Fig. 12-5). Thin skin is found covering the entire body, except for the

68 *epidermis*
69 *keratin*

70 *rete ridges (pegs)*

(70) _____

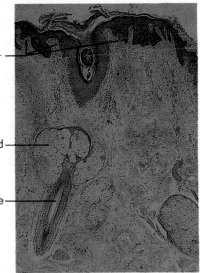

Sebaceous gland—

Hair follicle—

FIG. 12-5. Photomicrograph of an overall view of the skin, H and E stain (original magnification ×30).

71 *palms*
72 *soles*

(71) _____ and **(72)** _____. The skin of the eyelid is the thinnest in the body (about 0.5 mm), while the shoulders and back are covered by the thickest skin (about 5 mm). Thin skin has hair follicles, whereas thick skin does not. Hair is found in varying density throughout the body, but is lacking in one area covered by thin skin, the glans penis. Sweat glands are present, although not in as great a concentration as in thick skin. The stratum germinativum is similar in thin and thick skin; however, the outer layers—the stratum **(73)** _____, stratum **(74)** _____, stratum

73 *spinosum*

74 *granulosum*

75 *lucidum*
76 *corneum*
77 *lucidum*
78 *rete*
79 *yes*

80 *melanocytes*
81 *basal*

(75) _____, and stratum (76) _____—are all generally thinner. The clear layer, the stratum (77) _____, is very often missing. Are dermal papillae or (78) _____ ridges of the epidermis present? (79) _____.

Melanin and Melanocytes

Melanin, an important pigment in the skin, is produced by (80) _____ located in the (81) _____ (*basal, apical*) layers of the epidermis (Fig. 12-6). The importance of melanin lies in its ability to

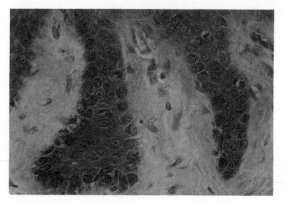

FIG. 12-6. Photomicrograph of a part of the epidermis and dermis, H and E stain (original magnification ×300).

82 *UV*

83 *brown black*

84 *epithelial (keratinocyte)*

85 *melanocytes*

86 *melanocyte*
87 *epithelial*

88 *macrophages*

89 *yes*

protect the skin and underlying structures from the effects of excessive (82) __ __ radiation. It is usually found as granules that often clump together. What color are the granules? (83) _____. The relative amount of melanin is responsible for the different colorations of skin.

In the epidermis, melanocytes are second in abundance to (84) _____ cells. Synthesis of melanin involves the rough endoplasmic reticulum (rER) Golgi, and the formation of membrane-bound vesicles, which eventually are transformed into melanin granules. These are released at the tips of the processes of the (85) _____, and are then phagocytized by the epithelial cells. Therefore, it is sometimes difficult to differentiate a (86) _____ that has just produced the melanin from an (87) _____ cell that has phagocytized it.

Langerhans' Cells

Langerhans' cells, found only in stratified squamous epithelia, probably function as migratory (88) _____. Usually located between epithelial cells, Langerhans' cells are very irregular in shape with a highly indented nucleus. Is this description similar to that of other macrophages described? (89) _____.

Sweat Glands

Eccrine

Eccrine sweat glands are the most common sweat glands in the body (Fig. 12-7). There are approximately 3 million in the skin. They are distributed throughout the body except on the lips and certain parts of the external genitalia. They are

Sweat Glands

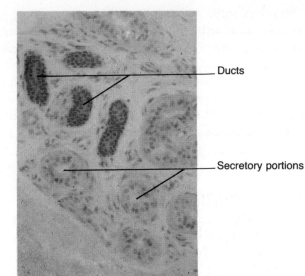

Ducts

Secretory portions

FIG. 12-7. Photomicrograph of the eccrine sweat glands and ducts, H and E stain (original magnification ×125).

more numerous in *(90)* _____ (*thin, thick*) skin. Morphologically, they are classified as simple, tubular glands, which implies a(n)
(91) _____ (*branched, unbranched*) duct system. The secretory portion of the gland is located beneath the dermis in the hypodermis, or
(92) _____ tissue. The cells of the secretory portion are
(93) _____ in shape, and the cytoplasm is *(94)* _____ (*pale, dark*)-staining.

Beneath the secretory epithelium, as with most epithelia, is a
(95) _____ _____. Between the secretory epithelium and the underlying basement membrane are spindle-shaped cells similar to smooth muscle cells. These cells, which completely surround the
(96) _____ portion of the gland, are called myoepithelial cells. Upon stimulation, these cells contract and aid in the expulsion of the secretion from the lumen into the ducts. Secretion is by exocytosis, also called
(97) _____ secretion.

The ducts of eccrine sweat glands are continuous with the secretory portion, although the lumen of the duct is generally narrower. The ducts are lined by a
(98) _____ _____ epithelium, and the cells stain *(99)* _____ (*darker, lighter*) than the secretory cells. The ducts follow a spiral course through the dermis and enter the epidermis at the tips of the ridges, or *(100)* _____ _____.

The secretion of sweat, which is modified by the cells lining the
(101) _____, contains Na, Cl, H₂O, and certain metabolites.

Apocrine

Apocrine sweat glands are not as numerous as *(102)* _____ sweat glands. The secretions of these glands give rise to distinctive body odors. Locations of these glands include the thin skin covering the axilla, pubic region, and areola of the breast. The secretory units are similar to those of eccrine sweat glands in that they are *(103)* _____ (*simple, compound*) tubular, lined by a *(104)* _____ _____ epithe-

90 thick

91 unbranched

92 subcutaneous
93 columnar (cuboidal)
94 pale

95 basement membrane

96 secretory

97 merocrine

98 stratified cuboidal
99 darker

100 rete pegs
101 ducts

102 eccrine

103 simple
104 simple columnar
    (cuboidal)

lium. Secretory units are surrounded by contractile *(105)* _____ cells. Secretion is continuous, but not abundant, and occurs by the same process as in eccrine sweat glands, *(106)* _____ secretion, as well as by the process of apocrine secretion. Apocrine secretion involves the release of a membrane-bound body containing the secretory product plus varying amounts of *(107)* _____. The ducts are also similar to eccrine ducts, lined by a *(108)* _____ _____ epithelium.

105 *myoepithelial*

106 *merocrine*

107 *cytoplasm*
108 *stratified cuboidal*

Hair

Hair is found in *(109)* _____ (*thick, thin*) skin but is lacking in the skin covering the *(110)* _____ _____ (Fig. 12-8). Hair functions in the repair of epidermis damaged by burns and abrasions, and in skin grafts. Hair develops, as do glands, as a downgrowth of *(111)* _____ cells into the *(112)* _____ and the hypodermis. The deepest part of the hair follicle becomes the germinal matrix, from which the actual hair grows. The external root sheath is a canalized structure that connects the deepest part of the follicle, the *(113)* _____ _____, with the thin skin on the surface. Consequently, it has the same components as thin skin, although the layers are thinned as the external *(114)* _____ _____ approaches the germinal matrix. The internal root sheath, produced by the germinal matrix, is also tubular and separates the hair from the surrounding *(115)* _____ root sheath. It extends only partly up the follicle. The keratohyalin granules (in hair referred to as trichohyalin granules) stain bright red. They are most prominent in the stratum *(116)* _____ of the skin. (You should finish #118 at this point.)

109 *thin*
110 *glans penis*

111 *epithelial*
112 *dermis*

113 *germinal matrix*

114 *root sheath*

115 *external*

116 *granulosum*

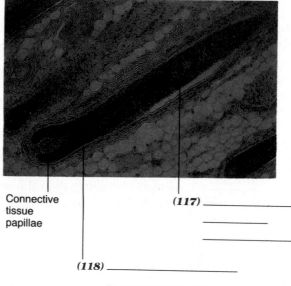

FIG. 12-8. Photomicrograph of a portion of a hair follicle, H and E stain (original magnification × 125).

Connective tissue papillae

(117) _____ _____

(118) _____ _____

117 *external root sheath*
118 *germinal matrix*

The hair itself develops from proliferation of cells of the *(119)* _____ _____. As the hair gets farther from the germinal matrix, the cells lose their nourishment and develop, by a process similar to that in skin, into *(120)* _____. The area of transition between live and dead cells is called the keratogenous zone. Pigmentation of the hair is due to *(121)* _____, produced by melanocytes in the germinal matrix.

119 *germinal matrix*

120 *keratin*

121 *melanin*

Hair

122 holocrine

123 basal

124 hair follicle

125 sebaceous gland
126 arrector pili muscle

127 dermis

128 sebaceous

Sebaceous Glands

Sebaceous glands are specialized glands found associated with hair. They develop from the external root sheath, and are usually located in the neck of the follicle, about one third of the way up. The glands secrete by a method in which whole cells, or contents of cells, are released, called *(122)* _____ secretion. The most proliferative cells of the gland are found on the *(123)* _____ (*basal, luminal*) surface. The oldest cells, which have acquired fatty material, are found closest to the lumen, as they have been pushed inward by proliferation. The most luminal cells eventually die, with the contents of the cells released as the secretion into the lumen. The secretion is referred to as sebum, an oily material that lubricates the skin and hair (Fig. 12-9).

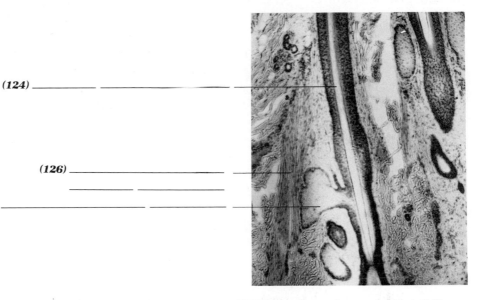

(124) _____ _____ _____

(126) _____ ____
_____ _____
(125) _____ _____

FIG. 12-9. Photomicrograph of hair follicle and associated structures (original magnification ×30).

Arrector Muscles of Skin

Arrector pili muscles are found associated with all hair except that of the beard and pubic region (Fig. 12-9). These are small, fan-shaped bundles of smooth muscle fibers that attach to the connective tissue sheath of the follicle and pass obliquely upward into the papillary layer of the *(127)* _____. Contraction of the muscle, stimulated by cold or intense emotion, straightens the naturally slanted follicle (so the hair stands up), and aids in the contraction and secretion of the *(128)* _____ glands associated with hair.

13 Oral Cavity and Associated Structures

After completing this chapter, you should be able to identify the following:

1 Hair follicles
2 Tongue
3 Tonsils
4 Salivary glands: parotid, submaxillary, and sublingual
5 Tooth structures: hard and soft
   tissues

Also, after completing this chapter, you should understand the following:

1 The histologic differences
   between salivary glands
2 The histologic similarities
   between teeth and bone

The oral cavity is the entrance to and is considered a part of the digestive system. The general boundaries of the oral cavity are the lips anteriorly and the communication of the pharynx with the esophagus posteriorly. The constituents of the oral cavity are the lips, teeth, glands, tonsils, and pharynx. In this chapter, knowledge concerning types of epithelium and glandular tissue is essential and review of those chapters would be helpful.

Lips

The surface of the lips is subdivided into the outer surface, the red free margin's transition zone, and the inner mucous membranes. The outer surface of the lip up to the red free margin is skin that contains hair follicles and sebaceous and sweat (1) _____. This surface is covered by
(2) _____ _____ epithelium that is
(3) _____ (highly, minimally) keratinized. Subdivided into the strata
(4) _____, (5) _____, (6) _____
and germinativum, this outer surface merges with the (7) _____ free
(8) _____ of the lip (Fig. 13-1). The (9) _____ free (10) _____
of the lip is covered by a highly modified epithelial surface called the transition zone. Covering the transition zone is a transparent stratified squamous epithelium that is minimally keratinized. The red color of this area is due to the rich blood supply of the area and the transparency of the epithelium. No glands or hair follicles are found in the (11) _____ free (12) _____ of the lip.

The red free margin as it passes onto the inner surface of the lip is transformed into a mucous membrane. The covering epithelium of this mucous membrane is nonkeratinized stratified squamous epithelium. Mucous mem-

1 glands
2 stratified squamous
3 highly
4 corneum
5 granulosum
6 spinosum
7 red
8 margin
9 red
10 margin
11 red
12 margin

branes are wet epithelial linings of the internal passages. The mucous membranes provide protection and ensure the integrity of the membranes by providing constant lubrication from the abundant **(13)** _____ (*mucous, serous*) glands in the epithelium. The term "mucous membrane" usually denotes an overlying epithelium, a thin connective tissue layer called the lamina propria, and often a thin muscular layer, the muscularis mucosa. These three layers are most highly developed in the gastrointestinal tract and a more detailed description can be found in Chapter 13. (You should finish #15 at this point.)

13 mucous

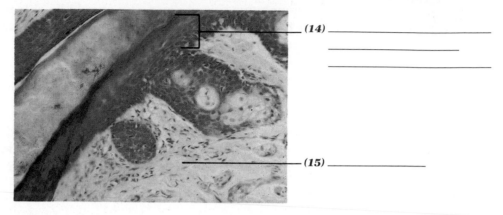

(14) _____

_____

_____

(15) _____

*14 stratified squamous
epithelium*

15 dermis

FIG. 13-1.   Lip, hematoxylin-eosin (H and E) stain (original magnification ×70).

Tongue

The tongue is a mass of interlacing striated muscle bundles covered tightly by an adherent mucous membrane (Fig. 13-2). The ventral (bottom) side of the tongue is

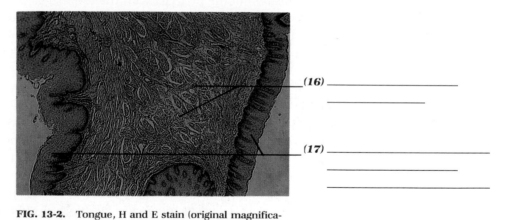

(16) _____

_____

(17) _____

_____

_____

16 striated muscle

*17 stratified squamous
epithelium*

FIG. 13-2.   Tongue, H and E stain (original magnification ×30).

smooth while the dorsal surface is covered by multiple small projections called papillae. Special nerve arrangements called taste buds are found in some of these small projections called **(18)** _____.

Papillae

There are three types of papillae found on the **(19)** _____ (*ventral, dorsal*) or **(20)** _____ (*bottom, top*) side of the tongue: filiform, fungiform, and vallate papillae. Filiform papillae are narrow conical papillae with a keratinized **(21)** _____ _____ epithelium. Fungiform

18 papillae

19 dorsal
20 top

21 stratified squamous

Tongue

22 *papillae*
23 *conical*

24 *nonkeratinized*
25 *stratified squamous*
26 *absence*

27 *vallate*

28 *nonkeratinized*
   stratified squamous
29 *circumvallate*
30 *papillae*
31 *filiform papillae*
32 *nerve*

(22) _____ are flat, not *(23)* _____, like filiform, and are also less numerous than the filiform. *Unlike* the epithelium of the filiform papillae, the covering epithelium of fungiform is *(24)* _____ (*keratinized, nonkeratinized*) *(25)* _____ _____. The *(26)* _____ (*absence, presence*) of keratin makes it possible for the rich blood supply beneath the epithelium of the fungiform papillae to produce the red color.

The last papillae, *(27)* _____ or circumvallate, are common at the base of the tongue. As in the fungiform papillae, the covering epithelium is *(28)* _____ _____ _____ epithelium.

Taste buds are found in all vallate or *(29)* _____ papillae and most fungiform *(30)* _____ but not in the *(31)* _____ _____. Essentially, taste buds are specialized *(32)* _____ endings that, when properly stimulated, send out nerve impulses that result in the sensation of taste.

Tonsils

There are two tonsils found at the root of the tongue, which are called the sublingual tonsils. The other oral cavity tonsils, pharyngeal and palatine, will be discussed later in this chapter. Lying behind the "wet" epithelium—mucous *(33)* _____ in the lamina *(34)* _____ layer are aggregates of lymphoid tissue. In each lingual tonsil one will find both primary and secondary *(35)* _____ _____.

33 *membrane*
34 *propria*
35 *lymphatic nodules*

Salivary Glands

Within the oral cavity, there are numerous small glands that continuously secrete a liquid, saliva (Fig. 13-3). These small glands or salivary glands are located in the

36 *mucus-secreting glands*

37 *secondary nodule*
38 *primary nodule*

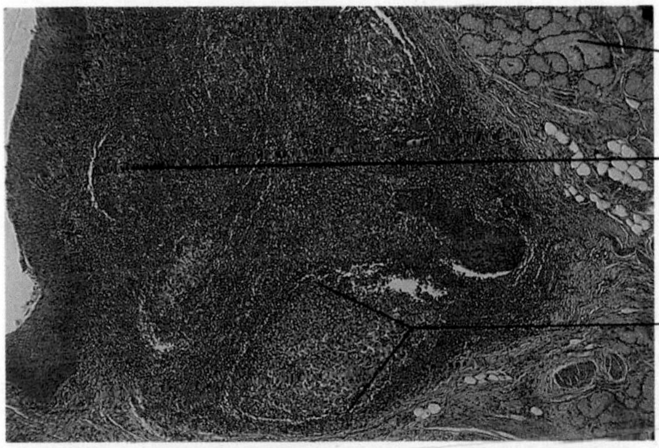

(36) _____
_____
_____
(38) _____
_____

(37) _____
_____

FIG. 13-3. Pharyngeal tonsil, H and E stain (original magnification ×35).

submucosal tissue layer and are named for their specific location within the oral cavity. The term "salivary glands" (or more correctly, "salivary glands proper") is most commonly used for the three largest paired glands of the oral cavity: parotid, submandibular or submaxillary, and sublingual. Each gland is categorized according to its type of secretory cell. Discussion of salivary glands will

39 *parotid*
40 *submandibular*
41 *submaxillary*

42 *serous*

43 *base*
44 *flattened*

45 *darker*
46 *protein*
47 *ribosomes*
48 *rough*
49 *endoplasmic reticulum*

50 *unlike*

51 *serous*
52 *mucous*

53 *demilune*

54 *serous demilune*

55 *serous*

56 *duct*

57 *mucous gland*

58 *mucous*
59 *serous*

60 *myoepithelial*
61 *cells*

concern only these three major glands, *(39)* _____,
(40) _____ or *(41)* _____,
and sublingual.

Saliva

Saliva is the mixture of all secretions of all the oral cavity glands whether they are mucus- or *(42)* _____-secreting. A colorless, viscous liquid that contains salivary enzymes and cellular debris, saliva functions in moistening the oral mucosa and the lips. Saliva also makes it easier to swallow food.

To review briefly: Mucous cells have a nucleus at the *(43)* _____ (*base, apex*) of the cell and it appears *(44)* _____ (*flattened, rounded*) because of the lipid droplets within each cell. Serous cells stain *(45)* _____ (*lighter, darker*) than mucous cells because of the large production of *(46)* _____ by the *(47)* _____ on the *(48)* _____ (*rough, smooth*) *(49)* _____ _____. An electron micrograph (EM) of a serous cell reveals secretory granules clustered between its rounded nucleus on the free surface. Also, serous cells, *(50)* _____ (*unlike, like*) mucous cells, contain a surface network of secretory canaliculi.

The cells of mixed glands, *(51)* _____ and *(52)* _____ cells, vary in proportion according to the specific salivary gland. Usually, the mucous cells of a mixed gland are located nearer the ducts, whereas the serous cells are found at the blind end of the terminal secretory portion. If mucous cells are the predominant cell type in a mixed gland, they often will be capped by serous cells forming a flattened moon-shaped serous *(53)* _____. The best way to identify mucus- or serum-secreting cells is by their different staining (Fig. 13-4).

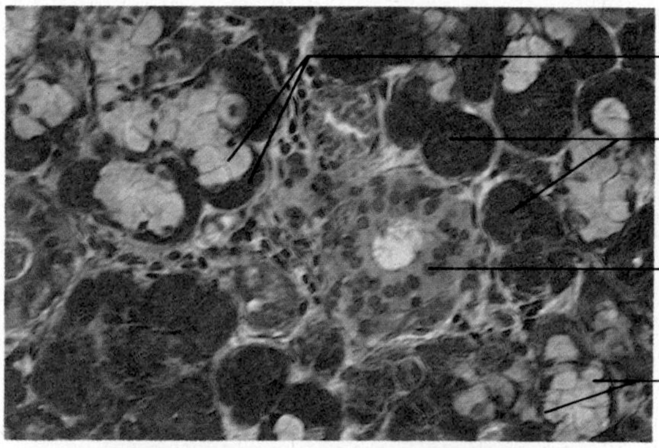

(54) _____
_____
(55) _____

(56) _____

(57) _____ _____

FIG. 13-4. Submaxillary gland, H and E stain (original magnification × 180).

All glands, whether *(58)* _____, *(59)* _____, or mixed, contain basket or basal myoepithelial cells. These cells, found primarily in the ducts and terminal portions between glandular cells, are stellate, spindle-shaped cells. Basal *(60)* _____ or basket *(61)* _____ have an ultrastructure similar to that of smooth muscle cells, and therefore function to facilitate the movement of secretion into and up the ducts.

Finally, the ducts of the glands of the oral cavity consist mainly of a low cuboidal epithelium. The epithelium can be columnar or pseudostratified columnar in the largest glands. At the ductal opening onto the mucous membrane *all* epithelial lining become stratified.

Parotid Gland

The parotid glands are situated subcutaneously and lie just in front of the ears (Fig. 13-5). Largest of all salivary glands, the parotid opens into the oral cavity by a duct called Stensen's duct. This gland is composed mainly of serous cells, and therefore stains **(62)** _____ (*darker, lighter*) than a mucous gland would. Since the terminal portion of the parotid gland's subunits assume an alveolar shape and the gland is composed of several simple glands emptying into one excretory duct, the parotid is called a **(63)** _____ (*simple, compound*) **(64)** _____ (*tubular, alveolar*) gland. Surrounding the gland is a fibrous connective tissue capsule that gives off incomplete septae, subdividing the gland. (You should finish #66 at this point.)

62 *darker*

63 *compound*
64 *alveolar*

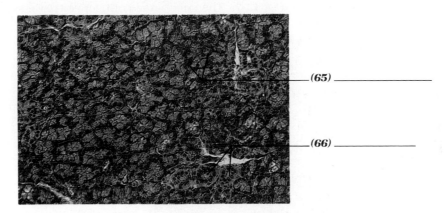

—**(65)** _____

—**(66)** _____

65 *serous*

66 *ducts*

FIG. 13-5. Parotid gland, H and E stain (original magnification ×100).

Submandibular Gland

Lying on the floor of the mouth is a paired salivary gland called the submandibular or **(67)** _____ _____ _____ gland. This gland empties into the oral cavity through Wharton's duct. Considered a mixed gland, the **(68)** sub_____ or **(69)** sub_____ contains both **(70)** _____ and **(71)** _____ cells (Fig. 13-6). Most of the

67 *submaxillary*
68 *maxillary*
69 *mandibular*
70 *serous*
71 *mucous*

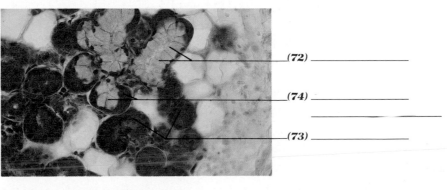

(72) _____

(74) _____
_____

(73) _____

72 *mucous*

FIG. 13-6. Identify the type of gland:
(75) _____. H and E
stain (original magnification ×250).

73 *serous*
74 *serous demilune*

cells stain dark; therefore the gland consists mainly of **(76)** _____ (*serous, mucous*) cells. Mucous cells, when found in the submandibular gland, are usually capped by a serous **(77)** _____. The terminal portion of the glandular subunit is either alveolar or tubular in shape, and the submandibu-

75 *submaxillary*

76 *serous*

77 *demilune*

78 *submaxillary*
79 *compound*
80 *alveolar*
81 *connective tissue*

82 *maxillary*
83 *mandibular*
84 *connective tissue*

85 *mucous*

86 *ducts*

87 *sublingual*

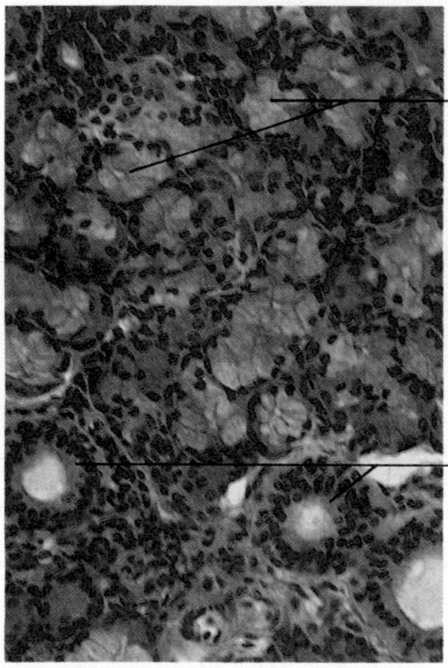

88 *parotid*
89 *serous*
90 *alveolar*
91 *compound*
92 *compound tubulo-alveolar*

lar or (*78*) _____ gland is considered a compound gland. Therefore, one can call the submaxillary gland a (*79*) _____ (*simple, compound*) (*80*) <u>tubulo</u>_____ gland. As is the parotid, the submandibular is surrounded by a fibrous (*81*) _____ _____ capsule.

Sublingual Gland

On the underside of the tongue lying on each side of the frenulum are the sublingual glands. Unlike the (*82*) <u>sub</u>_____ or (*83*) <u>sub</u>_____ and parotid gland, the sublingual gland does not have a well-defined fibrous (*84*) _____ _____ capsule (Fig. 13-7). The sublingual connective tissue septa are, however, far more

(*85*) _____

(*86*) _____

FIG. 13-7. Name of salivary gland:
(*87*) _____.
H and E stain (original magnification ×180).

prominent than the septa in the majority of salivary glands. Most cells in this mixed gland are mucous cells and therefore, the sublingual is a counterpart of the (*88*) _____ gland, which is mostly (*89*) _____ cells. As in the submandibular gland, the terminal portion of the sublingual gland sub-units is either (*90*) _____ or tubular, and the gland is also a (*91*) _____ (*compound, simple*) gland. Therefore, the sublingual gland is a (*92*) _____ _____-_____ gland.

Teeth

The gross structure of the tooth consists of a small internal cavity, pulp cavity, or chamber surrounded by hard tissue layers. The parts of the teeth are divided histologically into hard and soft tissues. The hard tissues are the dentin, enamel, and cementum layers; the soft tissues are the pulp, periodontal membrane, and the surrounding gingiva or gums.

Both soft and hard tissue form three distinct parts of the tooth: crown, root, and neck. The crown is that portion of the tooth projecting above the gingiva or

Teeth

93 *gums*

(93) _____, and consists mainly of enamel and dentin tissue layers, both hard tissue. The root is the long tapered part of the tooth inserted into the alveolus or socket of the jaw bone; it contains most of the pulp cavity, which is **(94)** _____ (*soft, hard*) tissue, and the cementum layer and a large portion of the dentin, both **(95)** _____ (*hard, soft*) tissue. Joining the root and the crown is a small nondistinct area called the neck of the tooth (Fig. 13-8).

94 *soft*
95 *hard*

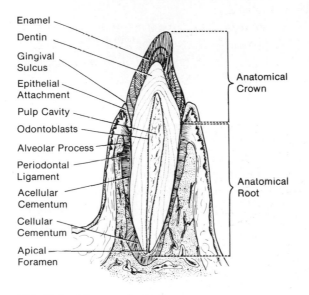

FIG. 13-8. Diagram of a tooth.

Two sets of teeth occur in humans. The first set of teeth, primary or deciduous teeth of childhood, are replaced by secondary or succedaneous teeth. Both sets of teeth have a similar histologic composition. Discussion of the three parts of the tooth and their soft tissues, the **(96)** _____, **(97)** _____ membrane, and **(98)** _____ or gums, and their hard tissues, **(99)** _____, **(100)** _____, and cementum composition will concern only the succedaneous or **(101)** _____ teeth.

96 *pulp*
97 *periodontal*
98 *gingiva*
99 *enamel*
100 *dentin*
101 *secondary*

Hard Tissue

DENTIN Dentin forms the bulk of the tooth and surrounds the pulp cavity. Thickest at the crown, the dentin tissue layer tapers as it forms part of the root of the tooth. Dentin, like bone but harder, consists of an organic and inorganic matrix. The inorganic matrix is the crystal **(102)** _____ apatite, which accounts for 80% of the dentin substance. The organic matrix of dentin is composed of mainly collagenous fibrils embedded in a glycosaminoglycan complex. The organic matrix is elaborated by odontoblasts, which are in teeth the counterpart of the **(103)** _____ of bone.

102 *hydroxy*

(104) Odonto _____ are long slender cells with attenuated cytoplasmic processes that extend throughout the entire **(105)** _____ (*dentin, enamel*) tissue layer (Fig. 13-9). Odontoblasts have abundant amounts of

103 *osteoblasts*
104 *blasts*
105 *dentin*

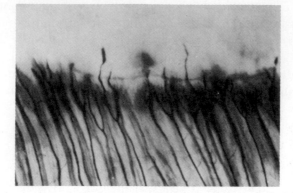

FIG. 13-9. EM of the odontoblastic process.

rough *(106)* _____ _____ surrounding a basally located nucleus. The *(107)* _____ on the endoplasmic reticulum synthesize the collagenous fibrils of the *(108)* _____ (*inorganic, organic*) matrix. The odontoblasts are found *only* along the pulp cavity side and not along any other dentin border. As the odontoblasts

(109) _____ (*produce, destroy*) dentin, they slowly

(110) _____ (*encroach on, enlarge*) the pulp cavity. Bone grows by addition of new layers by the *(111)* _____ on *(112)* _____ (*both, one*) side(s) of the bone.

    Odontoblasts lay down the *(113)* _____ matrix around its long slender *(114)* _____ processes. These processes extend outward to the dentin–enamel junction and, once the matrix is produced, they are enclosed in minute canals called dental tubules. Once the cytoplasmic process is surrounded by dentin, it is called an odontoblastic process. The layer of dentin immediately surrounding each dental *(115)* _____ is highly refractive; it is called the Neumann's (dental) sheath.

    As odontoblasts produce an *(116)* _____ matrix, forming *(117)* _____ tubules around the *(118)* _____ _____, two distinct zones can be readily identified. The first zone is that area immediately adjacent to the base of the odontoblastic process and closest to the cell body itself. Called the predentin or newly formed matrix, this is a zone of noncalcification. Immediately adjacent, and farther away from the cell body, is the calcified or dentin matrix, which is rich in *(119)* _____ crystals. This calcified area is not always complete or uniform (Fig. 13-10). Incomplete calcification in the dentin forms interlobular spaces. These spaces consist of only organic matrix and no *(120)* _____ crystals. Between the cementum and dentin layers, the dentocementum junction, are interlobular spaces called the granular layer of Tomes.

106 endoplasmic reticulum
107 ribosomes
108 organic

109 produce
110 encroach on
111 osteoblasts
112 both
113 organic
114 cytoplasmic

115 tubule

116 organic
117 dental
118 cytoplasmic processes

119 hydroxyapatite

120 hydroxyapatite

Teeth

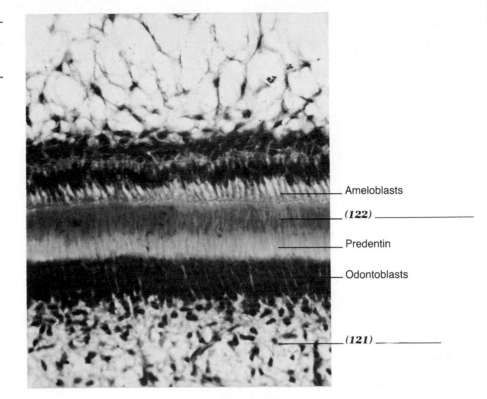

Ameloblasts

(122) _____

Predentin

Odontoblasts

(121) _____

FIG. 13-10. Dentinoenamel junction (high-power magnification).

121 *pulp*
122 *dentin*

ENAMEL Enamel, the hardest substance in the body, covers the visible tooth area (see Fig. 13-8). Enamel is composed almost entirely of the inorganic crystals called *(123)* _____. Cells that elaborate the enamel are called ameloblasts, and are therefore functionally similar to those cells that produce bone and dentin, the *(124)* _____ and *(125)* _____ respectively.

123 *hydroxyapatite*

Ameloblasts are tall columnar cells rich in mitochondria and rough *(126)* _____ _____ (Fig. 13-11). The distal

124 *osteoblasts*
125 *odontoblasts*

portion of the ameloblast is an elongate, vesicle-rich area called the Tomes' process. It is from the Tomes' *(127)* _____ that enamel is elaborated. Crystal rods composed of *(128)* _____ crystals are secreted by the *(129)* _____ process at the distal end of the

126 *endoplasmic reticulum*

127 *process*
128 *hydroxyapatite*
129 *Tomes'*
130 *amelo*

(130) _____ ^blast. The crystal rods calcify, forming hard long rods that run the full thickness of the enamel layer. Inside the rods is an inter-rod matrix of

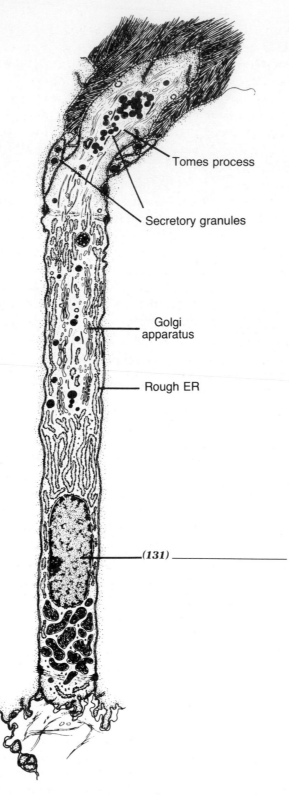

Tomes process

Secretory granules

Golgi
apparatus

Rough ER

(131) _____

FIG. 13-11.   Drawing of an ameloblast.

glycoprotein, and this too is elaborated by the cytoplasmic process in the
(132) _____ (*distal, proximal*) end of the
(133) _____ called the *(134)* _____
_____. Where the rods of neighboring areas cross, they form alter-

131 nucleus

132 distal
133 ameloblast
134 Tomes' process

Teeth

135 Schreger's
136 Retzius'

137 keratinized acellular

138 hard

139 soft

140 periodontal ligament
141 Sharpey's
142 blasts

143 bone
144 cementoblasts

145 periodontal ligament
146 pulp
147 gingiva
148 gums
149 periodontal
150 cementum
151 collagen
152 Sharpey's
153 periodontal
154 membrane
155 crown
156 collagenous
157 dense
158 regular
159 connective tissue
160 avascular
161 diffusion
162 pulp

163 mucoid
164 dentum

165 Weil

166 apical foramen

nating light and dark lines called Schreger's lines of enamel. In addition to
(135) _____, lines of enamel are called Retzius' lines or incremental lines. These (136) _____ lines are obliquely running lines reflecting the deposition and mineralization of growing enamel.

The free surface of enamel is covered by two thin layers, an inner enamel (Nasmyth's membrane) and an outer keratinized acellular layer (see Fig. 13-8). The outermost layer covering the enamel, the (137) _____ _____ layer is continuous with the cementum tissue layer and is histologically similar.

CEMENTUM Cementum is the (138) _____ (hard, soft) tissue layer that covers most of the root of the tooth, and also anchors the tooth to the periodontal ligament (139) _____ (soft, hard) tissue (see Fig. 13-8). Cementum is penetrated by coarse collagen bundles from the attaching (140) _____ _____. These fibers are analogous to (141) _____ fibers of the bone.

Remarkably similar to bone, cementum is formed by (142) cemento-_____ found in the apical region of the cementum tissue layer. Like osteoblasts, which elaborate (143) _____, (144) _____ form an avascular calcified connective tissue layer called cementum.

Soft Tissue

PERIODONTAL LIGAMENT The three soft tissues of the tooth are the (145) _____ _____, (146) _____, and the surrounding (147) _____ or (148) _____. The (149) _____ ligament or membrane penetrates the hard tissue layer, the (150) _____, by way of coarse (151) _____ bundles analogous to the (152) _____ fibers of bone, and therefore anchors the root of the tooth to the bony wall of the socket. The (153) _____ ligament or (154) _____ attaches from the root tip to the neck but not to the (155) _____ of the tooth. Composed of wavy (156) _____ fibers, the ligament is like other ligaments— (157) _____ (loose, dense) (158) _____ (irregular, regular) (159) _____ _____. Blood and lymphatic vessels run throughout the ligament. These vessels provide nourishment for the (160) _____ (vascular, avascular) cementum by (161) _____ (diffusion, capillaries).

PULP Dental pulp occupies the (162) _____ cavity of the tooth (see Fig. 13-8). The constituents of the pulp are an abundant metachromatic-staining ground substance, some free cells, and a multitude of collagenous fibrils not aggregated into bundles. The pulp cavity is therefore remarkably similar to (163) _____ (loose, dense, mucoid) connective tissue. Immediately surrounding the pulp cavity is the (164) _____ tissue layer. Between this tissue layer and the cavity is a relatively cell-free area called the zone of Weil or Weil's layer. The zone of (165) _____ contains bundles of reticular fibers only. Highly vascular, the pulp cavity receives vessels through a small opening at the tip of the root called the apical foramen. Nerves, lymphatics, and blood vessels both exit and enter through the tip of the root, the (166) _____ _____.

167 gum

168 mucous

169 membrane
170 stratified squamous

171 crown
172 root
173 enamel
174 dentin
175 pulp cavity
176 cementum
177 gingiva

178 pseudostratified ciliated
   columnar
179 membrane
180 lamina propria

181 pseudostratified ciliated
   columnar

182 respiratory

GINGIVA The gingiva or *(167)* _____ is a mucous membrane that surrounds each tooth. The base of this *(168)* _____ membrane is attached tightly to the tooth, and is called the epithelial attachment of Gottlieb or simply the epithelial attachment. The epithelium of the mucous *(169)* _____ is, typically, keratinized *(170)* _____ _____ (Fig. 13-12).

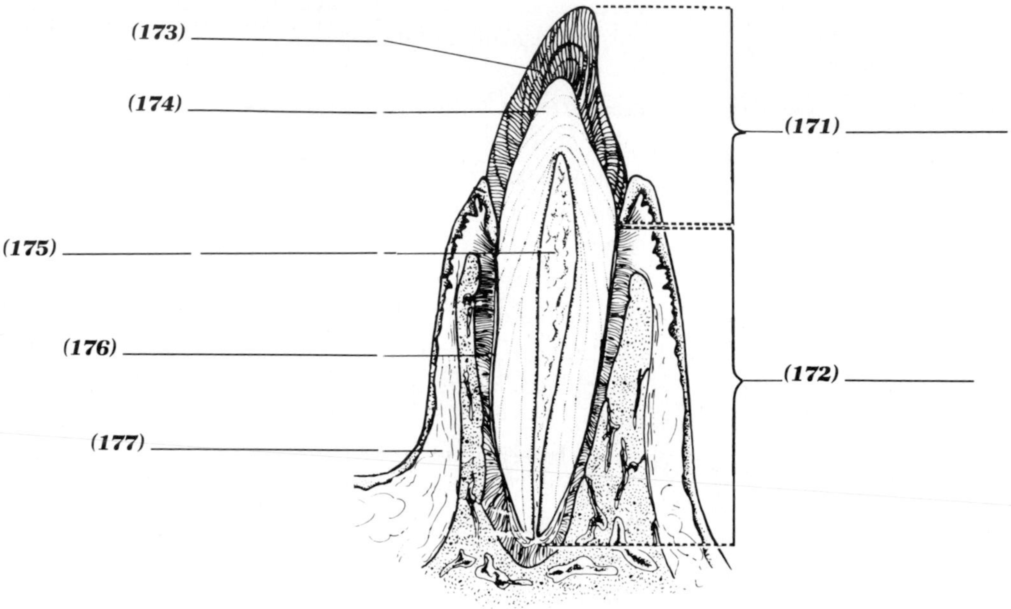

(173) _____

(174) _____

(171) _____

(175) _____

(176) _____

(172) _____

(177) _____

FIG. 13-12. Diagram of incisor tooth.

Pharynx

The pharynx is the posterior communication of the oral cavity, and it is divided anatomically into the upper pharynx or nasopharynx, the middle or oral pharynx, and the lower or laryngeal pharynx.

Nasopharynx

The nasopharynx is lined by a pseudostratified ciliated columnar epithelium rich in goblet cells; it is often called the respiratory epithelium. Essentially, the nasopharynx is part of the respiratory system. The lining epithelium, *(178)* _____ _____ _____ rests on a thin basement *(179)* _____, which in turn is supported by a highly elastic connective tissue layer, the *(180)* _____ _____. Beneath this layer is usually a bundle of striated muscle. Located in the nasopharynx is the solitary pharyngeal tonsil. Lying underneath the covering epithelium, which is *(181)* _____ _____ _____, the pharyngeal tonsil is separated by a thin connective tissue covering from the epithelium. Old, atrophic tonsils are not often covered by the overlying *(182)* _____ epithelium but by a stratified squamous epithelium.

Pharynx

183 *pseudostratified ciliated columnar*

184 *lamina propria*

185 *muscularis*

186 *secondary*

187 *connective tissue*
188 *epithelium*
189 *lymphatic*

Oral Pharynx and Laryngeal Pharynx

The oral and laryngeal areas of the pharynx belong more to the digestive system than to the respiratory system. Covered by a more "wear and tear" epithelium than respiratory epithelium or (183) _____ _____, the oral and laryngeal pharynxes are lined by stratified squamous epithelium. A connective tissue layer, the (184) _____ _____, is found immediately beneath the epithelium, and beneath that is a muscularis mucosa. A submucosal layer separates the (185) _____ mucosa from bundles, both longitudinally and circularly arranged striated muscle. The arrangement of these parts of the oral cavity are discussed in greater detail with its confluence with the upper esophagus in the next chapter.

Palatine Tonsils

The largest accumulations of lymphoid tissue in the oral cavity are the prominent palatine tonsils. Both primary and (186) _____ lymphatic nodules underlying stratified squamous epithelium are found in the palatine tonsils. As in the pharyngeal tonsils, a thin (187) _____ _____ layer separates the overlying (188) _____ from the (189) _____ tissue below.

14

Gastrointestinal System

After completing this chapter, you should be able to identify the following:

1 Esophagus
2 All areas of the stomach
3 Duodenum, jejunum, and ileum
4 Colon
5 Crypts of Lieberkühn
6 Appendix
7 Liver
8 Gallbladder
9 Islets of Langerhans and acinar tissue of the pancreas

Also, after completing this chapter, you should understand the following:

1 The histologic arrangement of the gastrointestinal system
2 The bile and blood flow in the liver
3 The different physiological arrangements of liver tissue
4 The histologic differences within the pancreas

Of all the body systems, the digestive system by far has the most histologic diversity. The discussion of the digestive system is divided into two parts: The first half of this chapter focuses on the gastrointestinal (GI) tract, which starts with the pharyngoesophageal border and continues through the esophagus, stomach, and small and large intestines. The second half of the chapter concerns itself with the ancillary organs of the digestive system: the liver, gallbladder, and pancreas.

General Outline of Gastrointestinal Tract

The general plan of the GI tract is similar from esophagus to large intestine, but the specific histology of each organ differs. Basically, the wall of the GI tract consists of four consecutive layers (Fig. 14-1). From the lumen outward, these four layers are the mucosa or mucous membrane, submucosa, muscularis or muscularis externa, and the adventitia or serosa.

Mucosa

The mucosa or (1) _____ _____ is subdivided into three components: the lining epithelium, (2) _____ propria, and muscularis mucosa. The type of epithelium varies according to the specific organ it lines: a protective layer in the esophagus, the superficial epithelium, becomes highly absorptive in the large intestine. The epithelium can have numerous mucus-secreting glands dispersed throughout it or none at all.

The lamina (3) _____ is a highly cellular (4) _____ _____ _____ layer. Very often, lymphatic tissue develops among the reticular, collagenous, and elastic fibers of the

1 mucous membrane
2 lamina

3 propria
4 connective tissue

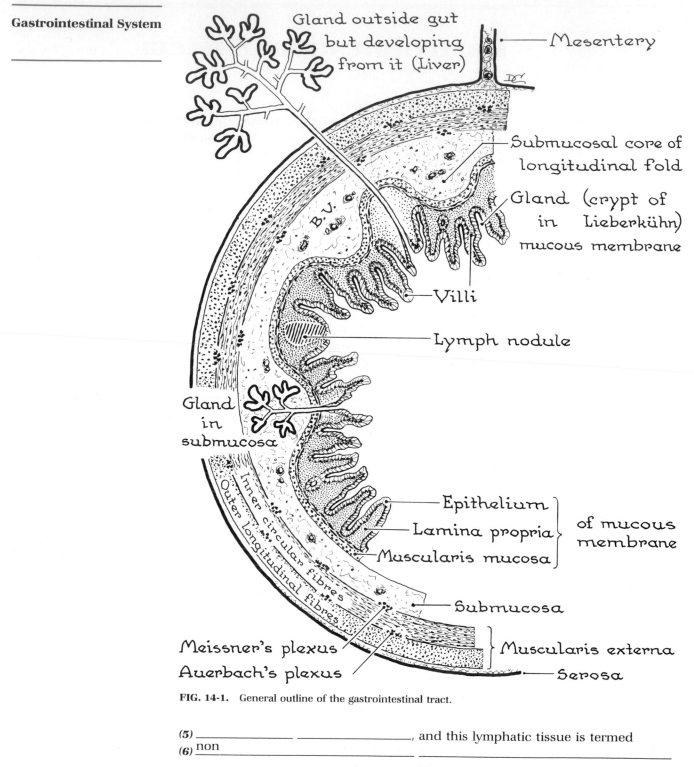

Gland outside gut but developing from it (Liver)

Mesentery

Submucosal core of longitudinal fold

Gland (crypt of Lieberkühn) in mucous membrane

B.V.

Villi

Lymph nodule

Gland in submucosa

Inner circular fibres

Outer longitudinal fibres

Epithelium
Lamina propria
Muscularis mucosa
} of mucous membrane

Submucosa

Meissner's plexus
Auerbach's plexus

} Muscularis externa

Serosa

FIG. 14-1. General outline of the gastrointestinal tract.

(5) _____ _____, and this lymphatic tissue is termed **(6)** non _____ _____

_____. The lamina propria is also highly vascular, enabling easy absorption of nutrients through the wall.

The third component of the mucosa and the **(7)** _____ (*outermost, innermost*) sublayer is the **(8)** _____

_____. This component consists of two (one circular and one longitudinal) thin layers of smooth muscle, and permits localized mucous membrane movement.

5 *lamina propria*
6 *encapsulated lymphatic tissue (gut associated with lymphoid tissue or GALT)*
7 *outermost*
8 *muscularis mucosa*

General Outline of Gastrointestinal Tract

The other three concentric layers of the GI tract—the
(9) _____, **(10)** _____ _____ or
(11) _____, and **(12)** _____ or serosa, do
not vary as much as the mucosa does from organ to organ.

9 submucosa
10 muscularis externa
11 muscularis
12 adventitia

Submucosa
Sandwiched between the outermost layer of the mucosa, the
(13) _____ _____ and the muscularis is the
(14) _____ layer (see Fig. 14-1). The submucosa is a fibrous
layer consisting of loose connective tissue that has abundant elastic fibers. This
elasticity of the submucosa enables the wall to form folds of the submucosa and

13 muscularis mucosa
14 submucosal

overlying **(15)** _____ or **(16)** _____ membrane. In addition to
blood vessel plexuses, the submucosa contains postganglionic fibers of the sympathetic division called the Meissner's or the submucosal plexus.

15 mucosa
16 mucous

Muscularis
The third major component is the highly muscular layer, the
(17) _____ externa. This layer consists of two substantial
layers of smooth muscle: an inner circular layer and outer longitudinal layer. The
(18) _____ externa is responsible for the propulsion of food
down the GI tract. This propulsion, peristalsis, is coordinated by nerve fibers
situated between the inner **(19)** _____ *(circular, longitudinal)* and
outer **(20)** _____ *(circular, longitudinal)* smooth muscle
layer. The plexuses, Auerbach's or myenteric, are mostly parasympathetic fibers
from the vagus nerve (see below).

17 muscularis

18 muscularis

19 circular
20 longitudinal

Adventitia
The **(21)** _____ *(outermost, innermost)* layer of the wall of the
gut is the adventitia or **(22)** _____, and consists of loose connective
tissue. When covered by a single layer of mesothelium or simple
(23) _____ cells the adventitia is then appropriately called serosa.
Nerves and blood and lymphatic vessels run through this layer to reach the outer
layers of the intestinal wall. When the connective tissue of one part of the GI
tract merges with adjacent connective tissue of another organ there is no covering mesothelium, and this connective tissue layer is called the adventitia;
(24) _____ *(serosa, adventitia)* ends with a covering mesothelium.

21 outermost
22 serosa

23 squamous

Esophagus
The esophagus is a long, 25-cm muscular tube that extends from the laryngo-
pharynx to the stomach. The esophageal wall consists of the four concentric
layers: **(25)** _____ or **(26)** _____ membrane,
(27) _____ or **(28)** _____ externa, and
adventitia (not **(29)** _____).

24 serosa

Mucosa
Esophageal epithelium is the same as that of the pharynx,
(30) non _____ _____
_____ epithelium (Fig. 14-2). At the esophageal–stomach junction,

25 mucosa
26 mucous
27 muscularis
28 muscularis
29 serosa

30 keratinized stratified
   squamous

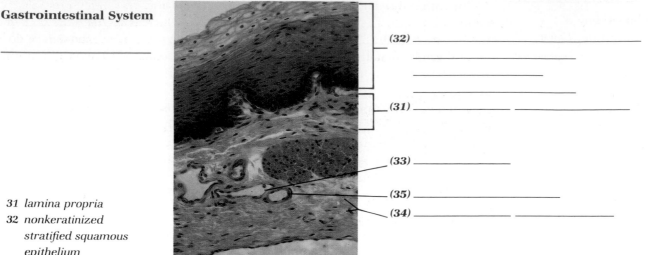

(32) _____ _____

_____

_____

_____

(31) _____ _____

(33) _____

(35) _____

(34) _____ _____

FIG. 14-2. Esophagus, H and E
stain (original magnification ×50).

31 *lamina propria*
32 *nonkeratinized
   stratified squamous
   epithelium*
33 *vessel*
34 *smooth muscle*
35 *arteriole*

the epithelium of the esophgus, *(36)* _____

_____ _____, abruptly changes to the epithe-
lium lining the stomach, which is simple columnar. Immediately beneath the
esophageal epithelium is the *(37)* _____ _____, which consists of a *(38)* _____ _____ _____ that is
composed of a fair amount of elastic fibers with a solitary lymph node. The
outermost subdivision of the mucosa, the *(39)* _____

_____, is a thin line of *(40)* _____ _____ fibers that
thickens as it approaches the stomach.

   There are some glands found in the mucosa, but only near the junction of
the esophagus and the stomach. Confined to the lamina *(41)* _____,
these glands—esophageal–cardiac glands—closely resemble those glands found
in the cardia portion of the stomach.

36 *nonkeratinized
   stratified squamous*

37 *lamina propria*
38 *loose connective tissue*

39 *muscularis mucosa*
40 *smooth muscle*

41 *propria*

Submucosa
The submucosal layer in the esophagus is mainly dense connective tissue rich in
blood vessels; it contains numerous small lymphocytes around specific glands.
Together with the muscularis layer, the submucosa forms the longitudinal folds
of the esophagus that flatten out during swallowing. Esophageal glands proper
are those specific glands unevenly distributed in the submucosa of the esophagus. Recognizable as very visible pale spots, the esophageal glands proper are
solely mucus secreting. These compound glands pierce the muscularis
(42) _____ and open through a small orifice.

Muscularis Externa
In the upper quarter to one third of the esophagus, the
(43) _____ externa consists solely of striated muscle in both
inner and outer layers. In the middle one third of the esophagus, the bundles of
striated muscles are gradually replaced by the usual *(44)* _____ muscle
fibers (Fig. 14-3). Areas of both *(45)* _____ and striated muscle fibers
lying adjacent to one another can be found in the middle one third of the
esophagus. In the lower one third, the externa consists only of

42 *externa*

43 *muscularis*

44 *smooth*
45 *smooth*

(46) _____ _____ fibers in both layers. The striated muscle found in the **(47)** _____ (*upper, lower*) part of the esophagus is unusual in that it is under **(48)** _____ (*voluntary, involuntary*) control rather than the usual **(49)** _____ (*voluntary, involuntary*) control. (You should finish #53 at this point.)

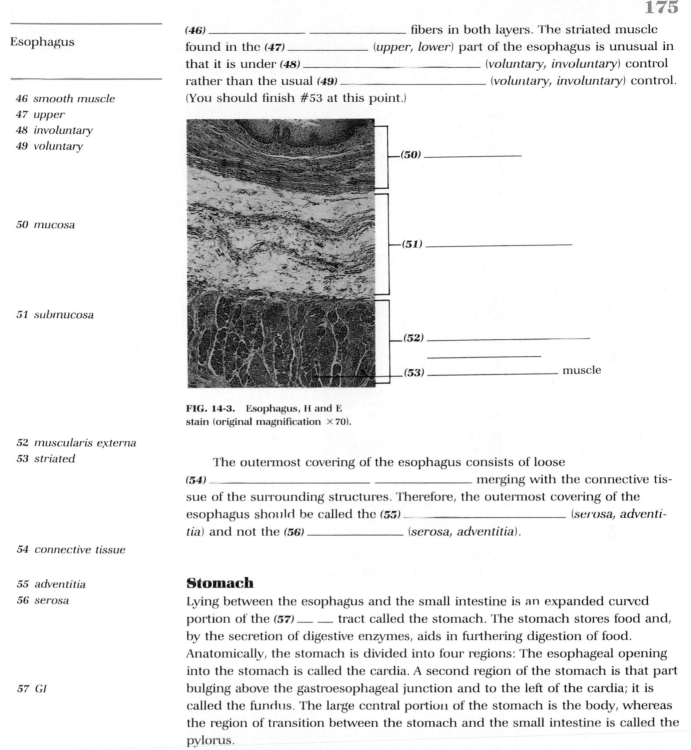

FIG. 14-3. Esophagus, H and E stain (original magnification ×70).

The outermost covering of the esophagus consists of loose **(54)** _____ _____ merging with the connective tissue of the surrounding structures. Therefore, the outermost covering of the esophagus should be called the **(55)** _____ (*serosa, adventitia*) and not the **(56)** _____ (*serosa, adventitia*).

Stomach

Lying between the esophagus and the small intestine is an expanded curved portion of the **(57)** __ __ tract called the stomach. The stomach stores food and, by the secretion of digestive enzymes, aids in furthering digestion of food. Anatomically, the stomach is divided into four regions: The esophageal opening into the stomach is called the cardia. A second region of the stomach is that part bulging above the gastroesophageal junction and to the left of the cardia; it is called the fundus. The large central portion of the stomach is the body, whereas the region of transition between the stomach and the small intestine is called the pylorus.

Histologically, only three different regions can be described in the stomach: the cardia, the fundus (which includes the anatomic body and fundus), and the pylorus.

All four major layers of the digestive tract make up the stomach wall as well. In order from the lumen outward, they are as follows: the **(58)** _____ or **(59)** _____ _____; the **(60)** _____; **(61)** _____ _____ or **(62)** _____ _____; **(63)** _____ or **(64)** _____. These layers are somewhat modified in that three instead of the usual two muscle

Esophagus

46 smooth muscle
47 upper
48 involuntary
49 voluntary

50 mucosa

51 submucosa

52 muscularis externa
53 striated

54 connective tissue

55 adventitia
56 serosa

57 GI

58 mucosa
59 mucous membrane
60 submucosa
61 muscularis
62 muscularis externa
63 serosa
64 adventitia

(50) _____
(51) _____
(52) _____
_____
(53) _____ muscle

65 *muscularis externa*

66 *serosal*

67 *cardia*
68 *pylorus*
69 *fundus*

70 *muscularis mucosa*
71 *outermost*

72 *foveolae or gastric pits*

73 *foveolae*
74 *gastric*

75 *body*
76 *pylorus*
77 *simple columnar*
78 *columnar*

layers make up the *(65)* _____ _____. The muscularis mucosa is also found to consist of three instead of two muscle layers. Unlike the esophagus, the stomach is covered by a *(66)* _____ (*serosal, adventitial*) outer layer.

Mucosa

There are a number of similarities among all three histologic regions of the stomach (the *(67)* _____, *(68)* _____, and *(69)* _____). Under the lowest power, an empty stomach exhibits numerous longitudinal folds of the mucosa called rugae. The plication of the mucosa is made possible by the contractile property of the *(70)* _____ _____, the *(71)* _____ (*outermost, innermost*) subdivision of the mucosa.

Closer examination of the mucosa reveals shallow furrows subdividing the mucosa into bulging gastric areas 1 mm to 6 mm in diameter (Fig. 14-4). These

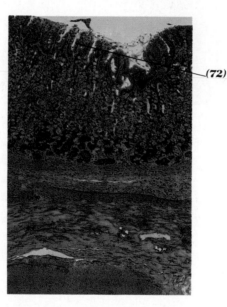

(72) _____

FIG. 14-4. Fundus of the stomach, H and E stain (original magnification ×50).

furrows or invaginations are termed gastric pits or foveolae.The gastric pits or *(73)* _____ have two to three gastric glands emptying into them. The secretions reach the lumen through the *(74)* _____ pits or foveolae. While the pits are uniform throughout the entire stomach, the glands that empty into them differ for each specific region of the stomach.

The epithelium lining the entire stomach wall, including the cardia, *(75)* _____, and *(76)* _____, is *(77)* _____ _____ epithelium. High-power magnification reveals that the simple *(78)* _____ epithelium of the stomach consists of mucus-producing cells (Fig. 14-5). Mucigen in vesicles is released at the cells'

Stomach

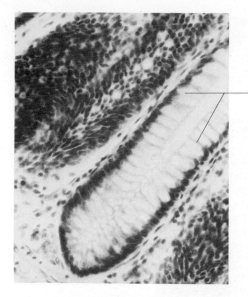

(79) _____ _____

_____

79 simple columnar
   epithelium

FIG. 14-5. Fundus of the stomach, H and
E stain (original magnification ×350).

(80) _____ (_apical, basal_) surface, and it protects the epithelium from corrosive enzymes also manufactured within the stomach. Also, electron microscopy (EM) reveals migration of newly formed cells in the deepest parts of the foveolae or **(81)** _____ _____ to the surface.

80 apical

Glands

81 gastric pits

The secretion of the stomach glands reaches the lumen through the **(82)** _____ _____ or **(83)** _____. Secretions from the three major histologic areas of the stomach, **(84)** _____, **(85)** _____, and **(86)** _____, aid in food digestion. The cardia and pylorus have glands named after their region, **(87)** _____ and **(88)** _____ glands, respectively. The glands of the fundus and body are called the gastric glands, and are both the most numerous and the most important glands in the stomch.

82 gastric pits
83 foveolae
84 fundus
85 pylorus
86 cardia
87 cardiac
88 pyloric

Gastric Glands

Found in the **(89)** _____ and **(90)** _____ of the stomach, gastric glands extend throughout the entire thickness of the mucosa up to its opening at the **(91)** _____ pits or **(92)** _____. Oriented perpendicularly to the mucosal surface, gastric glands have slightly coiled terminal ends and are composed of four cell types. The four cell types of the gastric glands are chief or zymogenic cells, parietal or oxyntic cells, neck mucous cells, and argentaffin cells. By identifying these types of cells and other histologic landmarks, one can properly identify the fundus and body of the stomach.

89 fundus
90 body
91 gastric
92 foveolae

CHIEF CELLS   Chief or **(93)** _____ _____ cells are simple cuboidal or low **(94)** _____ epithelia that line the base or lower one third of the lumen of the gastric glands. The chief or **(95)** _____ _____ cells are rich in secretory granules, which are often called zymogenic granules, and are located near the surface but do not stain dark (Fig. 14-6). Intense

93 zymogenic
94 columnar
95 zymogenic

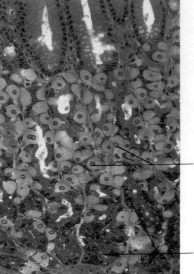

Parietal cells

Chief cells

FIG. 14-6. Pylorus, H and E stain (original magnification ×150).

(96) _____ philic staining is found at the base of the cell, caused by the large number of ribosomes and **(97)** _____ (*rough, smooth*) endoplasmic reticulum (rER). The granules are protein produced at the base of the zymogenic or **(98)** _____ cell (Fig. 14-7). This enzyme—pepsinogen not pepsin—is im-

96 *baso*
97 *rough*

98 *chief*

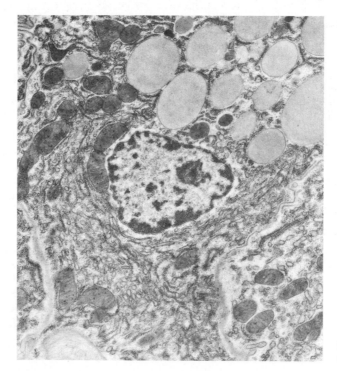

FIG. 14-7. Electron micrograph (EM) of a chief cell.

portant. Soon after secretion, pepsinogen is hydrolyzed to the active protein pepsin.

Fine microvilli line the surface of the **(99)** _____ or chief cell. Chief cells, which line the **(100)** _____ (*base, upper third*) of the lumen of the **(101)** _____ (*gastric, cardia*) glands, are

99 *zymogenic*
100 *base*
101 *gastric*

Glands

---

102 *cuboidal*
103 *baso*
104 *base*
105 *fundus*

106 *body*
107 *oxyntic*
108 *zymogenic*
109 *parietal*

110 *chief*

111 *unlike*
112 *endoplasmic reticulum*

113 *chief*
114 *zymogenic*
115 *pepsin*

116 *simple columnar*
117 *mucous*
118 *neck mucous*

119 *argyrophilic*
120 *argentaffin*

(102) _____ (*cuboidal, squamous*) with an intense
(103) _____ philic (104) _____ (*base, apex*) and are found only in the
(105) _____ and (106) _____ of the stomach.

PARIETAL CELLS Parietal or (107) _____ cells are scattered among the chief or (108) _____ cells, and some are found in the middle or neck of the gland, too. Pyramidal in shape, oxyntic or (109) _____ cells are often almost totally covered by surrounding zymogenic or (110) _____ cells. The most distinguishing feature of the parietal cell is a highly branching canal that forms an intracellular network around the nucleus and opens at the apex of the cell into the glandular lumen. Microvilli also line the surface of the cell. Parietal cells are rich in mitochondria (111) _____ (*like, unlike*) chief cells, but poor in rough (112) _____ _____ and secretory granules. The mitochondria are necessary to pump hydrochloric acid out of the cell and into the lumen. The acid makes it possible for the pepsinogen secreted by the (113) _____ or (114) _____ cells to be cleaved to its active form, (115) _____. Another substance, called intrinsic factor, is also secreted by the parietal cells.

NECK MUCOUS CELLS The neck mucous cells are relatively few in number (and very difficult to visualize on routine photomicroscopy). They are scattered between parietal cells in the neck of the gland but are virtually absent in the base. Staining positive with periodic acid–Schiff (PAS) stain, these mucous cells are deeply colored, indicating ovoid mucous droplets at their apexes. Neck mucous cells appear to be connected with the invaginating surface epithelium by a series of transitional epithelial cell forms. Between the surface epithelium, which is (116) _____ _____, and the neck (117) _____ cells are transitional cells that are neither fully developed epithelial cells nor (118) _____ _____ cells. Like most cells in the stomach, the neck mucous cells also have small microvilli on their surface.

ARGENTAFFIN CELLS Smallest in number, argentaffin cells are divided into two categories in gastric glands on the basis of the staining affinity for silver. Argentaffin cells are that category of cells that have specific granules that reduce silver salts without a reducing agent. Argyrophilic cells require a reducing agent before they react with silver. Both types of argentaffin cells, the (119) _____ and (120) _____ cells, are classified as enteroendocrine cells of the GI tract. The enteroendocrine cells have their granules at their base, indicating secretion into nearby blood vessels. These cells have been found to synthesize and secrete serotonin and other substances (Fig. 14-8).

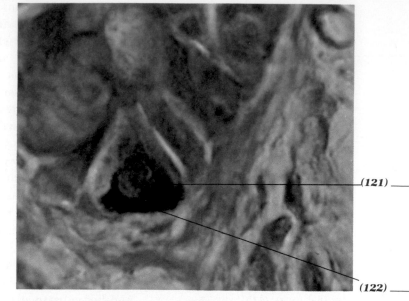

(121) _____

(122) _____

121 *nucleus*

FIG. 14-8.   Argentaffin cell (silver stain).

Pyloric Glands

122 *granules*

Pyloric glands are found in the *(123)* _____ of the stomach, and their foveolae or *(124)* _____ _____ are deeper than any other foveolae in the stomach. Also, the gastric *(125)* _____ or foveolae are quite wide, and this also aids in identifying the pyloric region (Fig. 14-9).

123 *pylorus*
124 *gastric pits*
125 *pits*

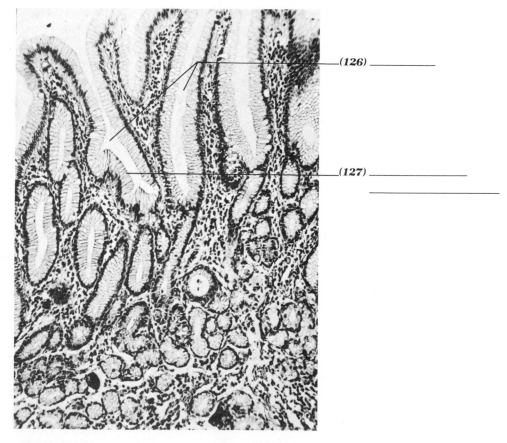

(126) _____

126 *pits*

(127) _____

_____

127 *simple columnar*

FIG. 14-9.   Pylorus of the stomach, H and E stain (low-power magnification).

Glands

_____

128 body
129 neck mucous

130 base

131 cardia
132 gastric pits
133 pylorus
134 simple columnar

135 do not need

136 fundus
137 body
138 pylorus
139 cardia
140 gastric pits
141 pylorus
142 gastric

143 stomach

144 mucosa
145 submucosa
146 muscularis
147 serosa
148 adventitia

149 plicae
150 valves

151 plicae
152 valves of Kerckring

Pyloric glands are the highly branched tubular type and are composed mainly of mucus-secreting cells. The cells of the pyloric glands are similar to those cells in the fundus and **(128)** _____, the **(129)** _____ _____ cells, yet pyloric cells release *both* pepsinogen (in very small amounts) and mucus. In addition to the pepsinogen-mucous–secreting cells, pyloric glands are also composed of (to a much lesser degree) enteroendocrine cells. The major enteroendocrine cell produces an important hormone, gastrin. Unlike the other enteroendocrine cells, those of the pylorus have granules dispersed throughout the cells, not at the **(130)** _____ (base, apex).

Cardiac Glands
Cardiac glands are found in the **(131)** _____ of the stomach. Foveolae or **(132)** _____ _____ of these glands are wide and deep but not to the extent they are in the **(133)** _____. The major cell component of the cardiac glands is the mucous cell, as in the lining **(134)** _____ _____ cells of the gastric gland and mucous cells of the pyloric gland. Scattered throughout cardiac glands are a few argentaffin cells, which **(135)** _____ (need, do not need) a reducing agent.

Review of Stomach Glands
Gastric glands include the glands of the **(136)** _____ and **(137)** _____, whereas the pyloric and cardiac glands are those glands of the **(138)** _____ and **(139)** _____, respectively. The widest and deepest foveolae or **(140)** _____ _____ are found in the **(141)** _____, while the **(142)** _____ glands are the narrowest of the three types.

Small Intestine
The small intestine is a tubular organ 7 m (20 ft) in length and situated between the **(143)** _____ and the large intestine. Divisible grossly and histologically into three distinct segments —duodenum, jejunum and ileum—the entire small intestine has the same basic wall organization as the stomach and esophagus. As in other sections of the GI tract, the wall of the entire small intestine is made of the four concentric layers: **(144)** _____, **(145)** _____, **(146)** _____, **(147)** _____ or **(148)** _____.

Mucosa
Using low power magnification one can see crescent folds extending about two thirds of the way around the intestinal lumen. These permanent structures are called plicae circulares or the valves of Kerckring. Composed of a mucosal lining and submucosal core the **(149)** _____ circulares or **(150)** _____ of Kerckring are absent in the first part of the duodenum, but reach the greatest development in the last part of the duodenum and first part of the jejunum. From the jejunum downward, the **(151)** _____ circulares or **(152)** _____ _____ _____ diminish until they are virtually absent beyond the middle of the ileum (Fig. 14-10).

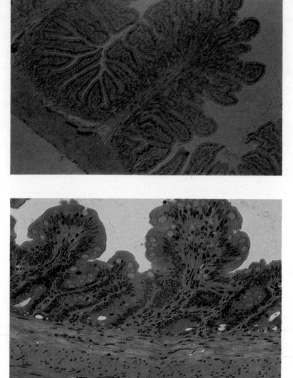

FIG. 14-10. Illustration shows *(153)* _____ *(jejunum, ileum).* H and E stain (original magnification ×25).

FIG. 14-11. Illustration shows *(154)* _____ *(jejunum, ileum).* H and E stain (original magnification ×25).

153 jejunum

154 ileum

Greater magnification reveals numerous minute fingerlike projections of the mucosa covering the entire surface of the mucosa (Figs. 14-10 and 14-11). Like the *(155)* _____ circulares, these fingerlike projections (called villi) are most numerous in the last part of the *(156)* _____ and the first part of the *(157)* _____. The cores of the villi are not submucosa like the plicae *(158)* _____ but consist of the *(159)* _____ propria.

The epithelial covering of the small intestine is simple columnar. There are three types of cells that can be distinguished in the covering epithelium—absorptive cells, goblet cells, and argentaffin or basal granular cells.

155 plicae
156 duodenum
157 jejunum
158 circulares
159 lamina

ABSORPTIVE CELLS Absorptive or columnar cells make up about 90% of the intestinal epithelium. The tall absorptive or *(160)* _____ cells have an ovoid nucleus lying at the bottom third of the cell. Organelles are abundant throughout the cell, except they are totally absent immediately beneath the cell's apical surface. The cell's free surface consists of closely packed microvilli. Microvilli *(161)* _____ *(increase, decrease)* the surface area, and therefore make it possible to *(162)* _____ *(increase, decrease)* absorption. Each microvilli is a bundle of longitudinally arranged *(163)* _____ *(microfilaments, microtubules)* in a cytoplasmic matrix enveloped by a typical plasma membrane. Detailed EM reveals a glycoprotein coat along the luminal surface of the microvilli. The coat has a dual purpose: to aid in digestion and to protect the epithelial lining from lytic agents. Because of the close and orderly arrangement of the microvilli on the *(164)* _____ columnar cell, the cell surface is often called a *(165)* _____ *(brush, striated)* border.

160 columnar

161 increase
162 increase

163 microtubules

164 simple
165 brush

Small Intestine

GOBLET CELLS Goblet cells are full of mucus and are shaped like a wine glass (Fig. 14-12). Almost 10% of the intestinal epithelium consists of goblet cells scattered

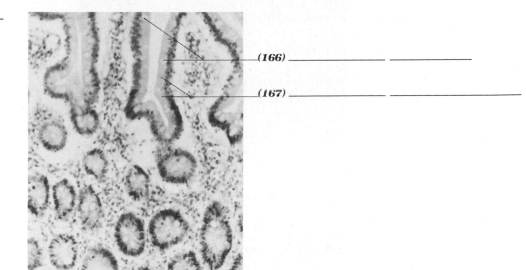

(166) _____ _____

(167) _____ _____

FIG. 14-12. Small intestine, H and E stain (original magnification ×225).

166 goblet cells

167 simple columnar

among the numerous *(168)* _____ or
(169) _____ cells. The goblet cell has a flattened
(170) _____ *(apically, basally)* located nucleus. Staining brilliant with
PAS, this *(171)* _____-secreting cell releases its product by a process called
(172) _____ cytosis. The released substance lubricates and protects the adjacent *(173)* _____ or absorptive cells.

BASAL GRANULAR CELLS Basal granular or *(174)* _____ cells
are very few in number, 0.5% (do not expect to locate them routinely), and are
found only at the base of the epithelium scattered beneath columnar cells.
Mainly pyramidal, basal granular or *(175)* _____ cells have
their granules located at their base like those of the *(176)* _____
(gastric, pyloric) glands. Secretion of these granules is into the adjacent
(177) _____ propria and not into the intestinal lumen. These cells are
called, as are those of the stomach, *(178)* entero _____ cells.
Finally, the *(179)* _____ granular or *(180)* _____
cells are in greatest number in the duodenum and least in the ileum and
jejunum.

Crypts of Lieberkühn

A set of glands found in the small intestine that extends from the submucosa to
the surface are called the crypts of Lieberkühn (Fig. 14-13). These are simple
tubular glands that secrete into the intestinal lumen between adjacent
(181) _____. The upper half of the crypts of
(182) _____ contain essentially the same epithelium lining as
the small intestine, *(183)* _____ or
(184) _____, goblet cells, and basal *(185)* _____
cells, which have an *(186)* _____ *(endocrine, exocrine)* function.
The production of new cells that migrate to the top of the villi to replace
exfoliated epithelia takes place in the lower half of the *(187)* _____ of

168 absorptive
169 columnar
170 basally
171 mucus
172 exo
173 columnar

174 argentaffin

175 argentaffin
176 gastric

177 lamina
178 endocrine
179 basal
180 argentaffin

181 villi
182 Lieberkühn
183 absorptive
184 columnar
185 granular
186 endocrine
187 crypts

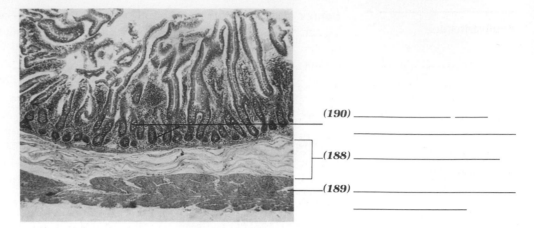

(190) _____ _____

_____

(188) _____

(189) _____

_____

188 *submucosa*

189 *muscularis externa*

190 *crypts of Lieberkühn*

FIG. 14-13.   Jejunum, H and E stain (original magnification ×25).

Lieberkühn. This process replaces cells every 3 days to 4 days. (You should finish #190 at this point.)

Paneth's cells are a group of cells found only in the crypts of Lieberkühn in the small intestine (Fig. 14-14). Pyramidal in shape, Paneth's cells have moder-

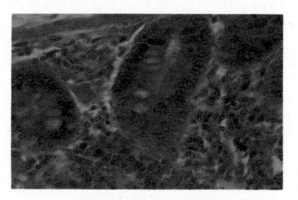

FIG. 14-14.   Paneth's cells, H and E stain (original magnification ×325).

ately sized, eosinophilic-staining granules in the apical cytoplasm. Most of the basophilic-staining basal cytoplasm of the Paneth's cell is composed of rER and other organelles.

Paneth's cells constitute a stable group of cells, and there is therefore little cell turnover. The specific function of the Paneth's cells is at present unknown.

Lamina Propria

Special attention must be paid to the tissue layer immediately beneath the epithelium, the *(191)* _____ _____. Forming the core of intestinal *(192)* _____ (*plicae circulares, villi*) and sandwiched between the lining epithelium and the *(193)* _____ _____, the lamina propria is highly cellular reticular tissue. Extensive elastic networks surround and support the penetrating crypts of *(194)* _____ within the lamina. A great number of lymphocytes, plasma cells, eosinophils, and macrophages function in protecting the body either by *(195)* _____ or the production of *(196)* _____. Lamina propria contains lymph vessels, often called lacteals.

191 *lamina propria*

192 *villi*

193 *muscularis mucosa*

194 *Lieberkühn*

195 *phagocytosis*

196 *antibodies*

Isolated lymphatic nodules called *(197)* <u>non</u>_____

_____ _____ are found in
the lamina. These small nodules are found throughout the intestine but are most
numerous in the distal parts. Small nodules occupy *only* the
(198) _____ _____ tissue layer. Large groups of nodules, as
often found in the ileum, extend throughout the *(199)* _____
mucosa and into the adjacent *(200)* _____ layer.

Aggregated lymphatic nodules or Peyer's patches *as a rule* are found in the
ileum (Fig. 14-15.) Numerous primary and secondary nodules with their

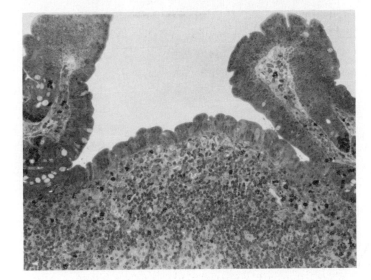

FIG. 14-15. EM of portion
of intestine (mouse) showing
a lymphoid follicle (original
magnification × 300). (Courtesy of Robert L. Owen,
M.D., Cell Biology Section, VA
Hospital, San Francisco, Cali-
fornia)

(201) _____ centers are found throughout the ileum in large
patches of lymphatic tissue. These patches, *(202)* _____

_____, are a histonomic area that should immediately signal to you
that you are examining the *(203)* _____ of the *(204)* _____ *(large,
small)* *(205)* _____.

Submucosa
Beneath the *(206)* _____ mucosa is the
(207) _____ layer. The submucosa consists of dense connec-
tive tissue with scattered lobules of adipose tissue. In the duodenum, situated in
the submucosal layer, are a set of glands called the duodenal glands or, more
commonly, Brunner's glands (Fig. 14-16). Brunner's glands or

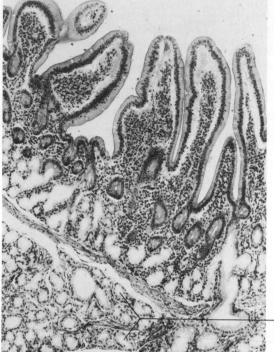

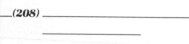

(208) _____

_____

FIG. 14-16. Name the specific area of the small intestine. **(209)** _____. H and E stain (low-power magnification).

208 *Brunner's glands*

209 *duodenum*

(210) _____ glands are encountered primarily in the first part of the duodenum and infrequently in the proximal area of the jejunum and the distal part of the stomach. These glands are largest in the **(211)** _____ of the duodenum. The ducts of **(212)** _____ or duodenal glands penetrate the muscularis **(213)** _____ and open into a **(214)** _____ of Lieberkühn. Brunner's glands are richly branched glands found only in the **(215)** _____ (*mucosal, submucosal*) layer of (usually) only the **(216)** _____ (*duodenum, ileum*) and infrequently in the proximal **(217)** _____ and distal **(218)** _____. The secretory cells of Brunner's or **(219)** _____ glands are mucous secretory cells with a basal nuclei. It is important to remember that **(220)** _____ _____ are indicative of the ileum while Brunner's glands are histonomonic for the **(221)** _____ (*duodenum, ileum*).

210 *duodenal*

211 *first part*
212 *Brunner's*
213 *mucosae*
214 *crypt*
215 *submucosal*
216 *duodenum*
217 *jejunum*
218 *stomach*
219 *duodenal*

220 *Peyer's patches*
221 *duodenum*

Muscularis and Serosa

The outer two layers of the small intestine, **(222)** _____ or **(223)** _____ _____ and the serosa, are well developed in the small intestine. The muscularis consists of the usual **(224)** _____ (*one, two, three*) **(225)** _____ (*striated, smooth*) muscle layers; an inner **(226)** _____ (*longitudinal, circular*) and an outer **(227)** _____ (*longitudinal, circular*) layer. Between the muscle layer is a nerve plexus called the **(228)** _____ or **(229)** _____ plexus. The serosal covering consists of simple

222 *muscularis*
223 *muscularis externa*
224 *two*
225 *smooth*
226 *circular*
227 *longitudinal*
228 *Auerbach's*
229 *myenteric*

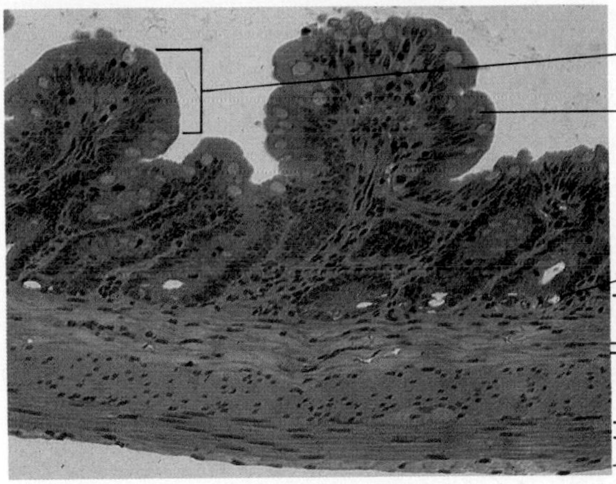

(231) _____ _____

(232) _____ , and _____

(233) _____ _____

(234) _____ _____

(235) _____ _____

(236) _____ _____ _____

FIG. 14-17. Name this organ. (230) _____
H and E stain (original magnification ×25).

(237) _____ or (238) _____ cells resting on a thin connective tissue layer (Fig. 14-17).

Review of Small Intestine

The small intestine is subdivided into three distinct regions: (239) _____ , (240) _____ , and (241) _____ . Consisting of the usual (242) _____ (two, three, four)-layer wall, the small intestine has a lining epithelium composed of (243) _____ (one, two, three, four) distinct cell types: simple (244) _____ or (245) _____ cells, the (246) _____ (least, most) prevalent; (247) _____ cells—(248) _____ -secreting cells; and basal (249) _____ cells or (250) _____ cells, which, in this case, are called (251) entero_____ cells and are the (252) _____ (least, most) prevalent of all epithelial cells.

Large folds of the mucosa and submucosa are absent in the first part of the duodenum but are best developed in the last part of the (253) _____ and first part of the (254) _____ . These folds diminish until they are virtually absent beyond the middle of the (255) _____ region of the small intestine.

Large Intestine

The large intestine is subdivided into the cecum; appendix; ascending, transverse, descending, and sigmoid colon; rectum; and anus. Absorption of water and storage of the feces are the major functions of the large intestine. The typical histologic organization of the GI wall is found throughout the entire large intestine.

Mucosa

The mucosa of the large intestine is thicker than that of the small intestine. While thicker, the mucosa of the large intestine does *not* form villi. The absence of villi is an important distinguishing feature between the two intestines. Also, the tremendous folding of the mucosa and adjacent (256) _____ found in the small intestine and called (257) _____ _____ are not evident in the large intestine except in the anal region (Fig. 14-18). Columns of mucosal folds, not as

230 ileum
231 plicae circulares
232 goblet cell
233 blood vessel
234 submucosa
235 inner circular muscle
236 outer longitudinal muscle layer
237 squamous
238 mesothelial
239 duodenum
240 jejunum
241 ileum
242 four
243 three
244 columnar
245 absorptive
246 most
247 goblet
248 mucus
249 granular
250 argentaffin
251 endocrine
252 least
253 duodenum
254 jejunum
255 ileal

256 submucosa
257 plica circulares

Gastrointestinal System

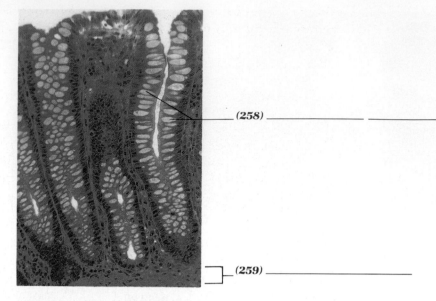

_____ (258) _____ _____

_____ (259) _____

FIG. 14-18. Colon, H and E stain
(original magnification ×170).

258 goblet cells

259 submucosa

distended as those in the *(260)* _____ (*duo-denum–jejunum, jejunum–ileum*), are found in the anal region of the
(261) _____ (*small, large*) intestine and are called the columns of Morgagni. These columns of *(262)* _____ help identify the
(263) _____ region of the large intestine.

Lining the large intestine's lumen is simple *(264)* _____

_____, which extends to 2 cm of the anal opening. Microvilli are
found as extensions of the epithelial border and form a *(265)* _____ border
(Fig. 14-19). A major distinguishing feature between this epithelium and that of

260 duodenum–jejunum

261 large
262 Morgagni
263 anal
264 columnar epithelium

265 brush

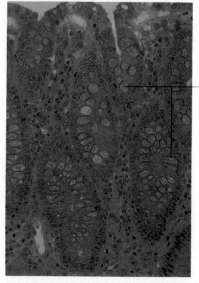

_____ (266) _____ _____

266 goblet cells

FIG. 14-19. The mucus-secreting
cells stain *(267)* _____-positive.
Colon, periodic acid–Schiff (PAS)
stain (original magnification ×170).

267 PAS

the small intestine is the greater number of goblet cells making up the large intestine's epithelium. Often the lining epithelium assumes a vacuolated appearance because of the large number of *(268)* _____ cells, which secrete *(269)* _____ (*dark, clear*)-staining *(270)* _____ (Fig. 14-20).

The epithelium at the end of the anal region represents a transition zone between the mucosa of the large intestine and the skin. This epithelium is

268 *goblet*
269 *clear*
270 *mucus*

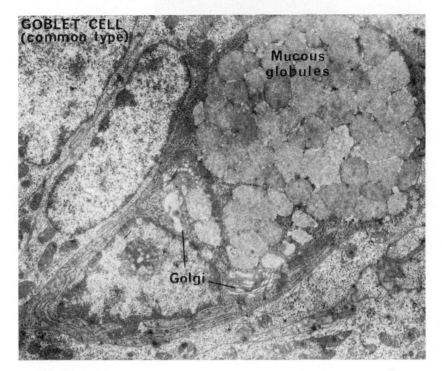

FIG. 14-20. EM of a goblet cell.

nonkeratinized stratified squamous and becomes confluent with the *(271)* _____ _____ _____ epithelium of the skin.

Since the mucosa of the large intestine is thicker, the crypts of *(272)* _____ are *(273)* _____ (*longer, shorter*). At the bottom of the crypts highly *(274)* _____ (*differentiated, undifferentiated*) cells are found, and these *(275)* _____ (*replace, do not replace*) exfoliated epithelial and *(276)* _____ cells. At the anorectal junction, where the simple *(277)* _____ epithelium abruptly changes to *(278)* _____ _____ _____ epithelium, the crypts will *not* be found.

271 *keratinized stratified squamous*

272 *Lieberkühn*
273 *longer*
274 *undifferentiated*
275 *replace*
276 *goblet*
277 *columnar*
278 *nonkeratinized stratified squamous*

Submucosa

The submucosa of most of the colon is typical intestinal submucosa. Often, scattered lymphatic nodules, which are found primarily in the *(279)* _____ propria, extend into the submucosa. This lymphoid tissue does not assume any organized or highly aggregated areas like Peyer's *(280)* _____ in the *(281)* _____ of the small intestine (Fig. 14-21).

279 *lamina*

280 *patches*
281 *ileum*

282 *goblet cells*

283 *primary nodule*

284 *smooth muscle*

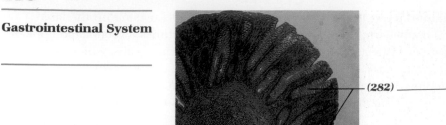

(282) _____ _____

(283) _____ _____

(284) _____ _____

FIG. 14-21. Colon, H and E stain (original magnification ×30).

Muscularis Externa

Surrounding the submucosa is the muscularis *(285)* _____. This layer differs somewhat from its arrangement in the other part of the GI tract. The outer *(286)* _____ *(longitudinal, circular)* layer is not organized as one continuous layer but from the cecum to the rectum is arranged into three longitudinal bands called the taeniae coli. These bands are responsible for gathering the bowel into sections or sacculations called haustra. In the rectum the *(287)* _____ coli merge and form one continuous outer *(288)* _____ *(longitudinal, circular)* sheath.

285 *externa*

286 *longitudinal*

Serosa

The serosa of the large intestine is *(289)* _____ _____ epithelium or *(290)* _____ cells resting on a thin *(291)* _____ _____ layer. The serosa is somewhat atypical in that it forms pendulous protruberances of adipose tissue that hang on the outside of the large intestine forming a distinctive gross anatomic feature.

287 *taeniae*
288 *longitudinal*

289 *simple squamous*
290 *mesothelial*
291 *connective tissue*

Appendix

The appendix is a blind-ending organ attached to the cecum of the *(292)* _____ intestine. The mucosa of the appendix is covered by the same epithelium as the intestine, *(293)* _____ _____. Few goblet cells, which secrete *(294)* _____ and are therefore PAS-*(295)* _____ *(negative, positive)*, are found in the appendix epithelium (Fig. 14-22). The lamina propria of the appendix forms an almost continuous layer of lymphatic nodules and makes identification of the appendix quite easy. The large amount of lymphatic tissue can occlude the lumen but most commonly only reduces its size. There are no villi, as in the *(296)* _____ (small, large) intestine, but small crypts of *(297)* _____ are evident.

292 *large*
293 *simple columnar*
294 *mucus*
295 *positive*

296 *large*
297 *Lieberkühn*

Appendix

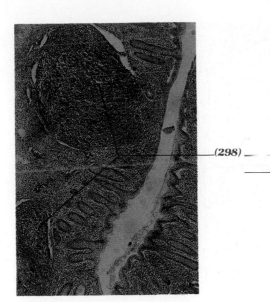

(298) _____ _____

_____

298 lymphatic nodules

FIG. 14-22. Name this organ.
(299) _____. H
and E stain (original magnification
×50).

299 appendix

The *(300)* _____ externa or *(301)* ___ _____
is present in the appendix and typically consists of *(302)* _____ muscle
layers surrounded by simple *(303)* _____ epithelium or
(304) _____, called the *(305)* _____.

300 muscularis
301 muscularis
302 smooth
303 squamous
304 mesothelium
305 serosa

Ancillary Organs

There are three major organs associated with the digestive system and are
directly connected to the GI tract. These organs are the liver and its closely
attached organ, the gallbladder, and the pancreas. All three of these organs aid in
the process of digestion by secretion of various enzymes and fluids.

Liver

The largest organ in the body, the liver is situated directly beneath the diaphragm on the right side of the body. Grossly, the liver is a reddish organ divided
into two main lobes, and covering both lobes is a thin but strong connective
tissue capsule called Glisson's capsule. Besides excreting enzymes for digestion,
the liver detoxifies toxic substances, synthesizes plasma proteins, and plays a
pivotal role in the maintenance of homeostasis in carbohydrate metabolism.

The Lobule

The liver consists of parenchymal tissue—hepatocytes and a supporting stroma.
The liver tissue is arranged in a tridimensional lattice network that is subdivided
into lobules. Lobules, more properly called hepatic lobules, represent the functional unit of the liver and are the focus of our histologic discussion.

There are three histiophysiological concepts used to describe the
(306) _____ lobule. Each concept—the classic lobule, portal lobule,
or acinar lobule— slightly overlap one another but need to be examined sepa-
rately (Fig. 14-23).

306 hepatic

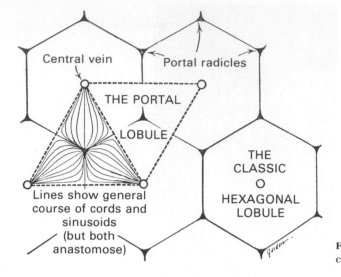

Central vein

Portal radicles

THE PORTAL

LOBULE

THE CLASSIC O HEXAGONAL LOBULE

Lines show general course of cords and sinusoids (but both anastomose)

FIG. 14-23. Diagram illustrating the concepts of liver tissue.

Classic Lobule

The classic hepatic lobule is the term most commonly used to describe the histologic makeup of the liver. Surrounding the liver is *(307)* _____ capsule, a *(308)* _____ _____ capsule that branches extensively throughout the parenchymal tissue, carrying blood vessels with it. At its largest subdivision, the connective tissue branch contains a branch of a blood vessel called the portal vein, plus the hepatic artery, bile duct (all described in greater detail below), and a very thin-walled and often difficult to see lymphatic duct. The hepatic artery, bile duct, and portal vein are often referred to as the *portal triad.* The central vein is a large vein that receives blood by way of sinusoids (also discussed below) and returns the blood by way of the sublobular vein to the hepatic vein. Hepatic veins eventually converge into the inferior vena cava. The central vein is not invested in connective tissue like the *(309)* _____ vein, *(310)* _____ artery, *(311)* _____ duct, and *(312)* _____ duct.

The classic lobule is defined by the *(313)* _____ triad and central vein (Fig. 14-24). With the central vein as the center of the lobule, the portal triad,

307 Glisson's
308 connective tissue

309 portal
310 hepatic
311 lymphatic
312 bile
313 portal

314 bile duct

315 hepatic artery

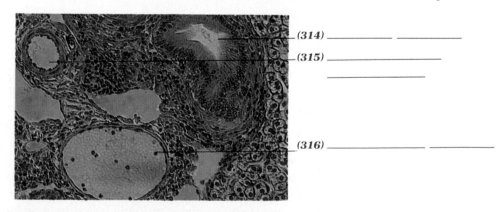

(314) _____ _____

(315) _____

_____

(316) _____ _____

FIG. 14-24. Liver, H and E stain (original magnification ×50).

316 portal vein

the *(317)* _____ _____, *(318)* _____ _____, and *(319)* _____ duct, forms the corners of a polygon. Physiologically, the classic lobule is defined by a direction of blood flow. Blood flows from the

317 hepatic artery
318 portal vein
319 bile

Liver

320 *portal*
321 *portal*

322 *vein*
323 *hepatic*

324 *portal vein*
325 *hepatic artery*
326 *bile*
327 *vein*

328 *opposite*

329 *hepatic*
330 *bile*
331 *portal*

332 *portal*
333 *acinar*
334 *classic*

branches of the hepatic artery and **(320)** _____ vein of the **(321)** _____ triad through portal sinusoids (see below), and is drained by the central vein. The central vein and its succeeding vessels are thought of as sinks and the portal **(322)** _____ and **(323)** _____ artery, as the sources.

Portal Lobule

The portal lobule concept is defined as the portal triad—**(324)** _____ _____, **(325)** _____ _____, **(326)** _____ duct at the *center* of the lobule, and the central **(327)** _____ at its periphery. This arrangement is dictated by the flow of a certain substance, bile. Bile is drained from the sinusoids to the bile duct—flow that is **(328)** _____ (*opposite, identical*) to blood flow through the sinusoids.

Acinar Lobule

The most difficult of all concepts of liver structure is that of an acinar lobule. Both portal and classic lobules are thought to be *not* the smallest unit of functional organization of the parenchymal liver tissue. The acinar lobule is not defined by the central vein, but it is a diamond-shaped area extending at right angles from the portal triad (Fig. 14-25). Essentially, the acinar lobule is tissue

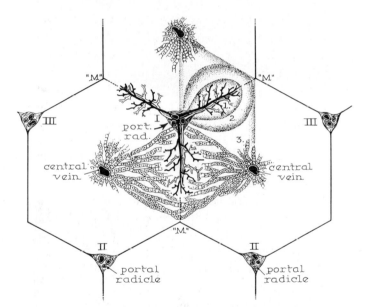

FIG. 14-25. Diagram illustrating the acinar lobule.

supplied by the terminal branches of the portal vein and of the **(329)** _____ artery and bile drained by a terminal branch of the **(330)** _____ duct. The vessels extend out at right angles from the **(331)** _____ triad and travel one third of the distance from the next directly diagonal canal. This concept states that this tissue area is the smallest functional unit and there are three units per portal canal. Further subdivisions of this acinar lobule are also proposed but greater detail on the exact nature of these subdivisions can be found in a textbook of histology.

Histology of the Liver

The histologic composition of the lobule, whether the **(332)** _____ lobule, **(333)** _____ lobule, or **(334)** _____ lobule theory, is basic and similar in many respects to the spleen. In histologic sections, the liver

335 *cells*

336 *hepatic artery*
337 *portal vein*
338 *central*

339 *hepato*

340 *lymph node*
341 *nodal*

342 *central vein*

343 *sinusoids*

344 *hepatocytes*

345 *fixed*

346 *phago*

347 *macrophages*
348 *Kupffer's*

349 *endothelial*
350 *hepatocytes*

351 *space*

352 *hepatocyte*
353 *Disse*
354 *hepatocytes*
355 *major*

356 *space of Disse*
357 *hepatocyte*

exhibits columns of hepatocytes—liver *(335)* _____, separated on either side by narrow vascular channels, the hepatic sinusoids. Blood flows through the sinusoids from the branches of *(336)* _____ _____ and *(337)* _____ _____ to the *(338)* _____ vein. Like the spleen, the sinusoids represent vascular channels into which blood is emptied. Lining the sinusoids and therefore adjacent to the columns of *(339)* _____ cytes is an endothelial cell wall (Fig. 14-26). The typical endothelial cell contains few organelles, and is greatly attenuated and therefore extremely difficult to see under the microscope.

Whether the sinusoidal endothelial cell wall is continuous or not is unresolved. Absent are tight cell junctions, very much like the *(340)* _____ _____ *(lymph node, splenic)* endothelium that lines the *(341)* _____ sinuses. Openings or fenestrae in the endothelium cells suggest some sort of filtering function.

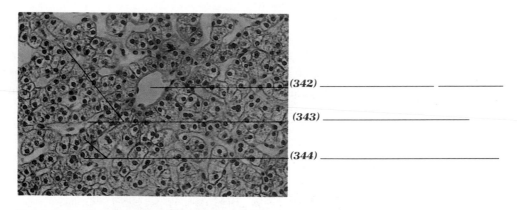

(342) _____ _____

(343) _____

(344) _____

FIG. 14-26. Liver, H and E stain (original magnification ×150).

Another type of cell found lining the sinusoids is larger but much fewer in number than the endothelial cells. These cells are the stellate Kupffer's cells and are fixed macrophages. Often, Kupffer's or *(345)* _____ macrophages are identifiable by colloidal particulate ingestion because of their highly *(346)* _____ cytic properties. Otherwise, Kupffer's cells in routine preparations are most difficult to visualize. One must realize that in humans the highly phagocytic *(347)* _____ or *(348)* _____ cells contribute to the endothelial wall and do not just rest on top of the endothelial cells.

There is a very narrow space that separates the sinusoidal *(349)* _____ cell lining from the columns of *(350)* _____. In fact this space, the space of Disse, is not an artifact but a true space containing plasma fluid with numerous microvilli projecting from the hepatocyte. The *(351)* _____ of Disse is thought to serve as a means of better exchange of metabolites between the microvilli of the *(352)* _____ and the blood. The space of *(353)* _____ is often called the perisinusoidal space.

The thick columns of *(354)* _____ make up a *(355)* _____ *(small, major)* part of the liver. The hepatocyte surface border consists of one of three different areas: adjacent to the perisinusoidal space or the *(356)* _____ ___ _____, adjacent to another *(357)* _____ column or line; or another, very narrow canal called the bile canaliculi (discussed below).

Liver

358 hepatocytes

359 smooth

360 space of Disse
361 perisinusoidal space
362 hepatocyte

363 cardiac muscle

364 hepatocytes
365 bile
366 opposite
367 hepatocytes
368 hepatocytes
369 bile
370 space of Disse
371 perisinusoidal space

372 portal
373 Hering

374 Hering

375 triad
376 duct
377 portal

378 columnar

Liver cells or *(358)* _____ are polyhedral and often binucleate, and greater than 70% are tetraploid. Each hepatocyte contains a plethora of organelles, mitochondria, rough and *(359)* _____ endoplasmic reticulum, Golgi, and free and fixed polysomes. Microvilli extend out into the *(360)* _____ ____ _____ or
(361) _____ _____ from each surface of the
(362) _____ adjacent to that area.

Both lipid droplets and glycogen granules are found in large numbers in the hepatocyte. Another type of granule or pigment easily identified in a light micrograph is a brown-staining pigment called lipofuscin. This pigment is often called age or "wear and tear" pigment and also found in *(363)* _____ _____ *(cardiac muscle, stomach epithelium)*. Essentially, lipofuscin is the residue of lysosomal digestion.

Bile Canaliculi

As a rule bile canaliculi run between adjacent pairs of
(364) _____ and carry *(365)* _____ in an
(366) _____ *(opposite, identical)* direction to the blood flow in the sinusoids. These canaliculi are expansions of the intercellular space between
(367) _____. Short microvilli from the lining
(368) _____ project into the *(369)* _____ canaliculi, similar to the longer microvilli of hepatocytes that project into the
(370) _____ ____ _____ or
(371) _____ _____ (Fig. 14-27).

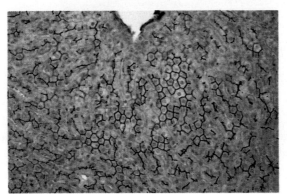

FIG. 14-27. Liver, reticular stain (original magnification ×130).

Bile canaliculi will empty into short canals called the canals of Hering as they approach the *(372)* _____ triad. The canals of
(373) _____ are unique in that both ductal epithelium and heptocytes border their lumen; however, this is not easily visualized (Fig. 14-28). Eventually the canals of *(374)* _____ connect with the slender bile ductules. Bile ductules then penetrate the connective tissue that surrounds the portal
(375) _____ and merge to form a bile *(376)* _____.

Bile ducts in the *(377)* _____ triad are composed of cuboidal epithelium. These ducts form a richly anastomotic network of interlobular ducts that follow the course of the portal vein. As the ducts merge to form larger ducts the epithelium becomes taller and therefore *(378)* _____, and the surrounding tissue becomes thicker and richer in elastic fibers. Eventually, the main hepatic bile duct merges with a duct of the gallbladder and empties into the duodenum.

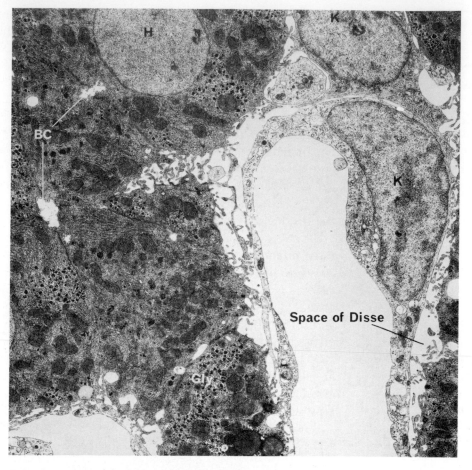

FIG. 14-28. EM of the bile canaliculi. A Kupffer's cell (*K*) is seen at top right.

The fluid coursing through these canals and ducts is *(379)* _____. This substance is an *(380)* _____ (*exocrine, endocrine*) secretion of the *(381)* _____ (*liver, gallbladder*) and is rich in pigments, cholesterol, enzymes, and metabolic wastes. Bile's primary function is to greatly facilitate the digestion of fat.

Supporting Structure

(382) _____ capsule, which surrounds the liver, branches into interlobular *(383)* _____ _____ septa that carry blood vessels throughout the liver parenchyma. Using silver staining technique, one can see a fine reticular fiber network between and around the sinusoids and hepatic cell columns. This network is a second component of the supportive structure of the liver.

Lymph Spaces

The liver is involved in the production of a tremendous amount of lymph fluid. Like bile ducts, lymphatic vessels found in the *(384)* _____ _____ follow the course of the *(385)* _____ vein. Lymphatic vessels have not been found around the sinusoids or *(386)* _____ cell columns. Where lymph is formed and by what means it is collected into lymphatic vessels have yet to be determined.

379 bile
380 exocrine
381 liver

382 Glisson's
383 connective tissue

384 portal triad
385 portal
386 hepatic

Gallbladder

Attached to the posterior side of the liver is a pear-shaped sac, the
(387) _____. The gallbladder serves as the site of concentration and storage of bile, which is continuously secreted by the
(388) _____. From various stimuli bile is released from the gallbladder; it is important in aiding fat *(389)* _____.

   The gallbladder is not arranged into the usual *(390)* _____ (*two, three, four*)-layer arrangement found in the rest of the GI tract (Fig. 14-29). Instead, the gallbladder wall consists of a mucosa without a *(391)* _____ mucosa, a layer of smooth muscle similar to the *(392)* _____ externa, and a perimuscular connective tissue layer followed by a serosal covering.

Mucosa

The mucosa has numerous folds or rugae that often seem to form glands. There are *no* glands in the gallbladder except in a small area at its neck. These folds or *(393)* _____ flatten out if the organ is distended. The lining epithelium consists of *(394)* _____ _____ just like that of the small and large *(395)* _____ except for 2 cm above the
(396) _____, where it is *(397)* _____
_____ _____ epithelium. Numerous microvilli extend from the epithelium and aid further in the gallbladder's ability to *(398)* _____ (*secrete, absorb*) and therefore
(399) _____ (*dilute, concentrate*) the *(400)* _____. This epithelium contains no mucus-secreting cells called *(401)* _____
_____, so common in the intestine, and even more common in the
(402) _____ (*small, large*) intestine. Basal *(403)* _____ cells or *(404)* _____ cells are also nonexistent in the gallbladder.

Lamina Propria

The lamina propria consists of *(405)* _____ (*dense, loose*) connective tissue that, instead of resting on the *(406)* _____ mucosa, is adjacent to a *(407)* _____ (*striated, smooth*) muscular layer. These muscle fibers are not necessarily organized into circular or longitudinal bundles as are most of the fibers of the *(408)* _____.

(415) _____

(416) _____
_____

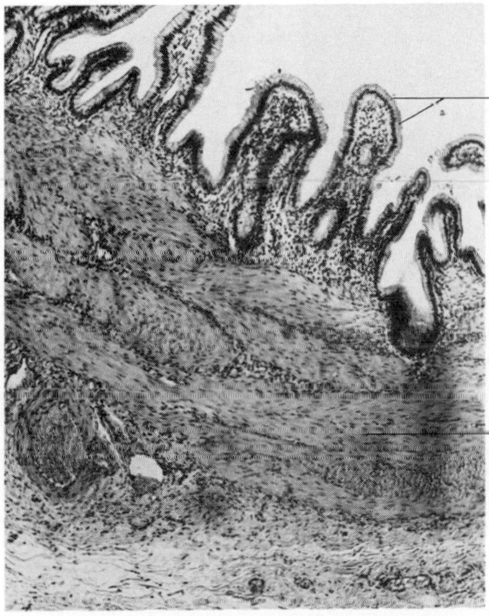

FIG. 14-29. Gallbladder, H and E stain
(original magnification ×50).

Subserosal Layer

Directly outside the **(409)** _____ muscle layer is a
(410) peri _____ or subserosal layer. This coat consists of loose
connective tissue rich in adipocytes and blood vessels. Finally, covering the
perivascular layer is the **(411)** _____, which is made up of
(412) _____ _____ epithelium or
(413) _____ resting on a thin
(414) _____ _____ layer. (You should finish #416
at this point.)

409 smooth
410 muscular

411 serosa
412 simple squamous
413 mesothelium
414 connective tissue
415 epithelium (cuboidal)
416 smooth muscle

Pancreas

Like the liver, the pancreas is an organ with complex and widely divergent
physiological functions. Under low power, the pancreas can be mistaken for the
parotid gland, which is a **(417)** _____ (salivary, GI) gland composed primarily of **(418)** _____ (mucus, serous)-secreting cells. One can
divide the pancreas into two easily differentiated histologic areas: the exocrine
pancreas or acinar tissue and the endocrine pancreas or the islets of Langerhans.

417 salivary
418 serous

Acinar Tissue

Acinar tissue or the **(419)** _____ pancreas forms most of the pancreas. Acinar tissue is essentially composed of acinous glands that are separated
into lobules, neatly bound together by connective tissue septa. The acini consist
of a single row of pyramidal cells surrounding a central lumen that leads to a
ductal system (Fig. 14-30).

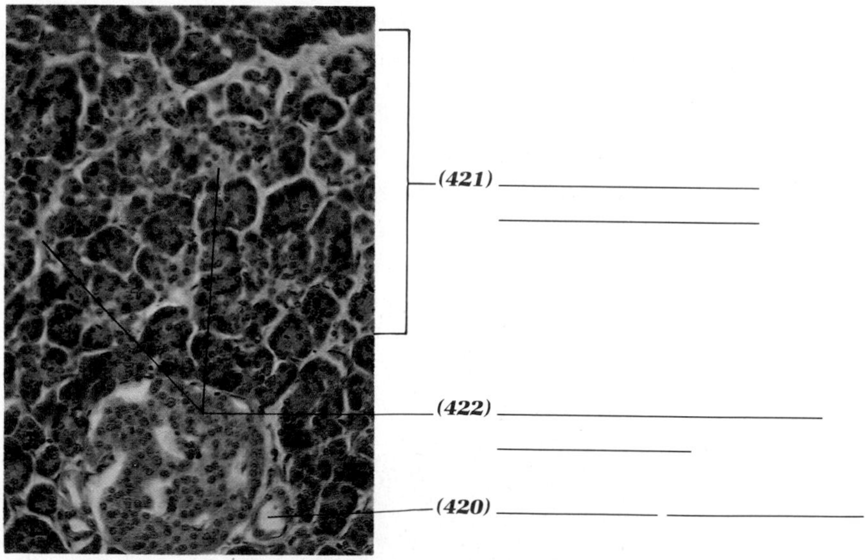

419 exocrine

(421) _____
_____

(422) _____
_____

(420) _____ _____

FIG. 14-30. Pancreas, H and E stain
(original magnification ×125).

420 blood vessel
421 exocrine pancreas or
acinar tissue
422 connective tissue

Pancreas

423 darker
424 islets of Langerhans
425 baso
426 rough

427 centrally

428 simple cuboidal

429 acinar
430 endocrine
431 islets of Langenhans
432 endocrine

433 ducts

434 circulatory

435 islets of Langerhans
436 acinar tissue

437 acinar

Acinar cells will always stain darkest in the basal portion of the cell and stain (423) _____ (lighter, darker) than the endocrine pancreas or (424) _____ _____ _____. The (425) _____ philic nature of the basal part of the cell is caused by the tremendous production of protein. A great number of (426) _____ endoplasmic reticulum and free and fixed polyribosomes are evident in this region of the cell. Well-developed Golgi apparatus and numerous mitochondria cluster in the middle portion of the cell.

The apical portion of the acinar cells consists of clusters of highly refractile granules or droplets. These granules, called zymogen granules, are a fluid mixture that is released into the (427) _____ (centrally, basally) located lumen. Difficulty in visualizing the lumen is due to sectioning and because the contents released from the cells create a blurring of the apical border and cell lumen. The surface of the acinar cell is lined by very short and highly irregular microvilli. The lumen of each individual acinus is continuous with the lumen of a small duct bounded by centri-acinar cells.

The terminal portion of the duct system drains proximally into intralobular ducts. These ducts are visible because their epithelium stains lighter than that of the acinar cells. Histologically, the ductal system does not resemble the rest of the pancreas but resembles ducts of a typical gland. Larger ducts, interlobular ducts, are more visible and are lined by (428) _____ _____ epithelium with a few muco-secreting cells. The ducts form a major duct that leaves the pancreas and drains into the duodenum.

Islets of Langerhans

As stated earlier, there are two distinct histologically different areas of the pancreas, the exocrine or (429) _____, and the (430) _____ pancreas or (431) _____ _____ _____. Closer examination of the islets reveals small numbers of different (432) _____ (exocrine, endocrine) cells. It is in this area that important hormones such as glucagon and insulin are produced; these hormones are not secreted into (433) _____ as happens in the exocrine portion of the pancreas, but are released into the capillaries of the (434) _____ system (Fig. 14-31).

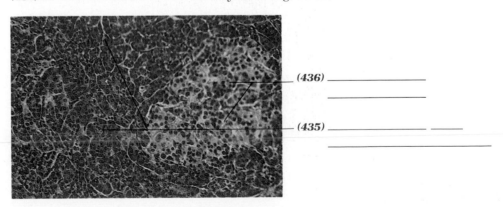

(436) _____
_____

(435) _____ _____
_____

FIG. 14-31. H and E stain (original magnification ×80).

The islets are not encapsulated but faintly demarcated from the (437) _____ tissue by thin connective tissue septa. Very little connective tissue is found within the islets themselves. It is often through special staining

438 islets of Langerhans

439 alpha

440 capillaries
441 beta

442 capillaries
443 delta
444 islets of Langerhans

445 A
446 glucagon
447 B
448 beta
449 capillaries
450 endocrine
451 capillaries
452 most
453 insulin
454 glucagon

techniques that the three different cell types of the *(438)* _____ _____
_____ can be distinguished easily. These three cell types are alpha or A cells, beta or B cells, and delta or D cells. The A or *(439)* _____ cells are the most striking of the cells because of their large numbers of bright-staining red granules. These granules are dispersed throughout the cell and contain glucagon, a hormone that is secreted into the smallest blood vessels, the *(440)* _____.

    B or *(441)* _____ cells have crystalloid granules that are difficult to differentiate. B cells are more numerous than A cells and contain more rough endoplasmic reticulum and free ribosomes. The B cell also secretes its hormone, insulin, into nearby *(442)* _____.

    D or *(443)* _____ cells have been studied the least and are also found in the smallest number in the *(444)* _____ _____
_____. Delta cells stain a pale blue, unlike the reddish staining of *(445)* __ cells that produce *(446)* _____. D cells do contain more rER than A cells but less than *(447)* __ or *(448)* _____ cells. The secretion of the D cells is also into nearby *(449)* _____, but its exact composition is unknown.

    All of these cells are *(450)* _____ (*endocrine, exocrine*) in function and secrete directly into *(451)* _____. B cells, the *(452)* _____ (*least, most*) numerous, secrete *(453)* _____, whereas A cells produce and secrete *(454)* _____.

15

Respiratory System

After completing this chapter, you should be able to identify the following:

1 True and false vocal cords
2 Trachea
3 Respiratory epithelium
4 Bronchi
5 Bronchioles
6 Alveolar bronchioles
7 Alveoli

Also, after completing this chapter, you should understand the following:

1 The changes in epithelium throughout the entire respiratory tract
2 The histologic differences between bronchioles and bronchi
3 The components of the intra-alveolar wall
4 The importance of the alveolar wall in gas exchange

The respiratory system is divided into two functional portions. The first part is the conducting portion, and this consists of the nose, pharynx, larynx, trachea, and bronchi of varying sizes. These "tubes" connect the outside environment to that portion of the lungs where gas is exchanged, the respiratory portion. The respiratory portion is the lung.

Nose

The nose is a hollow organ with two openings or nares separated by a cartilaginous epithelial-lined septum. Covering the outside of the nose is skin, which is
(1) _____ _____
_____ epithelium and is made up of the stratum
(2) _____, stratum (3) _____, stratum
(4) _____, and stratum (5) _____, but
missing the stratum (6) _____ usually found only in thick skin (Fig.

1 keratinized stratified squamous
2 corneum
3 granulosum
4 spinosum
5 germinativum
6 lucidum

Respiratory System

7 corneum

8 spinosum

9 germinativum

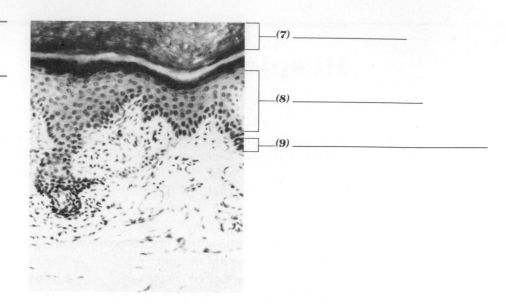

(7) _____

(8) _____

(9) _____

FIG. 15-1. Skin, hematoxylin-eosin (H and E) stain (original magnification ×150).

15-1). This skin continues into the nose for a short distance and has stiff hairs designed to filter large particles out of the inspired air. The nasal cavity is rich in goblet or *(10)* _____-secreting cells. Since this epithelium lines most of the conducting portion of the respiratory system, it is often called the respiratory epithelium.

Immediately beneath the *(11)* _____ epithelium of the nasal cavity is a *(12)* _____ propria rich in *(13)* _____ (*light, dark*)-staining mucus-secreting glands. These glands plus the *(14)* _____ cells in the epithelium help keep the epithelium lining moist. Certain areas of the nose have a lamina propria with a plethora of both *(15)* _____-secreting glands and blood plexuses. The plexuses serve to warm the inspired air while the glands *(16)* _____ the overlying epithelium.

A special type of epithelium, yellow in color, is located on parts of the roof high up in the nasal cavity. This epithelium is called the olfactory epithelium, and it forms the organ of olfaction (necessary for the sense of smell). Olfactory epithelium is nonkeratinized stratified squamous, and consists of three different types of cells, supporting or sustenacular, basal, and olfactory cells, which will not be discussed.

10 mucus

11 respiratory
12 lamina
13 light
14 goblet

15 mucus

16 moisten

Larynx

The larynx is an elongated tubal structure whose walls are made of hyaline and elastic cartilaginous rings, connective tissue, striated muscle, and an overlying mucosa (Fig. 15-2). The larynx framework is composed of thyroid, cricoid, corniculate, and cuneiform cartilage rings. (The names and muscle arrangements of the larynx need not be memorized.) Skeletal muscles pull on these cartilages from the outside; they are the extrinsic muscles of the larynx while the intrinsic muscles of the larynx, also *(17)* _____ muscle, join the cartilage rings. Through muscle tension, the lumen size is adjusted and the air passing through results in various sounds (phonation).

17 skeletal

Larynx

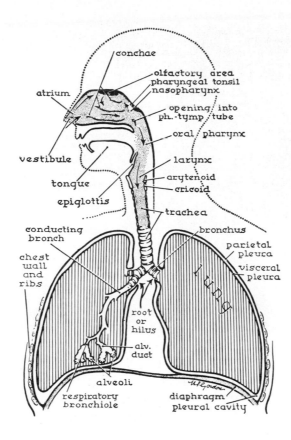

FIG. 15-2. Diagram of the respiratory system.

Histology of the Larynx

Humans are equipped with a flaplike structure, the epiglottis, which extends from the top of the larynx. It prevents food and liquid from passing from the (18) _____ pharynx into the larynx, instead of into the esophagus (the (19) _____ pharynx is continuous with both the respiratory and digestive systems). The epiglottis is in contact with the root of the tongue in the (20) _____ pharynx, and it is lined by oral pharyngeal epithelium, (21) _____ _____. Supported by an internal plate of elastic cartilage, the side of the epiglottis in contact with the larynx is covered by respiratory or (22) _____ _____ _____ epithelium. This epithelium at the base of the epiglottis clears mucus and debris away by (23) _____ beating up towards the pharynx.

The organ of sound production, the (24) _____, is composed of vocal cords (Fig. 15-3). At the top of the light micrograph is the base of the epiglottis, which is lined by (25) _____ _____ _____ or (26) _____ epithelium. Continuing downward is the first pair of folds, called the false vocal cord. The false vocal cord is covered by ciliated pseudostratified columnar epithelium with a connective tissue (27) _____ propria, and contains a fair amount of mucus-secreting glands.

18 *naso*

19 *naso*

20 *naso*

21 *nonkeratinized stratified squamous*

22 *ciliated pseudostratified columnar*

23 *cilia*

24 *larynx*

25 *ciliated pseudostratified columnar*

26 *respiratory*

27 *lamina*

28 *cartilage*

29 *false vocal cord*

30 *true vocal cord*

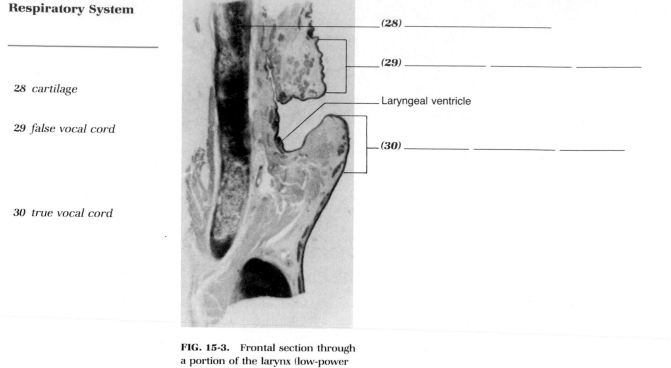

(28) _____

(29) _____ _____ _____

—— Laryngeal ventricle

(30) _____ _____ _____

FIG. 15-3. Frontal section through a portion of the larynx (low-power magnification).

Further down, there is a more prominent and histologically unique fold; this is the true vocal cord. Since the true vocal cord undergoes constant use in phonation, its covering epithelium is the "wear and tear"
(31) _____ _____
_____. Beneath this epithelium is a connective tissue layer, the
(32) _____ _____, which usually does not contain mucus-secreting glands, and is composed of elastic fibers that provide extra resiliency. Immediately below the connective tissue layer rich in **(33)** _____
fibers are **(34)** _____ muscle bundles connected to the
(35) _____ of the underlying cartilage. At the end of the true **(36)** _____ _____, the
(37) _____ _____
_____ epithelium abruptly becomes respiratory, or
(38) _____ _____
_____, epithelium, and **(39)** _____-secreting glands can be found again.

31 *nonkeratinized*
  stratified squamous
32 *lamina propria*

33 *elastic*
34 *skeletal*
35 *perichondrium*
36 *vocal cord*
37 *nonkeratinized*
  stratified squamous
38 *ciliated psuedostratified*
  columnar
39 *mucus*

Trachea

The larynx is confluent with the trachea, which divides into left and right smaller tubes called the bronchi. The trachea is roughly 2.5 cm wide in an adult. In an adult, U-shaped rings of cartilage prevent this tube from collapsing (Fig. 15-4). The U-shaped **(40)** _____ ring is seen easily on cross section, but on longitudinal view the ring appears as individual semicircular pairs of cartilage in a row. The area of trachea that has cartilage has a lining mucosa and a thin submucosa.

40 *cartilage*

Trachea

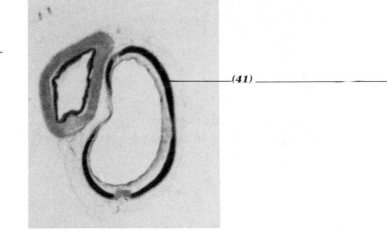

(41) _____

41 *cartilage*

FIG. 15-4. Cross-section through trachea and adjacent **(42)** _____.

Mucosa

Lining the tracheal lumen is **(43)** _____ _____ _____ or **(44)** _____ epithelium as in the **(45)** _____ (*true, false*) vocal cord. Rich in mucus-secreting **(46)** _____ cells, the trachea's epithelial cilia beat up toward the pharynx. The periodic acid–Schiff (PAS)–positive **(47)** _____ cells of the **(48)** _____ epithelium are slightly different in that after they have released their contents they will show visible microvilli in a "brush" pattern; therefore, they are often called brush cells (Fig. 15-5).

42 *esophagus*

43 *ciliated pseudostratified*
   columnar
44 *respiratory*
45 *false*
46 *goblet*
47 *goblet*
48 *respiratory*

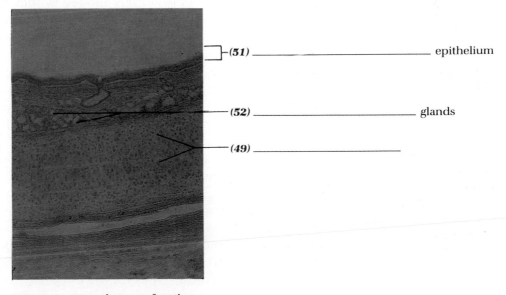

(51) _____ epithelium

(52) _____ glands

(49) _____

FIG. 15-5. Name the type of cartilage shown:
(50) _____. Name the type of glands shown:
(53) _____. Trachea, H and E stain (original magnification × 50).

49 *cartilage*
50 *hyaline*
51 *respiratory*
52 *epithelial*
53 *mucus*

Beneath the epithelium's basement membrane (which is the thickest basement membrane) is a very thin *(54)* _____ _____ layer rich in elastic fibers. Some lymphatic tissue is found here among the numerous small mucus-secreting glands.

54 lamina propria

Submucosa

The layer of tissue closest to the *(55)* _____ *(hyaline, elastic)* cartilage, aside from the immediately surrounding *(56)* _____ chondrium, is the submucosa. This contains the basal portions of some of the *(57)* _____- secreting cells of the overlying *(58)* _____ _____ layer.

55 hyaline
56 peri
57 mucus
58 lamina propria

Cartilage

The cartilage is *(59)* _____ *(hyaline, elastic)*, and is not a complete circle. The ends of the *(60)* __-shaped cartilage ring are joined at the posterior end of the trachea by bundles of regularly arranged *(61)* _____ muscle with interlacing fibroelastic connective tissue. This side of the tracheal lumen is *also* lined by *(62)* _____

_____ _____ epithelium, and has a lamina propria with *(63)* _____-secreting *(64)* _____. This arrangement of a *(65)* __-shaped *(66)* _____ ring joined by connective tissue and *(67)* _____ muscle bundles gives the trachea greater pliability than if it were a complete cartilaginous circle.

59 hyaline
60 U
61 striated

62 ciliated pseudostratified
  columnar
63 mucus
64 glands
65 U
66 cartilaginous
67 striated

Lungs

The trachea ends by dividing into right and left branches called the bronchi. The tubes directly off the trachea are called primary bronchi and enter the substance of the lungs. The right lung consists of three large lobes; the left is divided into two lobes. Each lobe is then further divided by thin connective tissue septa. The histologic examination of the lung starts with the primary *(68)* _____ and continues through progressively smaller tubes, concluding with the alveolar sacs and ducts.

68 bronchi

Primary Bronchi

Before the primary bronchi enter the lung (also called extrapulmonary bronchi) their histologic arrangement is virtually identical to that of the trachea: a *(69)* __-shaped *(70)* _____ *(hyaline, elastic)*, *(71)* _____ ring, lining *(72)* _____

_____ _____ epithelium; a thin *(73)* _____ propria; and an outer *(74)* _____ layer. Upon entering the lung tissue (at this stage the bronchi are now called intrapulmonary bronchi), the primary bronchi lose the *(75)* __ _____, and the cartilage becomes irregularly shaped, discontinuous plates (Fig. 15-6). Each

69 U
70 hyaline
71 cartilaginous
72 ciliated pseudostratified
  columnar
73 lamina
74 submucosal
75 "U" shape

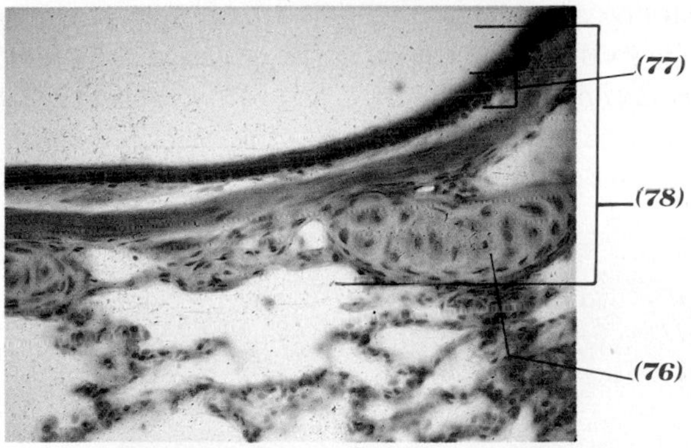

Lungs

FIG. 15-6. Portion of primary bronchus, H and
E stain (original magnification ×30).

76 hyaline cartilage
77 respiratory epithelium
 or ciliated
 pseudostratified
 columnar epithelium
78 intrapulmonary bronchi
79 pulmonary
80 pulmonary
81 respiratory
82 lamina propria
83 striated
84 discontinuous
85 more than one

86 pulmonary

87 smaller
88 mucus
89 respiratory

90 bronchi

91 primary

92 lung lobule

93 terminal
94 terminal
95 goblet
96 ciliated pseudostratified
 columnar
97 respiratory
98 ciliated columnar

99 endoplasmic

(79) __intra__ bronchus is lined by the same type of epithelium as the *(80)* __extra__ bronchi, that is,
(81) _____ epithelium. Beneath the lining epithelium is a
thin *(82)* _____ _____ that is surrounded by a
(83) _____ (*striated, smooth*) muscle layer. Since the cartilage of
the smaller bronchi is *(84)* _____ (*discontinuous, continuous*), one finds *(85)* _____ (*one, more than one*) area
of dense collagenous tissue connecting the cartilage. Lymph nodes and lymphatic nodules are scattered along the course of the bronchi.

The *(86)* __intra__ bronchi branch into smaller and
smaller bronchi. The bronchi differ only in the amount of cartilage in their wall,
which decreases as the bronchi become *(87)* _____ (*smaller, larger*).
(88) _____-secreting glands are found beneath the
(89) _____ epithelium of all bronchi. The smallest
branches of the bronchi are called bronchioles.

Bronchioles
Bronchioles arise from the smallest *(90)* _____ as they enter the
functional unit of the lung, the primary (or lung) lobule. The lung lobule is a
small pyramidal area of the lung parenchyma composed of bronchioles and the
respiratory portion of the lung: alveolar ducts, sacs, and alveoli with associated
blood vessels, lymphatics, and nerves. The lung lobule or *(91)* _____
lobule is the area of gas exchange.

After the bronchioles enter the primary or *(92)* _____ _____,
they are termed preterminal bronchioles; these in turn give rise to terminal
bronchioles. Bronchioles differ histologically and physiologically from bronchi.
Bronchioles, both *(93)* __pre__ and *(94)* _____,
are lined by ciliated *columnar* epithelium with mucus-secreting
(95) _____ cells, whereas bronchi are lined by *(96)* _____
_____ _____ epithelium or
(97) _____ epithelium (Fig. 15-7). The epithelium of the
bronchioles, *(98)* _____ _____, is thinner than
bronchial epithelium, and contains a few scattered nonciliated serum-secreting
tall columnar cells, Clara cells (not readily visible in a photomicrograph). Clara
cells are rich in smooth *(99)* _____ reticulum (sER) and
mitochondria, but the exact nature of their secretion is unknown. Bordering the
epithelium of the bronchioles is a lamina propria rich in elastic fibers, sur-

rounded by a very thin connective tissue layer. Also, the bronchioles *do not* have cartilage in their walls, **(100)** _____ (*like, unlike*) bronchi. Finally, bronchioles *do not* have **(101)** _____-secreting glands beneath the lining **(102)** _____ _____ epithelium. (You should finish #104 at this point.)

100 unlike
101 mucus
102 ciliated columnar

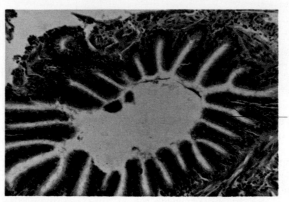

— **(104)** _____

_____

epithelium

FIG. 15-7. Illustration shows
(103) _____ (*bronchiole, bronchus*). H and E stain (original magnification × 225).

Preterminal bronchioles give rise to **(105)** _____

103 bronchiole
104 ciliated columnar

_____, and these in turn branch into respiratory bronchioles. These are short tubes proximally lined by the usual bronchiolar epithelium, **(106)** _____ _____ epithelium. The respiratory bronchiolar epithelium loses its cilia distally, and the epithelium becomes a low cuboidal type. The walls of the respiratory bronchioles are composed of collagenous **(107)** _____ _____ bundles with interlacing smooth muscle bundles and elastic fibers. A few delicate outpocketings of the respiratory bronchioles gives rise to the majority of the alveolar sacs (Fig. 15-8).

105 terminal bronchioles

106 ciliated columnar

107 connective tissue

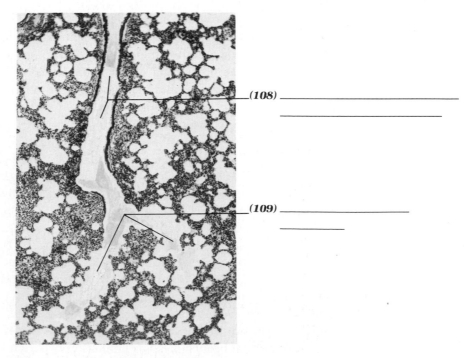

(108) _____

_____

108 respiratory bronchiole

(109) _____

_____

109 alveolar duct

FIG. 15-8. Lung, H and E stain (low-power magnification).

Lungs

The alveolar ducts, sacs, and the individual alveoli make up the respiratory portion of the lung, whereas the bronchi and bronchioles serve to conduct air from the trachea. The *(110)* _____ ducts and *(111)* _____ sacs are intimately involved in gas exchange.

110 alveolar
111 alveolar

Alveolar Ducts

Branches of the respiratory bronchioles, alveolar *(112)* _____ are difficult to distinguish precisely in a light micrograph (see Fig. 15-8). Because the alveolar duct is highly tortuous and its wall beset by closely packed sacs, a cross section will rarely show its tubular nature but will instead reveal an elongated empty space (Fig. 15-9). The wall of the alveolar duct between the openings of alveolar

112 ducts

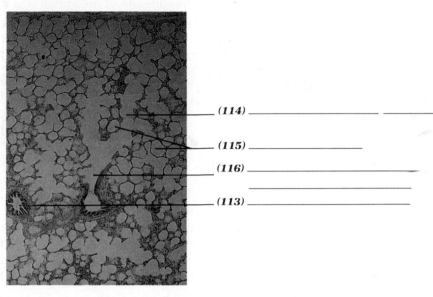

(114) _____ _____

(115) _____

(116) _____

_____

(113) _____

113 bronchiole
114 alveolar duct
115 alveoli
116 respiratory bronchiole

FIG. 15-9. Lung, H and E stain (original magnification ×15).

sacs consists of a thin lining squamous epithelium resting on a very thin strand of elastic and collagenous fibers with few smooth muscle cells. Alveolar ducts give rise to a single alveolar sac, which consists of two to four alveoli. The space between the ends of the duct and the beginning of the sac is the atrium. The histology of the sacs and individual alveoli is very important.

Alveoli

Alveoli, which make up the *(117)* _____ sacs, are thin-walled polyhedral sacs that are intimately involved in gas *(118)* _____. Before a discussion of the various cells lining the alveoli, an understanding of the supportive interalveolar wall is necessary (Fig. 15-10). Even under the highest

117 alveolar
118 exchange

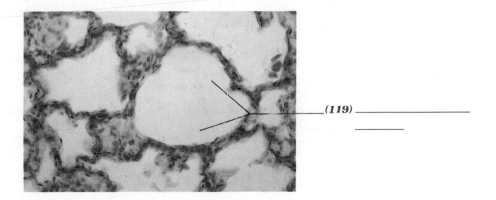

(119) _____

_____

119 alveoli sac

FIG. 15-10. Lung, H and E stain (original magnification ×75).

photomicrographic power, it is difficult to identify the various components of the interalveolar wall. The bulk of the wall is made up of a network of the thinnest and smallest blood vessels, *(120)* _____. These vessels (which have a few red blood cells in their lumina) bulge into the lumen of the interalveolar wall. Coursing through this *(121)* <u>inter</u>_____ wall, these blood vessels are supported by a thin elastic and reticular network. Elastic fibers compose most of the framework of the blood vessels and the rest of the wall. This wall is not continuous, and small pores are found connecting adjacent individual *(122)* _____. These minute openings, 7 μm to 9 μm, possibly provide collateral circulation throughout the lung lobule or *(123)* _____ _____.

Lining the respiratory lumina of the alveoli is a continuous epithelium resting on top of a basement *(124)* _____. The lining epithelium consists of two very different types of cells (Fig. 15-11). The most numerous cells,

120 capillaries

121 alveolar

122 alveoli

123 primary lobule

124 membrane

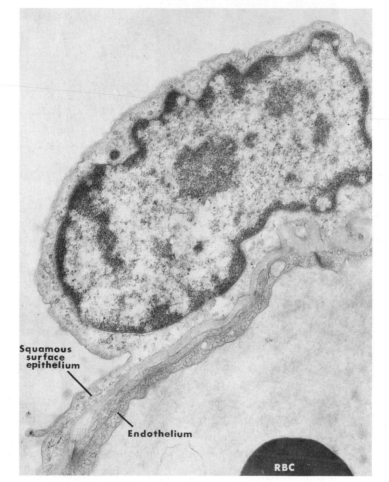

Squamous surface epithelium

Endothelium

RBC

FIG. 15-11. Electron micrograph (EM) of a squamous epithelial cell. Type I pneumonocyte of a cat. RBC = red blood cell.

type I pneumonocytes or pulmonary epithelial cells, are squamous epithelial cells.

Extremely thin—it is difficult to visualize the cytoplasm even with electron microscopy (EM)—type I *(125)* _____ or *(126)* _____ _____ _____ form a continuous lining, and are identified by their bright-staining flattened nuclei. Resting on a *(127)* _____ _____, type I *(128)* _____ can be properly visualized only with EM.

125 pneumonocytes
126 pulmonary epithelial cells

127 basement membrane

128 pneumonocytes

Lungs

The second type of cell lining the alveoli is the less numerous and larger type II pneumonocyte or secretory epithelial cell (Fig. 15-12). Often cuboidal in

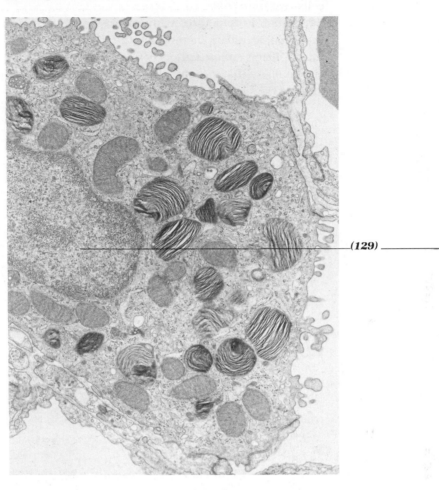

FIG. 15-12. EM of a secretory epithelial cell. Type II pneumonocyte of a cat.

129 nucleus

130 pneumonocytes

131 pneumonocytes

132 pulmonary epithelial
cells

133 desmosomes

134 pneumonocytes

135 secretory epithelial
cells

136 dust cell

137 cilia

138 respiratory

139 pneumonocytes

140 pulmonary epithelial
cells

shape, type II **(130)** _____ project into the alveolar space and are connected to adjacent type I

(131) _____ or **(132)** _____

_____ _____ by spot junctions or

(133) _____. The phospholipid secretion of type II

(134) _____ or **(135)** _____

_____ _____ plays an important role in respiration.

A third type of cell is found bulging into almost every alveolar space—the alveolar phagocyte or "dust cell." Because the cell is highly phagocytic, it engulfs particles (such as dust), and hence it is called the **(136)** _____ _____.
Eventually these cells migrate up to the bronchioles and bronchi and by the beating of the **(137)** _____ on the **(138)** _____ _____ epithelium, they are removed in sputum.

As the physiological importance of the alveoli is to transfer oxygen to the oxygen-depleted cells and remove carbon dioxide, the barrier between the blood vessel and alveolar space should be reviewed. Lining the alveoli space are the two types of cells, type I **(139)** _____ or

(140) _____ _____ _____, and type

Respiratory System

141 pneumonocyte
142 secretory epithelial
      cells
143 basement membrane

144 endothelial

II (141) _____ or (142) _____
_____ _____, which make up the first barrier. These
cells rest on a (143) _____ _____, the second bar-
rier, which in turn fuses with the basement membrane of the capillary, forming
the alveolocapillary membrane (the third barrier). The last barrier is the wall of
the capillary, composed of (144) _____ cells. Reticular and
elastic fibers that support the blood vessels are interspersed throughout these
four barriers.

16   Urinary System

After completing this chapter, you should be able to identify the following:

1 Cortex and medulla of the kidney
2 Glomeruli
3 Proximal and distal tubules
4 Loop of Henle
5 Macula densa area
6 Collecting tubules
7 Ureter
8 Bladder

Also, after completing this chapter, you should understand the following:

1 The histologic differences between proximal and distal tubules
2 The histologic aspects of filtration in the glomerulus
3 The blood supply throughout the kidney
4 The juxtaglomerular apparatus and its unique histologic aspects
5 The importance of transitional epithelium

The kidneys, ureters, and urinary bladder are the components of the urinary system. Functionally, the urinary system filters out the metabolic wastes found in the blood, regulates the concentrations of the body fluids (an endocrine function intimately involved in blood pressure and blood formation), and acts as a passageway for excreting body waste.

Kidney

There is no organ in the human body as complex, histologically or physiologically, as the kidney. Grossly, the kidney is a bean-shaped organ with an indentation called the hilus. At the hilus, there is a ureter and renal vein exiting and a renal artery entering. If one cuts away the thin but strong connective tissue capsule and superficial tissue of the kidney, one can see that this organ is divided into two chief zones. The cortex or outermost zone of the kidney follows the contour of the kidney. The second region of the kidney, the inner zone, is pyramidal and is called the medulla

Cortex

The cortex, the **(1)** _____ (outermost, innermost) region of the kidney, consists primarily of the main filtering apparatus of the kidney, the glomerulus (see below) and its associated tubules. Also, the cortex is penetrated by areas of medullary tissue that subdivide the area into separate regions. The medullary tissues or rays do not reach the surface of the kidney, but each ray and its immediately associated cortical tissue is called a renal lobule. Seen under

1 outermost

2 glomerulus

3 cortex

4 medulla

the lowest power, the cortex has a granular appearance caused by the
(2) _____ and its associated tubules (Fig. 16-1). This zone is
easily separated by the lighter staining and more striated appearing medullary
rays.

Medullary rays

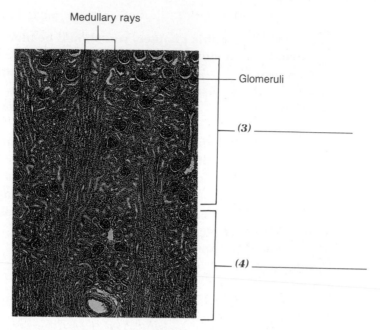

Glomeruli

(3) _____

(4) _____

FIG. 16-1. Kidney. Hematoxylin-
eosin (H and E) stain (original magnification ×30).

Medulla

5 inner

6 pyramid

7 medullary
8 medullary
9 cortex

On the other hand, the medulla or **(5)** _____most region of the kidney
consists of tubules running a straight course and no glomeruli. Essentially, the
medulla is made up of 8 to 18 lobes or conical subdivisions called renal pyramids, each projecting toward the hilus. Each renal **(6)** _____ is separated laterally by inward extensions of cortical substance. These extensions are
called renal columns of Bertin and can be thought of as cortical tissue in the
medulla; **(7)** _____ rays, however, can be thought of as
(8) _____ tissue in the **(9)** _____. Examining the me-
dulla under low power, one can easily identify the subdivisions (see Fig. 16-1). In
addition to its lateral subdivisions, the medulla is also divided horizontally; an
outermost zone next to the cortical tissue and a lighter staining inner region
nearest the hilus called the papillae. In the third zone of the medulla, the
collecting tubules coalesce and drain into specific collecting outpocketings at or
near the hilus. This region is noted by its light-staining characteristics and the
marked uniformity (see below).

 The kidney is therefore divided into a large outermost
(10) _____ region and an innermost **(11)** _____
region. The cortex is penetrated by medullary tissue called the
(12) _____ _____, and this tissue and its adjacent cortical
tissue are called the **(13)** _____ _____. Also, the granular appearance is due to the **(14)** _____; the medullary region is
(15) _____ in appearance and has **(16)** _____ (one, two, three)
horizontal zones.

 Each kidney is composed of 2 million to 3 million tubules. These tubules are
divided into two portions. The first portion is called the nephron, and it is

10 cortical
11 medullary
12 medullary rays
13 renal lobule
14 glomeruli
15 striated
16 three

Kidney

concerned with the filtering of waste and the ultimate formation of urine. The second portion is called the collecting tubule, and its function is to concentrate the urinary solution before it flows into the ureter.

Nephron

There are an estimated *(17)* ___ million to ___ million nephrons in each kidney. Each nephron consists of four physiologically and histologically distinct areas: renal glomerulus, proximal tubule, loop of Henle, and distal tubule. All four areas are continuous, starting with the renal *(18)* _____ and ending with the distal *(19)* _____.

17 2-3

At the tubule's most proximal end, there is a very thin-walled expansion called Bowman's capsule (Fig. 16-2). This capsule surrounds a tuft of capillaries that is called the glomerulus. The tubules plus the capillary tuft or *(20)* _____ is called the renal *(21)* _____ or renal corpuscle. Renal corpuscles are found for the most part in the *(22)* _____ of the kidney, giving that region its *(23)* _____ appearance. (You should finish #24 at this point.)

18 glomeruli
19 tubule

20 glomerulus
21 capsule
22 cortex
23 granular

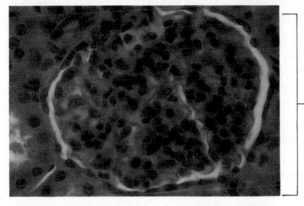

_ *(24)* _____

24 glomerulus

FIG. 16-2.   Kidney, H and E stain (original magnification ×350).

Closer examination of the corpuscle or renal *(25)* _____ reveals an intimate and very detailed relationship between the blood vessels and the urinary tubules (Fig. 16-3). Bowman's *(26)* _____, tubules that surround a tuft of *(27)* _____, is composed of a double wall of squamous epithelium. Since Bowman's *(28)* _____ is essentially a hollow tube, it has one layer of the *(29)* _____ epithelium applied to the *(30)* _____ tuft; this layer is called the visceral layer. The outer layer of the capsule is called the capsular epithelium or parietal epithelium, and this too is composed of *(31)* _____ epithelium. Between these two layers, the parietal or *(32)* _____ and the *(33)* _____ layers, is a space called the capsular or, more commonly, Bowman's space. (You should finish #37 at this point.)

25 capsule

26 capsule
27 capillaries
28 capsule
29 squamous
30 capillary

31 squamous
32 capsular
33 visceral

Urinary System

(36) _____

_____

_____

(34) _____

epithelium

(35) _____

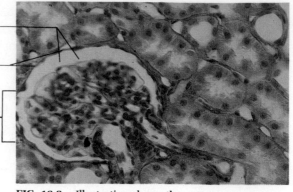

34 squamous
35 glomeruli
36 Bowman's space

FIG. 16-3. Illustration shows the
(37) _____ (cortical, medullary) area of
the kidney. Kidney, Mallory azan stain (original magnification ×220).

37 cortical

Examining the histology of the renal glomerulus, it is easiest to understand it in terms of how the filtration process works. Three layers compose the barrier: the endothelium of the glomerular capillary; the basement membranes of the capillary endothelium; and the (38) _____ (visceral, parietal) layers.

As mentioned in the chapter on the Cardiovascular System the endothelium of the capillaries in the kidney is (39) _____ (continuous, noncontinuous), and (40) _____ (is, is not) covered by a thin diaphragm. The (41) _____ (absence, presence) of the diaphragm allows for a tremendous (42) _____ (increase, decrease) in filtration through the capillaries.

38 visceral

39 noncontinuous
40 is not
41 absence
42 increase

An unusual component of this filtration barrier is the basement membrane. This membrane is unique in that it is quite thick and has three distinct layers. The three layers are appropriately named—the innermost to the capillary is the lamina rara interna, followed by a highly electron-dense line called the lamina densa, and the outermost, the lamina rare externa. The glomerular basement (43) _____, consisting of the (44) _____ _____ externa, (45) _____ _____, and the (46) _____ _____ _____, has a collagen component giving it tensile strength.

While the cells of the capsular or (47) _____ layer of Bowman's (48) _____ are typical (49) _____ epithelium, the cells of the outermost layer, the (50) _____ layer, are not. These cells are so modified that they assume the shape of a foot, and therefore are called podocytes. Podocytes assume an intimate relationship with the capillary's (51) _____ _____ (Fig. 16-4). The main body

43 membrane
44 lamina rara
45 lamina densa
46 lamina rara interna
47 parietal
48 capsule
49 squamous
50 visceral

51 basement membrane

Kidney

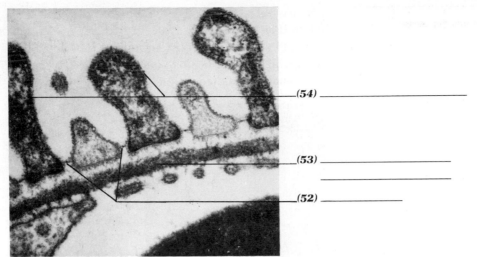

(54) _____

(53) _____
_____

(52) _____

FIG. 16-4. Electron micrograph (EM) of the glomerular filtration barrier.

52 *slits*
53 *basement membrane*
54 *podocytes*

of the podocyte is not in direct contact with the outermost segment of the capillary's (55) _____ _____, the (56) _____ _____ _____. The podocyte is separated from the membrane by a space filled with filtrate. This space (often called the subpodocyte space) is continuous with the main (57) _____ space, more commonly called (58) _____ space. Extending from the main cell body of the podocyte are minor processes interdigitating with small spaces visible between these processes, which are called filtration slits or slit pores. Covering each filtration slit is a slit diaphragm.

55 *basement membrane*
56 *lamina rara externa*

57 *capsular*
58 *Bowman's*

Associated with the capillary surface and not adjacent to the epithelial cells are mesangial cells. Mesangial cells are found in the areas between contiguous capillaries where there is the supporting epithelial wall of the (59) _____ (*capsular, visceral*) layer of the (60) _____ capsule. These mesangial cells lend support to the capillaries by the production of intercellular ground substance. Stellate in shape, the mesangial cells reveal that the cell is an undifferentiated smooth muscle cell like the (61) _____cytes of certain capillaries. Besides providing support, the mesangial cells are also phagocytic.

59 *visceral*
60 *Bowman's*

Blood vessels that enter the capsule and remove blood from it are called the afferent and efferent vessels, respectively. These vessels enter the capsule at what is called the vascular pole. Blood flowing *to* the capillary tuft by way of the (62) _____ arteriole will have its wastes filtered out. Waste must *first* pass through the (63) _____ and then through the three layers of the capillary (64) _____ _____: the (65) _____ _____, (66) _____ _____, and the (67) _____ _____ _____, and in that order.

61 *peri*

62 *afferent*
63 *endothelium*
64 *basement membrane*
65 *lamina rara interna*
66 *lamina densa*
67 *lamina rara externa*

Proximal Convoluted Tubules

The filtrate flows out of the glomeruli into the proximal (68) _____ tubule (PCT). Where the capsular or (69) _____ epithelium of (70) _____'s (71) _____ becomes confluent with the PCT is an area called the

68 *convoluted*
69 *parietal*
70 *Bowman's*
71 *capsule*

urinary pole. Capsular epithelium is *(72)* _____ while that of the PCT is *(73)* _____. The PCT is identified in two ways: First, the PCT will stain more eosinophilic than any other tubule; second, under high power a conspicuous border is found *only on* the PCT and not on the distal convoluted tubule (Fig. 16-5).

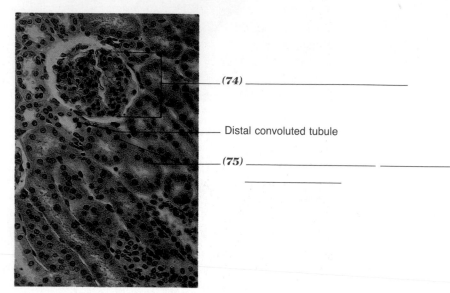

(74) _____

— Distal convoluted tubule

(75) _____ _____
_____

FIG. 16-5. Kidney, H and E stain (original magnification ×210).

The PCT is divided into two portions: a convoluted first portion and a distal straight portion. The first portion of the proximal tubule, the *(76)* _____ _____, pursues a tortuous course in the immediate vicinity of the glomerulus, and therefore the same PCT can be found numerous times in the same section. The proximal part of the PCT, the *(77)* _____ (*convoluted, straight*) portion (the PT), courses toward the medullary rays where it straightens out and runs toward the *(78)* _____ area of the kidney. The proximal tubules, which stain *(79)* _____ (*more, less*) eosinophilic than the distal tubules, are composed of *(80)* _____ epithelium. Each cell contains a single spherical nucleus with a normal complement of organelles. Extensive interdigitation between the cells of the PT makes it difficult to delineate individual cell borders. The microvilli that make up the *(81)* _____ _____ border are long and closely packed. Electron microscopy (EM) has revealed the existence of extensive tubular invaginations between the microvilli. These invaginations, apical canaliculi, are most probably involved in the reabsorption of filtrate that so characterizes the function of the tubule. From proximal to distal tubule, the microvilli decrease in number with less cell-to-cell interdigitation and less apical *(82)* _____, indicating a *(83)* _____ (*greater, lesser*) capacity for reabsorption of the filtrate.

Loop of Henle

The PCT originates at the *(84)* _____ pole and forms at its most distal segment the loop of Henle's thick descending limb. The loops of Henle are either short or long; 80% to 85% of all loops that extend from the cortical region are short. These short loops do not extend into the medulla. Loops that arise

Kidney

---

from glomeruli nearest the medullary area (called juxtamedullary glomeruli) have long loops that extend deep into the medulla. As the PCT travels toward the medulla (it is now called the PT), *(85)* _____ epithelium, with its short but evident microvilli forming the *(86)* _____ border, is abruptly terminated. Squamous epithelium replaces the *(87)* _____ epithelium of the PCT, and the lumen becomes quite narrow. Nuclei of the squamous epithelium bulge into the lumen and the loops of Henle are quite often mistaken for capillaries. This aforementioned area is the thin segment of the loop of Henle, its epithelium, *(88)* _____, contains *(89)* _____ *(many, no)* microvilli and *(90)* _____ *(flattened, bulging)* nuclei, and resembles the small blood vessel, the *(91)* _____ (Fig. 16-6). It is easiest to find the

85 cuboidal
86 brush
87 cuboidal

88 squamous
89 no
90 bulging
91 capillary

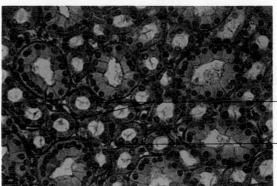

(93) _____

_____

(92) _____

FIG. 16-6. Kidney, H and E stain (original magnification ×220).

92 capillary (thin loop of Henle)
93 thick segment (of loop of Henle)

thin segment of the loop of Henle in the medullary area of the kidney. Often these loops are found to extend to the apex of each *(94)* _____ pyramid.

As the loop turns and begins an upward course through the medulla, the thin *(95)* _____ epithelium gives way to a wider tubule with thicker walls called the thick segment of the ascending limb of the loop of Henle. Usually, the place where the thin-walled loop gives way to the thicker segment marks the beginning of the outer or *(96)* _____ *(darker, lighter)* staining region. The outer zone stains the way it does because its constituents are thicker. The loop itself is composed of *(97)* _____ epithelium, but the thicker walls of the ascending segment of the *(98)* _____ ____ _____ are like those of the PCT, *(99)* _____ _____.
The thick ascending segment is confluent with the distal tubule and is essentially identical histologically.

94 renal

95 squamous

96 darker

97 squamous
98 loop of Henle
99 cuboidal epithelium

Distal Tubule
The distal tubule (DT) is shorter and thinner than the proximal tubule and *(100)* _____ *(has, does not have)* microvilli, and therefore *(101)* _____ *(does, does not)* have a brush border (Fig. 16-7). Composed of three parts—a straight portion, an area next to the glomeruli, and a convoluted portion—the DT functions in reabsorption but not to the degree the proximal tubule does.

100 does not have
101 does not

102 *distal*

103 *proximal*

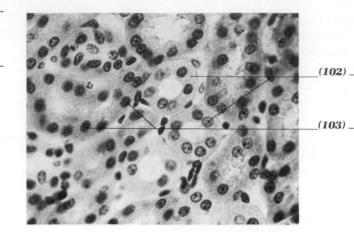

(102) _____ tubule

(103) _____ tubule

FIG. 16-7. Kidney, H and E stain (original magnification ×310).

The first portion of the DT, the **(104)** _____ portion, begins in the **(105)** _____ *(outer, inner)* zone of the **(106)** _____ region of the kidney and forms the thick ascending limb of the **(107)** _____ _____. As the DT travels up toward the granular portion or **(108)** _____ of the kidney, it passes the glomeruli and forms an area with the afferent arteriole that is crucial in human hemodynamics. This area is called the macula densa, and it is identifiable in a light micrograph (Fig. 16-8).

104 *straight*
105 *outer*
106 *medullary*
107 *loop of Henle*
108 *cortex*

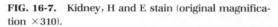

(110) _____
_____

(111) _____

(109) _____
_____

Macula densa

FIG. 16-8. Kidney. Macula densa. Mallory–Azan stain (original magnification ×220).

109 *proximal tubule*
110 *distal tubule*
111 *glomerulus*

Essentially, the macula densa consists of a modification of the DT's own cells. These cells are adjacent to special cells in the afferent arteriole's wall.

The afferent arteriole's tunica media consists usually of **(112)** _____ _____ cells, but it is different in the macula densa region. The cells are modified; filaments are replaced by granules and the nucleus is rounded. These cells are called juxtaglomerular cells or JG cells. JG cells are more basophilic than the surrounding cells and therefore rich in rough **(113)** _____ _____.

112 *smooth muscle*

Two other modifications of the arteriole wall are also evident. The intenal elastic lamina, the border separating the **(114)** _____ _____ and the **(115)** _____ _____, is absent when JG cells or **(116)** _____ cells are present. Also absent is the basement membrane of the adjacent DT. The macula densa of the DT and the JG

113 *endoplasmic reticulum*

114 *tunica interna*
115 *tunica media*
116 *juxtaglomerular*

Kidney

117 arteriole

118 macula
119 distal tubule

120 complex

121 JG
122 internal elastic lamina
123 interna
124 media
125 erythro

126 juxtaglomerular
127 convoluted tubule

128 nephron

129 collecting

130 cuboidal

131 lightly

132 loops of Henle
133 thick

cells of the afferent *(117)* _____ and its modifications together constitute the juxtaglomerular apparatus or complex. The intimate relationship between the *(118)* _____ densa of the *(119)* _____ _____ and the cells of the arteriole is evident by the *absence* of a basement membrane separating them (not visible in a photomicrograph).

The JG apparatus or *(120)* _____ is important physiologically. Changes in blood pressure and body fluids can lead to release of the granules in the *(121)* __ __ cells. Since there is no *(122)* _____ _____ _____ separating the tunica *(123)* _____ and tunica *(124)* _____, the JG cells easily secrete the granules into the bloodstream. The JG granules contain the hormone renin, and, as we have already learned, this hormone causes an increase in *(125)* _____poesis.

After the DT passes the glomeruli and forms the *(126)* _____ apparatus, it becomes contorted and forms the distal *(127)* _____ _____ (DCT).

Collecting Tubule

The DCT is short and descends into the medullary region of the cortex. The DCT coursing inward represents the last segment of the *(128)* _____ (*nephron, collecting apparatus*). The first part of the second system of tubules, the *(129)* _____ tubule, is the arch collecting tubule (Fig. 16-9). The arch collecting tubule is a tributary of the larger straight collecting tubules located in the medullary ray. These collecting tubules are composed of epithelium not unlike that of the DT, *(130)* _____ epithelium. Collecting tubular epithelial cells are far more distinctly outlined, and can be distinguished from the DT on this basis. While both the DT and collecting tubules (CT) stain *(131)* _____ (*lightly, heavily*) eosinophilic, the CT epithelia have a single flagellum on each cell. You should realize that the bulk of the inner zone and much of the outer zone of the medullary region consist mainly of the CTs and *(132)* _____ _____ with its thin and *(133)* _____ limbs. (You should finish #136 at this point.)

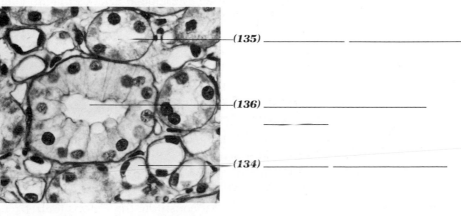

(135) _____ _____

(136) _____ _____

(134) _____ _____

FIG. 16-9. Kidney, H & E stain (high-power magnification).

134 thin segment
135 thick segment
136 collecting duct

As the straight collecting tubules run inward they merge and form larger ducts, 100 μm to 200 μm in diameter and are often called the papillary ducts of Bellini. The papillary ducts of (137) _____ are found mainly in the inner zone of the medullary region and can be identified by their large lumina. At the apex of each pyramid of the papilla, there is an area riddled with these large (138) _____ _____ _____ _____, and it is called the area cribosa. These large ducts contain epithelium of a columnar nature with nuclei in a row. The area cribosa stains (139) _____ (*light, dark*) because of the (140) _____ (*pale, dark*)-staining nature of the collecting tubules.

137 *Bellini*

138 *papillary ducts of Bellini*

139 *lightly*

140 *pale*

Finally, at the kidney's innermost region nearest the hilum, the collecting tubules empty into (141) _____ _____ _____ _____, and those in turn empty into minor calyces and then the major calyces. The calyces are large outpocketings lined by transitional epithelium; the large holes stand out in comparison to the very crowded nature of the rest of the organ. From the minor to the major calyces, the urine flows out of the kidney at the (142) _____ (region) by way of the ureter to the bladder.

141 *papillary ducts of Bellini*

142 *hilus*

Blood Supply of the Kidney

The blood supply of the kidney is intimately involved in the concentration of urine and the maintenance of body fluid homeostasis. The discussion of the histologic arrangement of the blood system will be discussed but not the important physiological implications.

The renal arteries enter the kidney at the (143) _____, and immediately divide into two branches that give off smaller arteries called interlobar arteries. As their name implies, the interlobar arteries travel between the (144) _____ pyramids and the (145) _____ lobes of the kidney. At the corticomedullary junction, arcuate arteries are formed, and these travel between the two *main* areas of the kidney, the (146) _____ and the (147) _____. Small interlobular arteries branch off from the arcuate arteries, and they course toward the kidney's surface.

143 *hilus*

144 *renal*

145 *renal*

146 *cortex*

147 *medulla*

It is from these interlobular arteries that an afferent arteriole arises, and this supplies the (148) _____. The efferent arteriole drains the (149) _____. These arteries are found at the (150) _____ pole. The efferent arterioles of the outer cortex immediately divide into cortical interlobular capillaries. The efferent arterioles of the juxtaglomeruli have a large lumen and, as they pass downward into the medulla, they form the counterpart to the (151) _____ _____ _____ and become known as the vasa recta.

148 *glomerulus*

149 *glomerulus*

150 *vascular*

Vasa recta are blood vessels larger than capillaries. They are found in the outer and inner zones of the (152) _____ area of the kidney. Penetrating deep into the (153) _____ region, the vasa recta then form hairpin loops and continue upward into the cortex. The vasa recta that turn backward constitute the venous limb. Except for the venous limb of the vasa recta in which the endothelium is fenestrated and not continuous like the capillaries in the kidney, the blood system of the kidney is histologically unremarkable (Fig. 16-10). *Do not* expect to be able to identify the specific veins and

151 *loops of Henle*

152 *medullary*

153 *medullary*

Blood Supply of
the Kidney

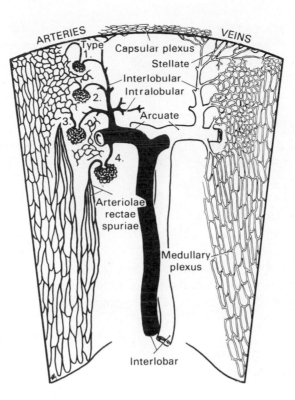

FIG. 16-10. Diagram of the blood supply to the kidney.

arteries, but realize that interlobular arteries coursing between renal

(154) _____ and lobes form arcuate arteries and the

(155) _____ arteriole that supplies the

(156) _____. Also remember that the *(157)* _____ recta

are found in the *(158)* _____ (*cortex, medulla*) and are the vascular

counterpart of the *(159)* _____ ___ _____.

154 *pyramids*
155 *afferent*
156 *glomerulus*
157 *vasa*
158 *medulla*
159 *loops of Henle*

Ureters

Urine formed in the kidney flows from the PT down through the *(160)* _____

____ _____ into the straight part of the *(161)* _____ tubule into

the *(162)* _____ tubules and then into the minor

(163) _____, then into the *(164)* _____ _____,

and finally into ureters at the *(165)* _____ of the kidney. The ureter wall is

made of three coats: a lining mucous membrane, a middle muscular coat, and an

outer adventitia.

160 *loop of Henle*
161 *distal*
162 *collecting*
163 *calyces*
164 *major calyces*
165 *hilus*

Mucous Membrane

The ureter is unlike the highly developed mucous membrane of the gastrointes-

tinal (GI) tract, which is composed of three layers, a lining

(166) _____, *(167)* _____ _____, and

(168) _____ _____. The ureter is missing the

outermost layer, the *(169)* _____ _____ (Fig. 16-11).

166 *epithelium*
167 *lamina propria*
168 *muscularis mucosa*
169 *muscularis mucosa*

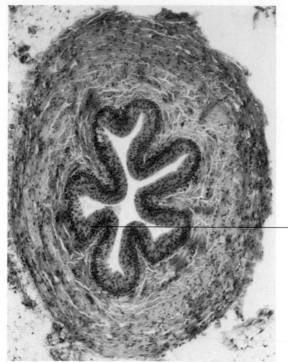

_____(170) _____
                  _____

170 *transitional epithelium*

FIG. 16-11. Ureter, H and E stain (low-power magnification).

From the calyces down to the bladder, all the structures are lined by
(171) _____ epithelium. The epithelium is four to five
cells thick in the ureter, and rests on a fairly dense connective tissue layer called
the *(172)* _____ _____. Not infrequently, one will find a
lymphatic nodule complete with a primary nodule and
(173) _____ nodule (identified by a *(174)* _____
center). Except where the ureter is in the renal pelvis, the mucous membrane is
thrown into numerous folds and gives a starfish appearance in cross section.
Transitional epithelium and the distensibility of the ureter make it possible to
increase the size of the lumen.

171 *transitional*

172 *lamina propria*

173 *secondary*
174 *germinal*

Muscular Coat
The muscular coat of the ureter consists of inner longitudinal
(175) _____ muscle fibers and outer circular *(176)* _____ muscle fibers. This inner and outer muscle arrangement is the exact opposite of that
found in the GI tract. This arrangement is only in the proximal two thirds of the
ureter. In the lower third, a third muscle layer is added on, and it is longitudinally arranged, as is the *(177)* _____ (*inner, outer*) layer of
(178) _____ muscle.

175 *smooth*
176 *smooth*

Adventitia
The adventitia is the *(179)* _____ (*innermost, outermost*) coat of
the ureter, and consists of fibroelastic connective tissue. At the region where the
ureter penetrates the bladder, both ureteral and bladder mucosal folds act as
valves in order to prevent retrograde flow of urine.

177 *inner*
178 *smooth*

179 *outermost*

Urinary Bladder

The urinary bladder is constructed for tremendous distension and easy relaxation. The bladder wall is made up of four layers: a mucous membrane, a submucosa, a muscular coat, and an adventitia.

Mucous Membrane

The lining epithelium of the bladder is *(180)* _____ _____ epithelium, and it is 11 to 14 cells thick. The epithelium stretches when the bladder is distended. Bladder distension causes flattening of the superficial cell layers to the point that they look like *(181)* _____ epithelium and the underlying cells become cuboidal (Fig. 16-12). EM reveals thickened plaques on the luminal surface of the cells. These plaques fill in the irregular contour of the bladder epithelium when the bladder is relaxed, and therefore prevent urine seepage. Tight junctions or *(182)* _____ _____ between epithelial cells of the bladder aid in further waterproofing of the lumen. (You should finish #185 at this point.)

180 transitional

181 squamous

182 zonula occludens

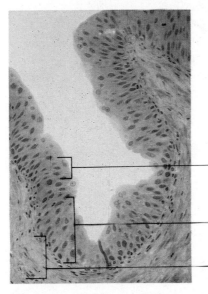

(183) _____ _____

(184) _____
_____

(185) _____ _____

183 squamous cell

184 transitional epithelium

185 lamina propria

FIG. 16-12. Bladder, H and E stain (original magnification ×175).

Submucosa

Beneath the epithelium lies the connective tissue layer, the *(186)* _____ _____, rich in *(187)* _____ fibers. This layer easily merges with the submucosal layer immediately below it. The submucosa of the bladder is rich in elastic fibers, and this is the *(188)* _____ *(least, most)* prominent layer in the bladder wall. The elastic fibers enable the bladder wall to assume great folds when the bladder is *(189)* _____ *(contracted, relaxed)*.

The bladder's muscular coat is clearly *not* organized into well-defined bundles. Instead, the muscular coat consists of three ill-defined muscle layers: an inner *(190)* _____ *(smooth, skeletal)* longitudinal band, a middle *(191)* _____ *(smooth, skeletal)* circular, and a prominent external *(192)* _____ *(smooth, skeletal)* longitudinal band. This layer arrangement is identical to that of the *(193)* _____ *(lower third, upper third)* of the ureter. As in the ureter, the adventitia of the bladder, lying

186 lamina propria
187 collagenous

188 most

189 relaxed

190 smooth
191 smooth
192 smooth
193 lower third

Urinary System

(194) _____ *(outside, inside)* the outermost *(195)* _____ *(smooth, skeletal)* muscle bundle, the *(196)* _____ *(circular, longitudinal)* layer, is composed of *(197)* _____ _____ _____.

194 outside
195 smooth
196 longitudinal
197 fibroelastic connective
    tissue

17

Endocrine System

After completing this chapter, you should be able to identify the following:

1 **Pituitary gland: posterior and anterior parts**

2 **Thyroid gland**

3 **Parathyroid gland**

4 **Adrenal gland: cortex and medulla**

5 **Pineal gland**

Also, after completing this chapter, you should understand the following:

1 **Hormones produced in specific organs**

2 **The interrelationship of endocrine organs**

3 **The differences between exocrine and endocrine glands**

There are two types of glands, exocrine and *(1)* _____. What is the major difference between the two? *(2)* _____ _____. Because endocrine glands *(3)* _____ *(have, do not have)* a duct system, at least one side of each secretory cell is in contact with a capillary. The capillaries found within endocrine glands are of the *(4)* _____ variety. These capillaries contain a discontinuous *(5)* _____ *(endothelial lining, basal lamina)* with small pores traversed by a thin *(6)* _____.

1 endocrine

2 endocrine secretes into capillaries, exocrine into ducts

3 do not have

4 fenestrated

5 endothelial lining

6 diaphragm

The secretion of endocrine cells is called a hormone—a substance secreted by a cell into the bloodstream that affects specific cells, called target cells, at a distant site. The hormones may be composed of amino acids, glycoproteins, or steroids. Endocrine glands include the pituitary, thyroid, parathyroids, adrenal, islets of Langerhans of the *(7)* _____, pineal, and the sex glands (to be discussed in Chaps. 18 and 19).

7 pancreas

Pituitary

The pituitary gland is a bilobed, ovoid structure (1.0 cm by 1.5 cm) that lies immediately below the base of the brain and is attached to it by the pituitary stalk (Fig. 17-1). The anterior lobe, called the adenohypophysis, is divided into three areas: The most anterior part is the pars anterior (or pars distalis); the projection of the pars anterior (or pars *(8)* _____) that extends up along side the stalk is the pars tuberalis; and the most posterior portion of the *(9)* _____ *(anterior, posterior)* lobe, which contains poorly developed glandular tissue, is the pars intermedia. The posterior lobe, called the neurohypophysis (or pars nervosa or pars posterior), contains tissue that is

8 distalis

9 anterior

10 *more*
11 *hypophysis*

12 *epithelial*

13 *adenohypophysis*

(10) _____ *(more, less)* fibrous than the tissue of the
(11) adeno _____, suggesting the presence of nerve fibers.
The neurohypophysis develops from nervous tissue, while the adenohypophysis,
like most glands, develops from *(12)* _____ tissue.

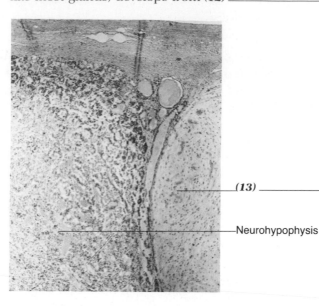

(13) _____

Neurohypophysis

FIG. 17-1. Photomicrograph of the overall
view of the pituitary gland (original magnification ×30).

Adenohypophysis (Anterior Pituitary)

14 *adeno*
15 *pars tuberalis*
16 *pars intermedia*
17 *no*
18 *fenestrated*

19 *ducts*

PARS ANTERIOR The pars anterior is part of the *(14)* _____ hypophysis, the
other parts being the *(15)* _____ _____ and the
(16) _____ _____. Does the arrangement of cells resem-
ble that of an exocrine gland? *(17)* ____. The cells are arranged as branching
cords with capillaries of the *(18)* _____ variety located
between the cords. The capillaries provide a means of transport for the secretions of these cells, a function served by the *(19)* _____ of exocrine glands.
The capillaries also supply the anterior pituitary with blood-containing secretions
from specialized nerve cells of the hypothalamus. These secretions may either
stimulate or inhibit the cells of the anterior pituitary, and thus are called releasing factors and inhibitory factors, respectively (Fig. 17-2).

The cells of the pars anterior are generally classified as either chromophils,
which attract stain, and chromophobes, which do not stain in hematoxylin-eosin
(H and E) preparations, and thus appear *(20)* _____.

20 *pale (clear)*

(21) _____

(23) _____

(22) _____

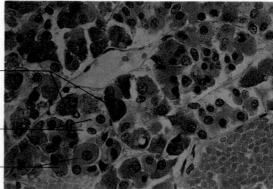

21 *acidophils*
22 *basophils*
23 *chromophobes*

FIG. 17-2. Photomicrograph of a part of the pars
anterior, hematoxylin-eosin (H and E) stain (original
magnification ×300).

Pituitary

Chromophils are either acidophils, which are periodic acid–Schiff (PAS)-negative, or basophils, which are PAS-positive. PAS stains for reactive carbohydrate groups.

Different types of basophils, each secreting specific hormones, may be distinguished using a PAS and aldehyde-thrionine stain. Thyrotrophs are cells that secrete thyroid-stimulating hormone (TSH), a glycoprotein. TSH is a trophic hormone; it stimulates the growth or function of another **(24)** _____ (*exocrine, endocrine*) gland. In this case, the stimulated gland is the **(25)** _____. Both follicle-stimulating hormone (FSH) and luteinizing hormone (LH) are secreted by gonadotrophs. These hormones, which are **(26)** _____ (*glycoproteins, steroids*) like TSH, stimulate the ovary (FSH) and the corpus luteum (LH) in the female, and the glandular cells of the testis (LH) in the male. Adrenocorticotropic hormone (ACTH) and melanocyte-stimulating hormone (MSH) are secreted by the same cell. ACTH is a trophic hormone like **(27)** ___ ___ ___, which stimulates the cortex of the **(28)** _____ gland. Melanocytes, found mainly in the basal layers of the **(29)** _____, are probably stimulated by MSH. Both ACTH and **(30)** ___ ___ ___ are composed of amino acids, and have a similar structure.

Acidophils are either mammotrophs (also called lactotrophs) or somatotrophs. The mammotroph (or **(31)** _____) secretes prolactin, which stimulates the production of milk in the breast of pregnant and lactating women. The other acidophil, the **(32)** _____, secretes growth hormone (GH; also called somatotropin), which is necessary for the growth of most tissues during development, especially the zone of proliferation in the **(33)** _____ disk of bones. Both acidophil hormones, **(34)** ___ ___ and **(35)** _____, are composed of amino acids (Fig. 17-3).

Chromophobes, the cells that **(36)** _____ (*stain, do not stain*), are of unknown function, but may represent degranulated acidophils or **(37)** _____. These are the **(38)** _____ (*least, most*) numerous of the cells of the pars **(39)** _____.

24 endocrine
25 thyroid
26 glycoproteins
27 TSH
28 adrenal
29 epidermis
30 MSH
31 lactotroph
32 somatotroph
33 epiphyseal
34 GH
35 prolactin
36 do not stain
37 basophils
38 least
39 anterior (distalis)
40 rER
41 Golgi
42 secretory granules

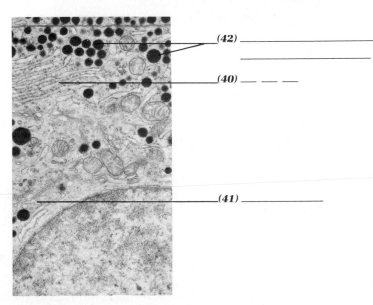

(42) _____

(40) ___ ___ ___

(41) _____

FIG. 17-3. Electron micrograph (EM) of a part of a somatotroph in the anterior pituitary (original magnification ×6900).

43 prolactin or GH
44 pancreas

45 exocytosis
46 hypothalamus

47 lysosomes
48 thyrotrophs
(gonadotrophs)

49 pars anterior (distalis)

50 stalk
51 basophilic

52 pale

53 microtubules

54 pars tuberalis
55 pars intermedia

56 distalis (anterior)
57 pars tuberalis
58 pars intermedia
59 pars nervosa
(posterior)

60 releasing
61 distalis (anterior)
62 hypophysis
63 synapses

64 neuro

Secretory-granule formation and release of amino acid hormones, such as *(43)* _____, from the pars anterior occur through the same process by which zymogen granules of the *(44)* _____ are formed and released. The release of granules is by the process of *(45)* _____. If release of the granules is inhibited by inhibitory factors of the *(46)* _____, the granules are enzymatically destroyed through fusion in the cytoplasm with membrane-bound *(47)* _____.

The cells such as *(48)* _____ that secrete glycoprotein hormones have an increased amount of sER and Golgi apparatus in the cytoplasm.

PARS TUBERALIS   The pars tuberalis is the upward extension of the *(49)* _____ _____, and is located along the pituitary *(50)* _____. The cuboidal cells are organized into small clusters or cords, and have mildly *(51)* _____-staining cytoplasm (Fig. 17-4). The function of the cells of the pars tuberalis is unknown.

PARS INTERMEDIA   The pars intermedia is composed of an irregular row of follicles containing *(52)* _____ *(pale, dark)*-staining colloid material. The cells lining the follicles are pale and have cilia (which contain a core of orderly arranged *(53)* _____). (You should finish #55 at this point.)

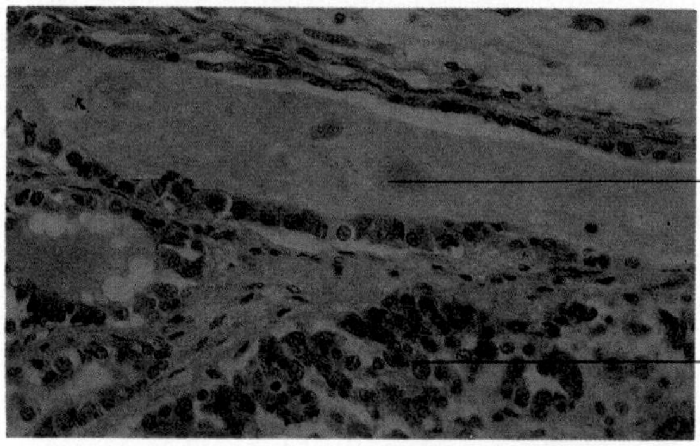

(55) _____

_____

(54) _____

_____

FIG. 17-4.   Photomicrograph of the pars tuberalis and pars intermedia of the anterior pituitary, H and E stain (original magnification ×200).

Neurohypophysis

The two parts of the pituitary gland are the adenohypophysis, composed of the pars *(56)* _____, *(57)* _____ _____, and *(58)* _____ _____; and the neurohypophysis, or *(59)* _____ _____. The neurohypophysis contains the axons of nerve cells whose cell bodies lie in two specific areas of the hypothalamus. These nerve cells differ from those secreting the *(60)* _____ factors and inhibitory factors affecting the pars *(61)* _____. The nerve fibers of the *(62)* neuro _____ are unique because their axons do not form *(63)* _____ with other nerve cells. The axons of the nerve cells pass from the hypothalamus through the hypothalamic–hypophyseal tract to terminate as axon terminals near capillaries in the *(64)* _____ hypophysis.

Pituitary

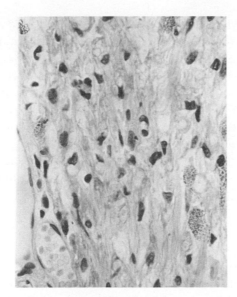

FIG. 17-5. Photomicrograph of a section of the neurohypophysis (original magnification ×300).

The neurohypophysis is divided into lobules by connective tissue septa, which contain the blood vessels (Fig. 17-5). The central part of each lobule contains the unmyelinated nerve fibers of the *(65)* _____–
_____ tract. Neurosecretory granules may be seen within the axoplasm of the fiber. Pituicytes are also found in the center of the lobules. These cells have an oval-round nucleus and long cell processes that serve a supporting function similar to the *(66)* _____ cells of the central nervous system (CNS). Hering bodies (specifically stained with the Gomori technique) probably represent terminal bulb formations of the axons containing numerous neurosecretory *(67)* _____ (Fig. 17-6).

65 *hypothalamic-*
   hypophyseal

66 *neuroglial*

67 *granules*

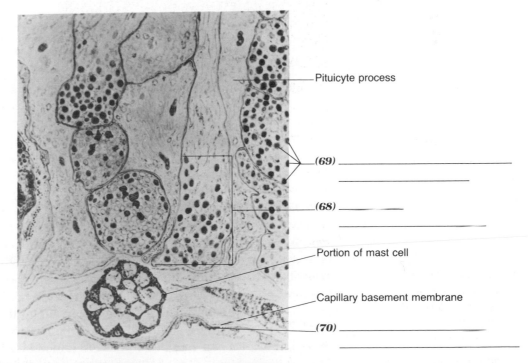

Pituicyte process

(69) _____
_____

(68) _____
_____

Portion of mast cell

Capillary basement membrane

(70) _____
_____

68 *axon terminal*
69 *neurosecretory*
   granules

70 *capillary endothelium*

FIG. 17-6. Diagram of portion of pars nervosa (original magnification × approximately 8000). (Modified from original drawing of Elinor Bodian in Weiss RO, Greep L: Histology, 2nd ed. New York, McGraw–Hill, 1966)

Antidiuretic hormone (ADH or vasopressin) is the neurohormone produced by the cell bodies in the supra-optic nucleus of the *(71)* _____. Its effect is to increase water retention in the distal tubules of the kidney. Oxytocin is produced by the cell bodies in the paraventricular nucleus of the hypothalamus. It acts to increase contractions of the pregnant uterus and to aid in evacuation of milk by the lactating breast through stimulation of the myoepithelial cells surrounding the milk gland.

Although these two neurohormones, *(72)* __ __ __ and *(73)* _____, are produced by cell bodies found in the *(74)* _____, they are released by axons that terminate near capillaries found in the *(75)* _____ _____ _____.

71 hypothalamus

72 ADH (vasopressin)
73 oxytocin
74 hypothalamus
75 pars nervosa (posterior)

Thyroid

The thyroid gland has two lobes of reddish brown glandular tissue joined by an isthmus that lies over the second and third tracheal cartilages (Fig. 17-7). Two

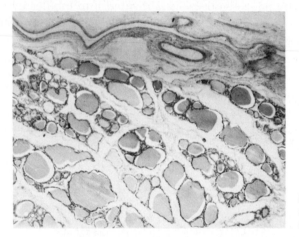

FIG. 17-7. Photomicrograph of the thyroid gland, H and E stain (original magnification ×30).

capsules cover the gland. The outer layer of *(76)* _____ _____ connective tissue is continuous with the fascia of the trachea; the inner layer is the true capsule. The inner layer is continuous with the *(77)* _____ that divide the gland into lobules. The septa provide support for the gland and carry the nerves, lymphatics, and blood vessels that supply the gland.

76 dense irregular

77 septa

Follicles

Follicles are the structural unit of the thyroid gland. Each is composed of simple *(78)* _____ cells arranged in a sphere (appears as a ring on section) with a central lumen containing the secretion of the gland, called colloid. The follicles vary in size from 0.05 mm to 0.5 mm in diameter. The follicular cells, like most epithelial cells, are surrounded by a *(79)* _____ _____. The follicular cells have microvilli on the surface facing the colloid, that aid in the resorption of material from the lumen. To prevent any leakage of colloid, the apical surfaces of the cells are joined by zonula *(80)* _____. Macula adherens and nexus are also present.

The colloid appears as a structureless *(81)* _____ *(acidophilic, basophilic)*, homogeneous material. Thyroglobulin, a glycoprotein with a high carbohydrate content, is the main component of *(82)* _____.

78 cuboidal

79 basement membrane

80 occludens
81 acidophilic

82 colloid

Thyroid

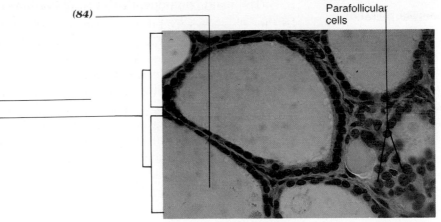

(84) _____

Parafollicular
cells

(83) _____

83 *thyroid follicles*
84 *colloid*

FIG. 17-8. Photomicrograph of thyroid follicles, H and E stain (original magnification ×300).

The other cells present in the thyroid are the parafollicular (C or light) cells (Fig. 17-8). These larger cells are found on the outer aspect of the follicles, so that contact with the follicular lumen is avoided. Both the cytoplasm and nuclei stain *(85)* _____ (*paler, darker*) than those of follicular cells. Parafollicular, or *(86)* _____, cells secrete a hormone much different from *(87)* _____ produced by the follicular cells (Fig. 17-9).

85 *paler*
86 *C (light)*
87 *thyroglobulin*

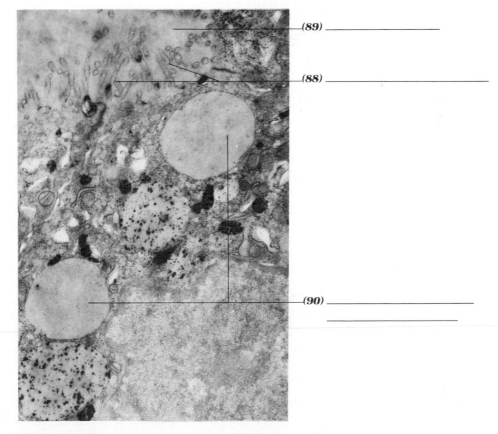

(89) _____

(88) _____

88 *microvilli*
89 *colloid*

(90) _____

90 *secretory granules*

FIG. 17-9. EM of portion of follicular cell of thyroid gland. (Wetzel BK, Spicer SS, Wollman S: Changes in fine structure and acid phosphatase localization in rat thyroid cells following thyrotropin administration. J Cell Biology 25:593, 1965)

The main components of thyroid hormone are the glycoprotein **(91)** _____ and iodine. Iodide is removed from the blood by the follicular cells and is converted to iodine; then it is secreted into the follicular **(92)** _____ where it is bound to the thyroglobulin. When stimulated by the anterior pituitary hormone **(93)** __ __ __, the follicular cells phagocytize a small droplet of colloid; once in the cytoplasm the colloid fuses with a lysosome to form a **(94)** _____. Thyroid hormone is produced, and then secreted into the bloodstream. Thyroid hormone acts on most cells of the body to increase the metabolic activity, and is very important in growth and development.

TSH, released by the **(95)** _____ hypophysis, stimulates the overall activity of the thyroid follicles. The follicular cells increase in size and number so that they may appear columnar, and the volume of the colloid decreases. With no stimulation, the gland stores colloid and the cells appear as low cuboidal epithelium.

The light (or **(96)** _____) cells, which are **(97)** _____ (*larger, smaller*) than follicular cells, secrete calcitonin directly into the bloodstream. Calcitonin acts on the multinucleate cells in bone, the **(98)** _____. Because the activity and size of osteoclasts is decreased by calcitonin, less calcium will be released into the blood from the breakdown of bone. Thus, calcitonin acts to **(99)** _____ (*increase, decrease*) blood levels of calcium.

91 *thyroglobulin*

92 *lumen*

93 *TSH*

94 *phagolysosome*

95 *adeno*

96 *parafollicular (C)*

97 *larger*

98 *osteoclasts*

99 *decrease*

Parathyroid

There are four parathyroid glands, two located on the posterior aspect of each lobe of the thyroid. They lie immediately outside the true capsule of the thyroid but within the outer capsule. Each parathyroid gland is yellow brown and has a flattened oval shape, approximately 0.5 cm in diameter.

A thin connective tissue capsule covers each gland that, as in the thyroid, sends **(100)** _____ into the gland to divide it into lobules (Fig. 17-10). Two types of glandular cells exist. The chief (or principal) cells are the most numerous. These cells appear smaller than the cells of most endocrine glands, and the staining of the cytoplasm is dependent upon the amount of stored glycogen. Storage granules are not present, although chief, or **(101)** _____, cells have the normal complement of organelles. How are the cells arranged? **(102)** _____.

Chief cells secrete parathyroid hormone (PTH). The effects of PTH upon bone are the opposite of those of calcitonin. PTH will **(103)** _____ (*increase, decrease*) the size and activity of **(104)** __osteo_____, increasing bone resorption and liberating **(105)** _____ (*more, less*) calcium into the bloodstream. PTH also affects the kidney and small intestine to increase blood calcium levels. Is there a tropic hormone from the anterior pituitary that primarily stimulates chief cells? **(106)** _____. Activity of chief cells is regulated directly by blood levels of calcium.

Oxyphils are much **(107)** _____ (*less, more*) common than chief cells. They are **(108)** _____ (*larger, smaller*) than chief cells, and have a **(109)** _____-staining cytoplasm, which is due to the large number of **(110)** _____. These cells are usually found in small groups. Their function is unknown.

100 *septa*

101 *principal*

102 *cords or small clumps*

103 *increase*

104 *clasts*

105 *more*

106 *no*

107 *less*

108 *larger*

109 *eosinophilic*

110 *mitochondria*

Parathyroid

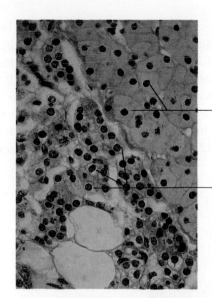

111 oxyphils

_(111)_ _____

Chief (principal) cells

FIG. 17-10. Photomicrograph of the parathyroid gland, H and E stain (original magnification ×300).

Adrenals

The adrenal glands are paired glands, one found lying on top of each kidney. Each gland is about 5 cm by 3.5 cm and 1 cm in thickness. There is an outer cortex of glandular tissue that develops from _(112)_ _____ tissue and an inner medulla that develops from nervous tissue. What other endocrine gland has both glandular and nervous components? _(113)_ _____.

The adrenal gland is covered by a thick _(114)_ _____ of connective tissue containing elastic fibers and a network of reticular fibers that supports the glandular parenchyma. The center of the gland contains large veins, and the hormones produced enter the bloodstream by passing through the fenestrated endothelium of _(115)_ _____ (Fig. 17-11).

112 epithelial

113 pituitary
114 capsule

115 capillaries

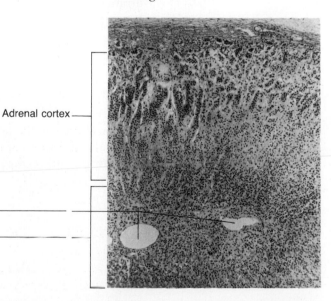

Adrenal cortex

_(116)_ _____

_(117)_ _____

116 central veins

117 adrenal medulla

FIG. 17-11. Photomicrograph of an overall view of the adrenal gland (original magnification ×30).

118 adrenal

119 irregular clusters

120 zona
121 large

122 zona glomerulosa

123 zona fasciculata

124 zona fasciculata
125 lipofuscin

126 zona fasciculata

127 zona reticularis

Adrenal Cortex

There are three layers to the cortex of the *(118)* _____ gland (Fig. 17-12). Immediately beneath the capsule is the zona glomerulosa. How are these columnar cells arranged? *(119)* _____.
Varying amounts of lipid appear in the cytoplasm. The largest layer is the zona fasciculata. These polyhedral cells are arranged in fairly straight cords, one to two cells thick. Also called spongiocytes, the cells of the *(120)* _____ fasciculata contain a very *(121)* _____ (*large, small*) amount of lipid and appear pale.

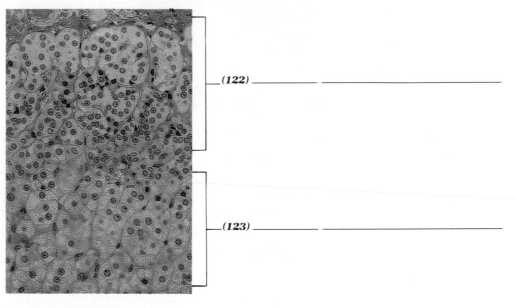

(122) _____ _____

(123) _____ _____

FIG. 17-12. Photomicrograph of a part of the adrenal cortex, H and E stain (original magnification ×160).

The third layer of the cortex is the zona reticularis (Fig. 17-13). The cells are arranged into cords that run in various directions. The staining characteristics of this layer are variable, although the lipid content of the cells is less than that of the *(124)* _____ _____. Wear and tear pigment, called *(125)* _____, is also present in the cytoplasm of these cells.

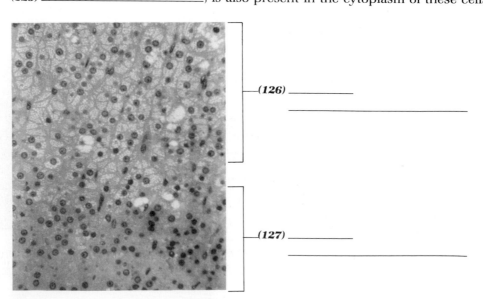

(126) _____

_____

(127) _____

_____

FIG. 17-13. Photomicrograph of a portion of the adrenal cortex (original magnification ×200).

Adrenals

128 *glomerulosa*
129 *fasciculata*
130 *reticularis*
131 *sER*

132 *middle*

133 *plasma*
134 *ACTH*

135 *zona glomerulosa*

136 *zona reticularis*

137 *pars nervosa*
    (posterior)

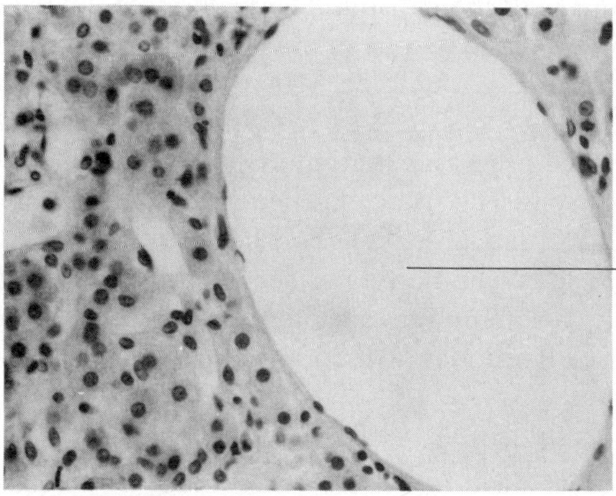

138 *central vein*

139 *Golgi*

The hormones produced by the three layers, the zona **(128)** _____, zona **(129)** _____, and zona **(130)** _____, all have a steroid backbone. What organelle is basically responsible for the production of steroid compounds? **(131)** __ __ __.

Glucocorticoids are secreted by the cells of the zona fasciculata, the **(132)** _____ (*outer, middle, inner*) layer. Cortisol, the major glucocorticoid, is catabolic in nature in that it promotes glucose formation and will increase blood glucose levels. It also suppresses the immune response by decreasing the proliferation and activity of antibody-producing **(133)** _____ cells. The stimulatory hormone from the anterior pituitary is **(134)** __ __ __ __.

Aldosterone, a mineralocorticoid, is secreted by the cells of the outer layer, the **(135)** _____ _____. This hormone functions at the kidney to increase sodium and water retention. Stimulation of the zona glomerulosa is independent of ACTH.

The cells of the inner layer, the **(136)** _____ _____, secrete weak sex hormones called androgens, clinically significant in certain disease states.

Adrenal Medulla

The adrenal medulla develops from nervous tissue, as does the **(137)** _____ _____ of the pituitary gland, yet the adrenal medulla is of the autonomic nervous system and the pituitary is of the CNS. The cells are large and ovoid, grouped together in small clusters (Fig. 17-14).

_____ **(138)** _____ _____

FIG. 17-14. Photomicrograph of the adrenal medulla (original magnification × 200).

The granules within the cytoplasm contain the neurosecretory product, and stain brown with chromaffin salts. Because of this chromaffin reaction, these cells are referred to as chromaffin cells. There are two types of chromaffin cell: an epinephrine-secreting cell and a norepinephrine-secreting cell. The formation of mature granules involves the transformation and modification of the amino acid tyrosine, and occurs both inside and outside the granule. Because packaging is so important in the formation of these granules, large amounts of **(139)** _____ _____ are found in the cytoplasm.

Capillaries and venules are numerous in the adrenal medulla. The venules, arising from capillary beds of the cortex, carry blood-containing hormones from

Endocrine System

140 cortisol (aldosterone)

141 epinephrine
142 norepinephrine

143 septa

144 nucleolus
145 basophilic

146 pinealo
147 flattened

the cortex, such as *(140)* _____. The venules eventually empty into the large central veins in the center of the medulla.

Secretion of the neurohormones of the medulla,

(141) _____ and

(142) _____, is stimulated by general stimuli of the sympathetic nervous system. The adrenal medulla acts to augment the effects of the sympathetic nervous system.

Pineal

The pineal gland is cone shaped and 0.5 cm to 1 cm in length, and lies dorsal to the midbrain (Fig. 17-15). It is divided into lobules by irregular *(143)* _____

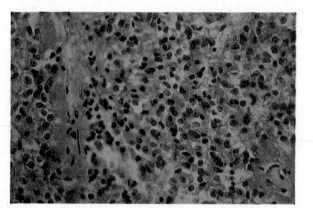

FIG. 17-15. Photomicrograph of the pineal gland, H and E stain (original magnification × 125).

continuous with the capsule. The majority of the cells present are pinealocytes. These large cells have a large nucleus with a prominent

(144) _____. The cytoplasm contains

(145) _____ (*basophilic, acidophilic*) material, and there are extensive cell processes that intertwine with the processes of the supporting neuroglial cells. The triangular neuroglial cells are smaller than

(146) _____cytes and have a *(147)* _____ (*flattened, round*) nucleus. The hormones secreted by the pinealocytes are melatonin and serotonin. Melatonin may play a regulatory role in the secretion of the gonadotropins (sex hormones), which are involved in the onset of puberty.

18

Male Reproductive System

After completing this chapter, you should be able to identify the following:

1 Testes   5 Seminiferous tubules
2 Leydig's cells   6 Prostate
3 Sertoli's cells   7 Urethra
4 Spermatozoon   8 Penis

Also, after completing this chapter, you should understand the following:

1 The stages of maturation of spermatozoa

2 The endocrine system's association with the male reproductive system

Four parts make up the male reproductive system. The two gonads or testes produce both the male germ cells called spermatozoa and the male sex hormones (androgens). Thus, part of the testes function as an
(1) _____ gland. The penis functions in copulation to deliver sperm to the female. There is a long set of tubes that connect the testes with the penis and provide a place for the spermatozoa to mature. The accessory glands produce a fluid to nourish and carry the sperm, and contractions of the smooth muscle in the walls of these glands aid in ejaculation.

1 endocrine

Testes

The testes are found in a pouch called the scrotum. The scrotum is covered by
(2) _____ *(thin, thick)* skin with a **(3)** _____ *(keratinized, nonkeratinized)* stratified squamous epithelium. Intermixed with the subcutaneous tissue is an incomplete layer of smooth muscle (the dartos muscle) that contracts when stimulated. Each testis is 4-cm to 5-cm long and covered by a thick connective tissue capsule, the tunic albuginea. This capsule thickens posteriorly to form the mediastinum, an area that contains the rete testis, the beginning of the tubes that carry the sperm out of the testes. Connective tissue septa from the mediastinum divide each testis into approximately 250
(4) _____.

2 thin
3 keratinized

Seminiferous Tubules and Spermatocytogenesis

The major component of the testes are the numerous glandlike structures called seminiferous tubules. These are a series of tubules (over 0.5-mile long) lined by the germ cells in various stages of maturation. The most apical cells differentiate into spermatozoa, which are released into the lumen where they travel to the beginning of the transport tubes, the **(5)** _____ of the me-

4 lobules

5 rete testis

Male Reproductive System

6 basement membrane
7 tubule

8 actin

9 basement membrane

10 chromatin

11 mitosis

12 spermatogonia
13 lumen

14 spermatocytes

15 seminiferous

16 type A
   spermatogonia

17 type B
   spermatogonia
18 myoid cells

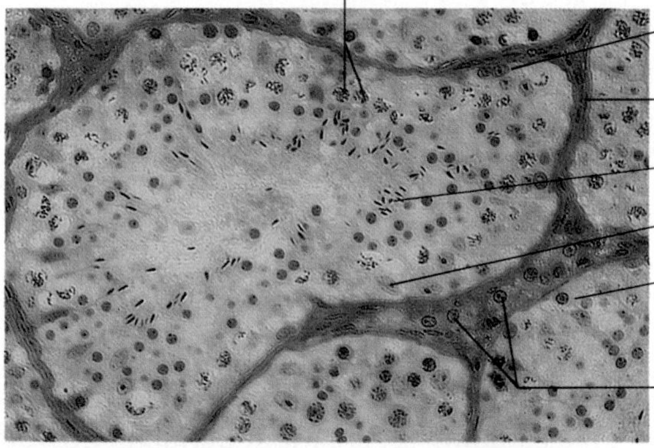

19 acrosome

diastinum. As in most gland-type structures, the basal germ cells rest on a *(6)* _____ _____. Each seminiferous *(7)* _____ is surrounded by loose connective tissue and a single continuous layer of squamous-appearing myoid cells. Although contractile in function, these cells bear little resemblance to smooth muscle cells except for the presence of the thin contractile filaments, *(8)* _____ filaments (Fig. 18-1).

Spermatocytogenesis, the maturational process of germ cells, begins with the mitotic proliferation of basal spermatogonial cells into primary spermatocytes. Two types of spermatogonial cells can be found resting on the *(9)* _____ _____. Type A spermatogonia have an ovoid nucleus with dark or pale nucleoplasm, depending upon the amount of condensed *(10)* _____. The nucleolus rests against the nuclear membrane, and cytoplasm is scarce. When these cells divide, half of the daughter cells develop into type A spermatogonia and one half develop into type B spermatogonia. Type B spermatogonia have a round nucleus with heavily staining chromatin and a centrally located nucleolus. These divide by the process of *(11)* _____ and develop into primary spermatocytes.

Primary spermatocytes appear similar to type B *(12)* _____, but have a large nucleus and an increased amount of cytoplasm. They are located closer to the *(13)* _____ *(lumen, basement membranes)* than type B cells. Primary spermatocytes pass through the first meiotic division to become secondary spermatocytes. Secondary *(14)* _____ are rarely observed because they rapidly pass through the second meiotic division and result in spermatids. These cells are now located on the luminal border of the *(15)* _____ tubule. Spermiogenesis is the cytologic transformation of spermatids into mature spermatozoa.

Primary spermatocytes

(16) _____ __

_____

(18) _____ _____

Spermatids

(48) _____ _____

(17) _____ __

_____

(49) _____

_____

FIG. 18-1. Photomicrograph of the seminiferous tubule of the testis, hematoxylin-eosin (H and E) stain (original magnification ×125).

The acrosome (or head cap) of the spermatozoon is formed through secretion by the Golgi apparatus of mucopolysaccharides into a membranous saccule, which then sits on top of the apical pole of the nucleus. Hyaluronidase, an enzyme that facilitates penetration of the ovum by the sperm, is found within the saccule. The nucleus, located beneath the *(19)* _____, undergoes condensation of both the nucleoplasm and the chromatin. Two centrioles move behind the caudal pole of the nucleus. An elongate flagellum referred to as the axoneme, which composes the core of the tail of the mature

Testes

20 spermatozoon
21 organized

22 energy
23 microtubules

24 chromatin
25 acrosome
26 fibrils
27 mitochondria

28 head cap

29 nucleus

30 mitochondria

31 middle piece

32 spermatocytogenesis

33 spermiogenesis

34 tubules

(20) _____, develops at the distal end. The flagellum has the normal **(21)** _____ (_organized, random_) arrangement of microtubules. A series of thick longitudinal fibrils form peripherally to the axoneme and fuse into a sheet at the base of the tail. These provide support for the tail. Throughout the middle of the tail, elongate mitochondria surround the fibrils. The mitochondria provide **(22)** _____ for movement of the tail, which also involves the **(23)** _____ of the flagellum.

Thus, a mature spermatozoon is an elongate structure 65 μm in length. It consists of the head (5 μm) containing the nucleus with condensed **(24)** _____, which is covered by the **(25)** _____. The beginning of the tail, called the middle piece (7 μm), contains the coarse **(26)** _____ that are surrounded by numerous elongate **(27)** _____ (Fig. 18-2). The principal portion of the tail

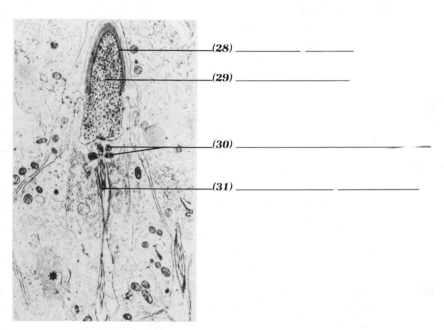

(28) _____ _____

(29) _____ _____

(30) _____ ___

(31) _____ _____

FIG. 18-2. EM of late spermatid. (Courtesy of Dr. Martin Dym, Department of Anatomy, Georgetown University, Washington, DC)

(45 μm) contains the fibrils and an extra supporting fibrous sheet surrounding the axoneme. The end-piece (5 μm) contains only microtubules and the closely applied cell membrane. No other organelles are found in a mature spermatozoon, and excess cytoplasm is cast off as a residual body to be phagocytized.

Thus, the maturation of spermatogonium into spermatid is called **(32)** _____, while the cytologic transformation into a mature spermatozoon is called **(33)** _____.

Sertoli's Cells

A cell found within the seminiferous tubules that does not produce germ cells is the Sertoli's (sustentacular) cell. These elongate cells have an irregular-shaped and indented nucleus with basophilic structures around the prominent nucleolus (see Fig. 18-1). The cells of the seminiferous **(34)** _____ are divided into two compartments by the Sertoli's cells. The basal compartment contains only the cells in contact with the basement membrane, the **(35)** _____ cells. This compartment is bathed by tissue fluid. The adluminal compartment contains the more differentiated germ-cells, such as **(36)** _____ _____, which are protected by fitting into indentations in the cytoplasm of the Sertoli's cells. A "blood–testes barrier" is accomplished through the fusion of the plasmalemmas of the Sertoli's cells by watertight **(37)** _____ _____ . Sertoli's cells also function to phagocytize the excess cytoplasm released in the process of spermiogenesis, called **(38)** _____ _____. Sustentacular, or **(39)** _____, cells are stimulated by follicle-stimulating hormone (FSH), a gonadotropin released by **(40)** _____ (basophils, acidophils) of the **(41)** _____ pituitary gland.

Leydig's Cells

Interstitial cells (Leydig's cells) are found singly or in clumps in the connective tissue separating the **(42)** _____ _____. These cells are large (20 μm in diameter), with a pale-staining oval-round nucleus. More than one nucleolus may be present (see Fig. 18-1). Endocrine in nature, these cells produce the male sex hormones called **(43)** _____, testosterone being the principal secretion. Lipid droplets in the cytoplasm reflect the steroid backbone of these hormones. Which organelle should be in abundance in these cells? **(44)** __ __ __.

Unlike the cells stimulated by FSH (the **(45)** _____ cells), the Leydig's cells are stimulated by the other gonadotropin, **(46)** _____ _____, which in the male is also called interstitial cell–stimulating hormone (ICSH). Testosterone, produced by the **(47)** _____ cells, stimulates the development of the seminiferous tubules and is responsible for the appearance of secondary sex characteristics at puberty. (You should finish #49 at this point; see Fig. 18-1.)

Rete Testis and Epididymis

The seminiferous tubules become straight as they approach the mediastinum, and are referred to as tubuli recti. At the mediastinum, all tubuli recti empty into the **(50)** _____ testis. The tubuli recti are lined by all Sertoli-like cells, and the rete testis is lined by a cuboidal epithelium. The rete testis empties into 15 to 20 efferent ductules that are part of the epididymis, a crescent-shaped structure that caps the upper part of each testis and covers one side. Thus, the head of the epididymis is composed of the **(51)** _____ _____. The efferent ductules are cone-shaped structures with a pseudostratified lining, an underlying **(52)** _____ _____, and a thin layer of smooth muscle cells and elastic tissue. Functionally, the **(53)** _____ ductules remove excess fluid and materials from the secretion of the testes.

The body and tail of the **(54)** _____ is formed by the ductus epididymis, an extremely convoluted set of tubules (Fig. 18-3). The epithelial lining is a **(55)** _____ epithelium, with apical stereocilia. Stereocilia are structurally similar to

---

35 spermatogonial

36 primary or secondary spermatocytes, spermatids

37 zonula occludens (tight junction)

38 residual bodies

39 Sertoli's

40 basophils

41 anterior

42 seminiferous tubules

43 androgens

44 sER

45 Sertoli's

46 luteinizing hormone (LH)

47 interstitial (Leydig's)

48 Sertoli's cells

49 Leydig's (interstitial) cells

50 rete

51 efferent ductules

52 basement membrane

53 efferent

54 epididymis

55 pseudostratified

Testes

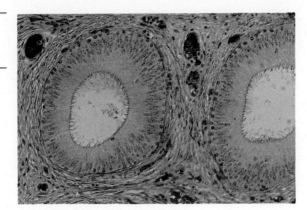

FIG. 18-3. Photomicrograph of a portion of the epididymis, H and E stain (original magnification ×30).

(56) _____, except much *(57)* _____ (*longer, shorter*). Besides acting as a conduit to the penis, this set of tubules also functions as previously mentioned, as a site for final *(58)* _____ of the spermatozoa. The tubules of the ductus *(59)* _____ eventually converge and exit the epididymis as the vas (ductus) deferens (Fig. 18-4). The epithelial lining is pseudostratified

56 microvilli
57 longer

58 maturation
59 epididymis

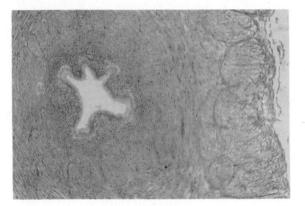

FIG. 18-4. Photomicrograph of the vas (ductus) deferens, H and E stain (original magnification ×30).

columnar with stereocilia, beneath which is a lamina propria (Fig. 18-5). There is a very thick layer of *(60)* _____ _____ surrounded by an adventitia composed of loose connective tissue. The smooth muscle layer is divided into three layers: the outer and inner layer are arranged *(61)* _____, while the middle layer is *(62)* _____.

60 smooth muscle

61 longitudinally
62 circular

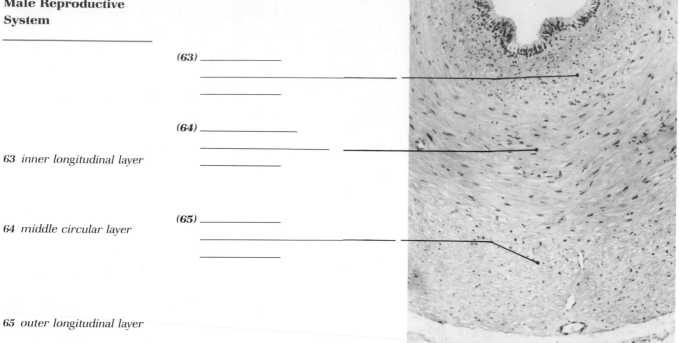

(63) _____

_____ _____

_____

(64) _____

63 _inner longitudinal layer_

_____ _____

_____

(65) _____

64 _middle circular layer_

_____ _____

_____

65 _outer longitudinal layer_

FIG. 18-5. Photomicrograph of the wall of the vas (ductus) deferens.

Spermatic Cord

As the vas deferens passes upward to the inguinal canal, the loose connective tissue of the outer **(66)** _____ joins with connective tissue covering associated arteries, veins, nerves, and skeletal muscle fibers. These structures together constitute the spermatic cord. Before the vas is joined by the seminal vesicles, accessory glands, it becomes dilated and is referred to as the ampulla. In this region, the smooth muscle coat is thinner, the lumen is larger, and the mucosal lining is thrown into numerous folds. The pseudostratified columnar epithelium, however, lacks apical **(67)** _____.

66 _adventitia_

67 _stereocilia_

Seminal Vesicles

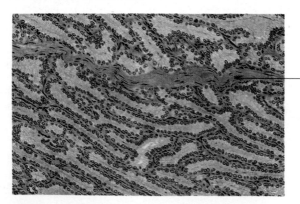

_____ **(68)** _____

_____

68 _smooth muscle_

FIG. 18-6. Photomicrograph of a portion of the seminal vesicles, H and E stain (original magnification × 125).

Seminal Vesicles

69 *vas (ductus)*

70 *thinner*

71 *spermatozoa*

72 *seminal*

73 *bladder*

74 *branched*

75 *straight*

76 *basement membrane*

77 *smooth muscle*
78 *seminal*
79 *nutrients*

The seminal vesicles grow as out-pocketings of the *(69)* _____ deferens (Fig. 18-6). Each tubelike structure is 5-cm to 7-cm long and extremely convoluted; multiple secretions appear in a cross-sectional view. The epithelium is composed of tall columnar cells with occasional small cells resting on the lamina propria. The muscle layer is *(70)* _____ (*thicker, thinner*) than that of the vas deferens. The epithelial cells produce a thick yellowish proteinaceous secretion that provides nourishment and a fluid vehicle for the maturing *(71)* _____. During ejaculation, the secretion is expelled from the lumen of the gland into the ejaculatory ducts. The ejaculatory ducts course through the prostate gland, and connect the vas deferens and *(72)* _____ vesicles with the urethra.

Prostate

The prostate gland is the size and shape of a chestnut, with a firm consistency. The urethra passes through the gland immediately after originating in the *(73)* _____. The capsule of the gland is thin, composed of connective tissue and smooth muscle fibers. The two ejaculatory ducts divide the glands into three lobes. The secretory units are compound tubulo-alveolar and thus the duct system is *(74)* _____ (*branched, unbranched*). Tall columnar cells with microvilli and, occasionally, small round cells line the glandular portion and ducts. The mucosal lining appears *(75)* _____ (*highly folded, straight*), and projections of the epithelial lining intrude into the lumen. A *(76)* _____ _____ lies under the epithelial lining and the remainder of the supporting tissue is connective tissue and *(77)* _____ _____. The secretion of the gland is a thin milky fluid that, like the secretions of the *(78)* _____ vesicles, acts as a fluid vehicle and provides *(79)* _____ for the spermatozoa. Very commonly found in the lumen of the gland are pink homogeneous bodies, called concretions, which may be calcified (Fig. 18-7).

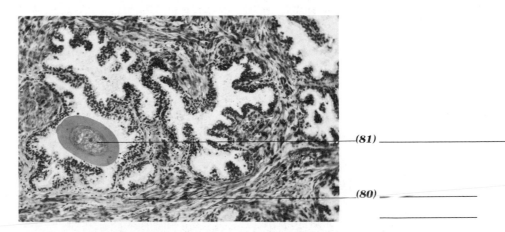

(81) _____

(80) _____

FIG. 18-7. Photomicrograph of a portion of the prostate gland.

80 *smooth muscle*
81 *concretion*

82 *interstitial (Leydig's)*

83 *vesicles*

Testosterone, produced by *(82)* _____ cells, is necessary for the development and maintenance of the seminal *(83)* _____ _____ and prostate gland.

Penis

The penis is characterized by three cylindrical erectile (cavernous) bodies: two corpora cavernosa on the dorsal side; and the corpus cavernosum urethrae (spongiosum) on the ventral side, which contains the urethra and expands directly into the glans penis. Each cavernous body is surrounded by a sheet of **(84)** _____ _____ called the tunica albuginea. The tunica albuginea surrounds the urethra-containing **(85)** _____ _____, and is highly elastic to prevent compression of the urethra. The three cavernous bodies are bound together by loose connective tissue called the fascia penis. The skin covering the penis is **(86)** _____, and hair **(87)** _____ (is, is not) found at the base of the shaft (Fig. 18-8).

84 *connective tissue*
85 *corpus spongiosum*

86 *thin*
87 *is*

88 *corpus cavernosum*

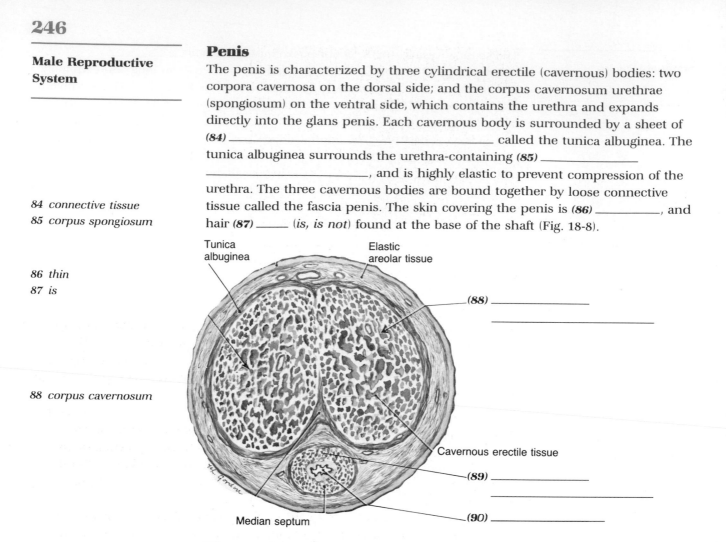

Tunica albuginea

Elastic areolar tissue

(88) _____
_____

Cavernous erectile tissue

(89) _____

(90) _____

Median septum

FIG. 18-8. Diagram of a cross section of the penis.

89 *corpus spongiosum*
90 *urethra*

91 *endothelial*

The cavernous bodies are composed of trabeculae containing connective tissue and smooth muscle fibers covered by an **(91)** _____ lining. The arteries that supply the cavernous bodies branch in the trabeculae and empty into the spaces between these numerous trabeculae. These helicine arteries have an increased amount of smooth muscle, and are usually very coiled in the flaccid penis. Upon excitement, the smooth muscle of the arteries relaxes, increasing the blood flow into the spaces between the **(92)** _____. The **(93)** _____ bodies become turgid, resulting in erection. The **(94)** _____ spongiosum, because of the elasticity of its tunica albuginea, does not become as turgid (Fig. 18-9).

92 *trabeculae*
93 *cavernous*
94 *corpus*

Penis

95 smooth muscle

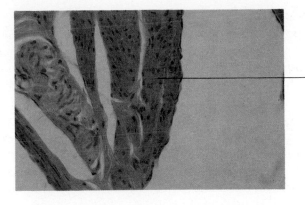

(95) _____

_____

FIG. 18-9. Photomicrograph of a portion of the cavernous body of the penis, H and E stain (original magnification ×200).

Urethra

The urethra is an 8-inch long tube divided into three parts that conveys both urine and semen (spermatozoa and fluid) to the external environment. The prostatic part contains the openings for the continuation of the vas deferens, the **(96)** _____ _____. The epithelial lining of the prostatic portion is typical for urinary tract structures, **(97)** _____ epithelium. As the urethra leaves the prostate and courses through the urogenital diaphragm, the epithelium becomes pseudostratified or columnar. This portion is referred to as the membranous urethra. Mucous glands called bulbo-urethral glands are located beneath this portion, but empty into the beginning of the third part, the cavernous portion. The cavernous portion runs through the **(98)** _____ _____ of the penis and is lined by stratified cuboidal or columnar epithelium. Distally, the epithelium is keratinized stratified squamous, continuous with the epithelium covering the glans penis. Mucous glands called the Littre's glands found within and beneath the lamina propria are scattered throughout the urethra but are most numerous in the third part, the **(99)** _____ portion (Fig. 18-10).

96 ejaculatory ducts

97 transitional

98 corpus spongiosum

99 cavernous

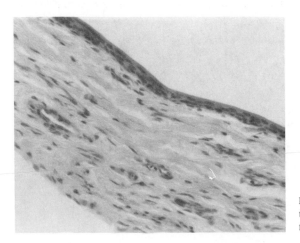

FIG. 18-10. Photomicrograph of a portion of the penile urethra (original magnification ×200).

19

Female Reproductive System

After completing this chapter, you should be able to identify the following:

1 Ovary
2 Oocyte
3 Corpus luteum
4 Oviduct
5 Uterus

6 Menstrual changes of the uterus
7 Placenta
8 Vagina
9 Breast

Also, after completing this chapter, you should understand the following:

1 The histologic aspects of the changes of the endometrium during menses

2 The endocrine association with the female reproductive system

---

The female reproductive system consists of two ovaries, two oviducts (fallopian tubes), the uterus, vagina, external genitalia, and two mammary glands.

Fertilization

The ovaries contain the germ cells in epithelial vesicles called follicles. The counterpart of the oocyte (the female germ cell) in the male is the *(1)* _____. Ovulation is the process by which one oocyte matures and ruptures through the surface of the *(2)* _____ every 28 days. The oocyte and some covering epithelial cells are released into the peritoneal cavity, and are drawn into the infundibulum of the open-ended oviduct through the actions of the fimbriae (fringes) that project from its end. Fertilization of the ovum occurs in the midportion of the tubelike *(3)* _____, which connects the ovary with the uterus. The ovum moves into the uterus, and if fertilization occurs in the *(4)* _____, it implants into the mucous membrane (endometrium) of the uterus. A placenta then develops to support the endometrium and nourish the developing embryo. In anticipation of implantation, the *(5)* <u>endo</u>_____ of the *(6)* _____ thickens and its glands proliferate. If fertilization does not occur, the superficial layer of the endometrium breaks down and exfoliates. This is accompanied by bleeding and constitutes the menstrual flow, which occurs once every 28 days unless pregnancy intervenes.

Ovaries

The ovaries are flattened, ovoid bodies ranging from 2.5 cm in length to 1.5 cm to 3 cm in width and 0.5 cm to 1.5 cm in thickness. Supported by various ligaments and *(7)* _____ (*loose, dense*) connective tissue, ovaries are found in the peritoneum. Histologically, ovaries are divided into an outer covering surface, a cortex, and a medullary area.

1 spermatozoon

2 ovary

3 oviduct

4 oviduct

5 metrium

6 uterus

7 loose

Female Reproductive System

8 simple squamous

GERMINAL EPITHELIUM Unlike other peritoneal structures, the ovaries are not covered by a serosal covering, *(8)* _____ _____ epithelium. Instead, ovaries are covered mainly by cuboidal epithelial cells. This covering epithelium is referred to as germinal epithelium, because it was mistakenly thought to give rise to the primordial oocyte (Fig. 19-1).

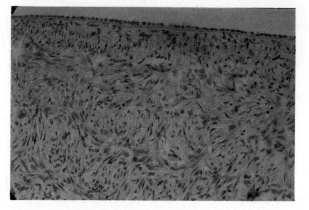

FIG. 19-1. Photomicrograph of a portion of the ovary, outer surface, hematoxylin-eosin (H and E) stain (original magnification ×160).

9 cuboidal

10 albuginea

CORTEX Immediately beneath the germinal epithelium, *(9)* _____ (*cuboidal, columnar*) epithelium, there is a layer of dense connective tissue called the tunica albuginea. The tunica *(10)* _____ is a thin layer that immediately surrounds the area of the ovary called the cortex. The cortical area consists of spindle-shaped cells similar to connective tissue fibroblasts, plus extracellular fibers loosely organized into a swirling pattern. The cortex immediately beneath the tunica *(11)* _____, a layer of dense *(12)* _____ _____, contains the follicles that have the oocytes or ova within them.

11 albuginea
12 connective tissue

MEDULLA The medulla is different histologically from the surrounding *(13)* _____. Consisting mainly of loose connective tissue, the medulla has a mass of very large and contorted blood vessels but no follicles.

13 cortex

Primordial Follicles
The germ cells of the female, *(14)* _____, are found in epithelial vesicles called follicles (Fig. 19-2). Embedded in the stroma of the

14 oocytes

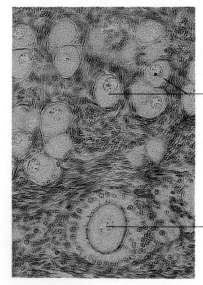

(15) _____ _____

15 cuboidal cells

Nucleus of oocyte (primary follicle beginning to grow)

FIG. 19-2. Photomicrograph of a close-up of a portion of the ovary, H and E stain (original magnification ×200).

Ovaries

16 *cortex*
17 *albuginea*
18 *dense connective tissue*

19 *mordial*
20 *laminar*
21 *cortical*

22 *unilaminar*

23 *majority*
24 *cortical*
25 *ovary*
26 *unilaminar*

27 *ovum*
28 *follicular*
29 *ovum*

30 *unilaminar*

31 *follicular*
32 *one*
33 *simple cuboidal*

(16) _____ (*cortex, medulla*) and deep to the tunica *(17)* _____, a thin layer of *(18)* _____ _____ _____ are the follicles. The majority of follicles found in the ovary are the primordial follicles (the others are the primary, secondary, and mature follicles).

Primordial follicles, or unilaminar follicles, are found in the female fetus and remain throughout her entire life. Thousands of *(19)* <u>pri</u>_____ or *(20)* <u>uni</u>_____ follicles exist in the *(21)* _____ (*cortical, medullary*) stroma, and once puberty is reached, each month several of these are stimulated to begin to form the mature follicle. Usually only one primordial or *(22)* _____ follicle will mature fully and be released with each ovulatory cycle.

The primordial follicle is unique in its histology. Constituting the *(23)* _____ (*majority, minority*) of all follicles within the *(24)* _____ (*cortical, medullary*) area of the *(25)* _____, primordial or *(26)* _____ follicles are the smallest of all ovarian follicles. Primordial follicles consist of a one-cell-layer covering of flattened follicular cells that surround the oocyte or primordial ovum. The oocyte's nucleus is eccentric in location and, like its cytoplasm, stains very light. The surfaces of the oocyte or *(27)* _____ and the surrounding *(28)* _____ (*follicular, granulosa*) cells are in close apposition.

The primordial oocyte or *(29)* _____ remains in the first meiotic division until properly stimulated by follicle-stimulating hormone (FSH). Upon stimulation, cytologic changes take place within the oocyte, follicular cells, and adjacent connective tissue stroma that transform the primordial or *(30)* _____ follicle into the primary follicle.

Primary Follicle

The primary follicle is a maturing primordial follicle, and is considerably different histologically. As the oocyte enlarges, the surrounding *(31)* _____ cells change from *(32)* _____ (*one, two, three*)-cell layer(s) thick, *(33)* _____ _____ _____ (*simple cuboidal, simple squamous*) in type to stratified cuboidal cells called granulosa cells (Fig. 19-3).

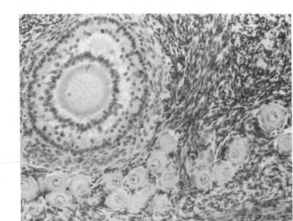

FIG. 19-3. Photomicrograph of a primary follicle of the ovary (original magnification ×125).

Changes within the oocyte consist of redistribution and proliferation of organelles as the cell increases in size. Dense lipid droplets, in addition to the increased number of ribosomes, mitochondria, and Golgi, are found in the cytoplasm of the oocyte (or primary *(34)* _____). As the oocyte enlarges, it pushes away the surrounding *(35)* _____ cells, which are *(36)* _____ _____ in type. Microvilli are found projecting from the oocyte's surface into the space between the oocyte and the *(37)* _____ cells. Material deposits in this space, and a thick dark-staining membane is formed called the zona pellucida. The zona *(38)* _____ is thought to be formed mainly by the granulosa cells.

Granulosa cells, *(39)* _____ _____ in type, project slender processes into the zona *(40)* _____, intermingling with the *(41)* _____ of the oocyte or *(42)* _____ ovum. As the follicle grows, these cells move deeper into the *(43)* _____ (*cortex, medulla*) and closer to the *(44)* _____ (*cortex, medulla*). The sheath of the surrounding stromal cells starts to develop into a two-layered theca. The thecae are two readily identifiable areas: theca interna, a highly cellular and vascular inner layer and the theca externa, the outer zone composed mainly of connective tissue. It is estrogen, a *(45)* _____, that is produced by the *(46)* _____ interna, which is the *(47)* _____ (*avascular, vascular*) area. Estrogen is involved in regulating pituitary hormones and preparing the endometrium of the *(48)* _____ for implantation.

Secondary Follicles

As the granulosa cells continue proliferating, the oocyte becomes eccentric in position and the follicle oval in shape (Fig. 19-4). When the granulosa cells are 6 to 12 cell layers thick or the follicle is almost 0.2 mm in diameter, clear fluid appears between the cell layers of *(49)* _____ cells. The fluid, termed liquor folliculi, increases with follicular enlargement. As the fluid, *(50)* _____ _____, increases between the *(51)* _____ cells, now *(52)* _____ cell layers thick, it will eventually become confluent, forming a single cavity, the antrum. At this point, the follicle is called a secondary follicle or antral follicle. As a secondary or *(53)* _____ follicle, the oocyte has attained its full size but the follicle will grow up to 10 mm to 12 mm in diameter.

The antral or *(54)* _____ follicle is described as having a cavity filled with *(55)* _____ called *(56)* _____ _____ with 6 to *(57)* ___ layers of *(58)* _____ cells. It typically displays a local thickening of granulosa cells called the cumulus oophorous. This thickened edge, *(59)* _____ _____, protrudes into the fluid-filled antrum and communicates with the oocyte or *(60)* _____. (You should finish #63 at this point.)

---

34 ovum
35 granulosa
36 stratified cuboidal

37 granulosa

38 pellucida

39 stratified cuboidal
40 pellucida
41 microvilli
42 primary
43 cortex
44 medulla

45 hormone
46 theca
47 vascular
48 uterus

49 granulosa

50 liquor folliculi
51 granulosa
52 6 to 12

53 antral

54 secondary
55 liquid
56 liquor folliculi
57 12
58 granulosa
59 cumulus oophorous
60 ovum

Ovaries

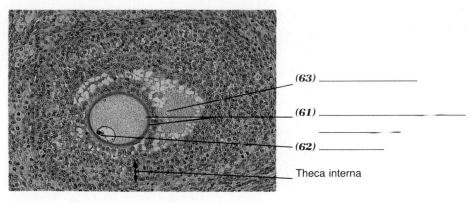

(63) _____

(61) _____
_____

(62) _____

Theca interna

FIG. 19-4. Photomicrograph of a mature secondary follicle of the ovary, H and E stain (original magnification × 125).

61 *granulosa cells*
62 *ovum*
63 *antrum*

Mature Follicle

The follicle before ovulation is called the mature or graafian follicle. As the follicle approaches maximum size, it consumes most of the **(64)** _____ (*medullary, cortical*) area and bulges from the free surface of the organ. The granulosa cells stop proliferating at this point, and the intercellular spaces become more prominent, too. The theca interna, the **(65)** _____ (*inner, outer*), **(66)** _____ (*avascular, vascular*), **(67)** _____ -producing hormonal layer, and the **(68)** _____ externa reach their greatest development in the mature or **(69)** _____ follicle.

As the follicular cells loosen, now called **(70)** _____ cells, the cumulous **(71)** _____ with its connection to the **(72)** _____ or **(73)** _____ starts to break up, too; one or more of these granular layers remain attached to the ovum, forming the corona radiata. It is the corona **(74)** _____ that remains as a loose investment around the ovum after ovulation.

Before the **(75)** _____ (or graafian) follicle, which bulges from the surface of the **(76)** _____, is released in the process of **(77)** _____, the oocyte completes the first **(78)** _____ (*meiotic, mitotic*) division. The second meiotic division begins but it is not completed unless fertilization occurs. The final stimulus for the follicle to burst through is supplied by luteinizing hormone (LH). When the ovary ruptures, the oocyte is released with the surrounding corona **(79)** _____ (composed of **(80)** _____ cells).

64 *cortical*

65 *inner*
66 *vascular*
67 *estrogen*
68 *theca*
69 *graafian*
70 *granulosa*
71 *oophorous*
72 *ovum*
73 *oocyte*
74 *radiata*

75 *mature*
76 *ovary*
77 *ovulation*
78 *meiotic*

79 *radiata*
80 *granulosa*

Corpus Luteum

The remains of the follicle collapse, and the ruptured ovary seals over the wound to form a scar. The corpus luteum develops through infolding of remaining follicular cells and the theca interna (Fig. 19-5). The theca externa does not change its shape. The granulosa cells enlarge and are referred to as follicular lutein cells. Cells of the infolded theca **(81)** _____ enlarge and are called theca-lutein cells. Stimulus for the cytologic transformation comes from the hormone responsible for ovulation, **(82)** _____. The cytoplasm of both the follicular **(83)** _____ cells and the smaller theca-lutein cells appears very pale, suggesting the presence of lipid. (You should finish #85 at this point.)

81 *interna*

82 *LH*
83 *lutein*

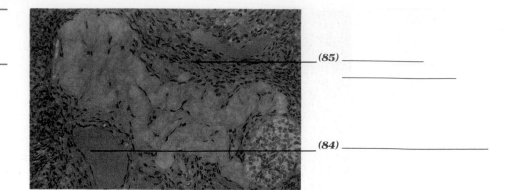

(85) _____
_____

(84) _____

FIG. 19-5. Photomicrograph of a corpus luteum, late stage, H and E stain (original magnification ×125).

84 *capillary*
85 *theca externa*

Progesterone, the product of these modified endocrine cells, is similar to testosterone in that both are steroids. If implantation occurs, progesterone from the corpus luteum will support the *(86)* _____metrium until the *(87)* _____ develops and takes over this function. If implantation does not take place, the *(88)* _____ luteum breaks down within 10 days to 12 days, and is replaced by a connective tissue scar called the corpus albicans. Without *(89)* _____ to support the endometrium, this too will break down and result in the *(90)* _____ flow.

86 *endo*
87 *placenta*
88 *corpus*

89 *progesterone*
90 *menstrual*

Oviduct

The oviduct, also called the *(91)* _____ or uterine tube, is 12-cm long and divided into four parts (Figs. 19-6 and 19-7). The infundibulum is the flared, open-ended portion that receives the *(92)* _____ once it has ruptured from the ovary. Movement of the fingerlike *(93)* _____ attract the oocyte into the lumen. The ampulla, the longest portion, connects the infundibulum to the isthmus. The isthmus is the narrowed portion that approaches the uterus, and the intramural portion penetrates the uterus. Fertilization of the oocyte normally occurs in the longest portion, the *(94)* _____. The simple *(95)* _____ epithelium lining the mucous membrane is of two types, ciliated and secretory. Both increase in height until the time of ovulation, after which the ciliated cells decrease in height while the *(96)* _____ cells remain relatively unchanged. The mucosal membrane is thrown into numerous folds, most extensive in the ampullary region. The secretion of the cells is both nutritive and protective to the egg and sperm. The cilia are not involved in moving the egg or sperm; this is accomplished through peristalticlike contractions of the *(97)* _____ _____ in the wall of the oviduct. An adventitia covers the outer, longitudinal and inner, circular smooth muscle layers, the latter of which is thickest in the *(98)* _____ (*ampulla, isthmus*). (You should finish #99 and #100 at this point.)

91 *fallopian*

92 *ovum (oocyte)*

93 *fimbriae*

94 *ampulla*
95 *columnar*

96 *secretory*

97 *smooth muscle*

98 *isthmus*

Oviduct

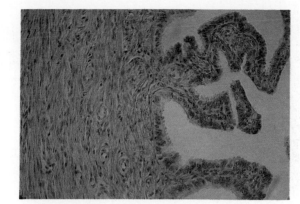

FIG. 19-6. Photomicrograph of the **(99)** _____ (ampulla, isthmus) of an oviduct, H and E stain (original magnification ×125).

99 ampulla

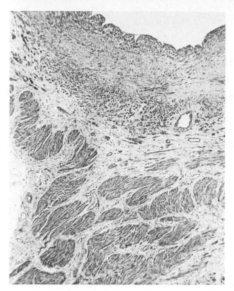

FIG. 19-7. Photomicrograph of the **(100)** _____ (ampulla, isthmus) of an oviduct (original magnification ×30).

Uterus

100 isthmus

The uterus is a hollow muscular organ, the shape of an inverted pear with a slitlike central cavity. The part that ends in a blind pouch is called the fundus; the narrow part is the body; and the uterus terminates in the cervix, which projects into the vagina. Covering the uterus is an external **(101)** _____ composed of a mesothelium. The muscular layer is called the myometrium, and the mucous membrane is called the **(102)** _____.

The smooth muscle layer, or **(103)** _____, is composed

101 serosa

of smooth muscle and connective tissue separated into three ill-defined layers. During pregnancy, the smooth muscle cells increase in both size and number

102 endometrium

owing to stimulation by estrogen. The endometrium is composed of a columnar

103 myometrium

epithelium and a **(104)** _____ propria containing simple tubular glands. The endometrium can be divided into two layers: a superficial functional layer and a deep basilar layer. During the menstrual cycle, the superficial

(105) _____ layer undergoes several changes while the

104 lamina

(106) _____ layer remains fairly unchanged (Fig. 19-8).

105 functional
106 basilar

**Female Reproductive
System**

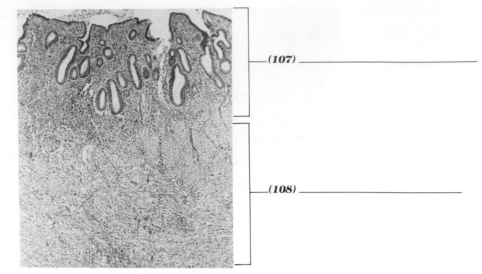

FIG. 19-8. Photomicrograph of a part of the wall of the uterus (original magnification ×30).

107 endometrium

108 myometrium

Menstrual Cycle

The menstrual cycle, approximately 28 days long, begins with the first day of menstrual bleeding. This sloughing of the functional layer of the **(109)** _____ usually lasts from day one to day four. From day four until ovulation, the **(110)** _____ layer is regenerated due to stimulation by estrogen. The estrogen is produced by the **(111)** _____ cells covering the oocyte and by the cells of the theca **(112)** _____. This period is referred to as the follicular, estrogenic, proliferative, or reparative phase. The period from approximately the time of ovulation until day 28 is called the progestational, progravid, or secretory phase. The last few days of this period are called the ischemic phase because the blood vessels supplying the **(113)** _____ layer begin to close off.

Follicular Phase

During the follicular (also called the **(114)** _____) phase, the thickness of the endometrium increases from approximately 1 mm to 3 mm (Fig. 19-9). The epithelial cells of the surface and of the glands are very

109 endometrium
110 functional

111 granulosa (follicular)
112 interna

113 functional

114 estrogenic
(proliferative,
reparative)

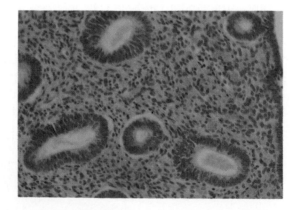

FIG. 19-9. Photomicrograph of the uterine wall, follicular phase, H and E stain (original magnification ×160).

Menstrual Cycle

115 *simple tubular*

116 *estrogen*
117 *ovary*

118 *progravid*
    (progestational)

119 *simple tubular*

120 *pale*
121 *wide, coiled, tortuous,*
    sacculated

122 *ovulation*
123 *28*
124 *progesterone*
125 *luteum*

126 *secretory (progravid,*
    progestational)

actively proliferating and even appear stratified in places. The glands are of the *(115)* _____ _____ variety. The small amount of mucus secreted during this phase is thin and watery. The stimulatory hormone for this phase is *(116)* _____, secreted by the *(117)* _____ (oviduct, ovary).

Secretory Phase

The secretory phase is also called the *(118)* _____ phase (Fig. 19-10). During this phase, the endometrium doubles in thickness owing to an

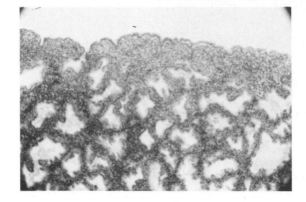

FIG. 19-10. Photomicrograph of the uterine wall, secretory phase (original magnification ×30).

increased amount of tissue fluid, an increased amount of secretion by the *(119)* _____ _____ glands, and an increase in the size of the lamina propria. The epithelial cells accumulate glycogen, which is reflected by the *(120)* _____-staining cytoplasm. How do the glands appear in this stage? *(121)* _____ _____.
The secretion is much thicker and is secreted in great quantities. The secretory phase, which lasts from the time of *(122)* _____ until day *(123)* _____, is under the influence of *(124)* _____ secreted by the corpus *(125)* _____.

Ischemic Phase

The ischemic phase occurs during the last few days of the *(126)* _____ phase (Fig. 19-11). The coiled arteries that supply the cells of the functional layer

**Female Reproductive
System**

127 functional layer

128 basalis

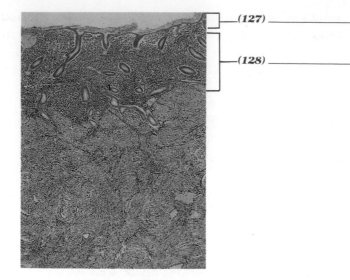

(127) _____ _____

(128) _____

FIG. 19-11. Photomicrograph of the uterine wall, ischemic phase, H and E stain (original magnification ×30).

periodically close off during this period. Consequently, parts of the functional layer of the (129) _____ die and are sloughed off. As this layer is sloughed off, accompanied by bleeding from exposed vessels, the (130) _____ layer becomes exposed. This deeper layer has an independent blood supply and is not affected by the spasms of the coiled arteries. By the end of this phase, which is accompanied by the (131) _____ flow, the entire (132) _____ layer is lost. Regeneration of the functional layer occurs in the (133) _____ phase. Proliferation occurs in the cells of the (134) _____
layer and in the cells lining the remaining portions of the glands.

129 endometrium

130 basal

131 menstrual
132 functional
133 follicular
134 basalis

Placenta

The placenta develops during pregnancy in association with the fetus, and the site of implantation is in the (135) _____. When fully developed, it has the shape of a pancake 15 cm in diameter and 3 cm thick. The function of the (136) _____ is to transfer nutrients from the mother to the fetus, and to aid in the elimination of waste by the fetus.

The outer layer of cells of the embryo that have implanted into the endometrium are responsible for most of the placental development. There are two layers involved: an inner layer of well-defined cells called the cytotrophoblast, and an outer cell layer composed of a mass of cytoplasm with numerous nuclei and no discernable cell borders called the syncytiotrophoblast. These two cell layers together, the (137) _____ and the (138) _____, constitute the trophoblast. Extensions of the trophoblast burrow into the endometrium and erode the walls of vessels. These extensions are called primary trophoblastic villi, and they become surrounded by maternal blood that flows from the eroded vessels. Thus, the spaces between the (139) _____ trophoblastic villi are filled with (140) _____ (maternal, fetal) blood and are called lacunae. As the villi develop, connective tissue and blood vessels grow into them and they are then referred to as secondary (141) _____ villi.

135 endometrium

136 placenta

137 cytotrophoblast
138 syncytiotrophoblast

139 primary
140 maternal

141 trophoblastic

Placenta

Each villus is a branching structure, and 8 to 15 villi together constitute a lobule (or fetal cotyledon) of the placenta (Fig. 19-12). The two-cell-layer thick

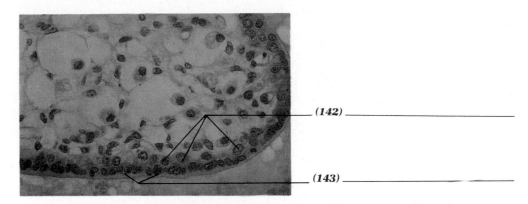

(142) _____

(143) _____

FIG. 19-12. Photomicrograph of an immature placental villus, H and E stain (original magnification ×300).

142 *cytotrophoblast*
143 *syncytiotrophoblast*

covering of the villus is the *(144)* _____. The cells of the cytotrophoblast, the *(145)* _____ (*inner, outer*) layer, are large pale-staining cells with large nuclei. These cells rest on a basement membrane. The outer layer, the *(146)* _____ , stains

144 *trophoblast*
145 *inner*

(147) _____ (*paler, darker*) than the cells of the cytotrophoblast. Are cell borders discernable in this layer? *(148)* _____. The connective tissue supporting the villus appears to be *(149)* _____ connective

146 *syncytiotrophoblast*
147 *darker*
148 *no*
149 *areolar (loose)*
150 *endothelium*
151 *basement membrane*

tissue. The fetal capillaries are lined by an *(150)* _____ and an underlying *(151)* _____ _____.

In a fully developed placenta, the cells of the cytotrophoblast have disappeared. Thus, the "placental barrier" through which the nutrients from the maternal blood must pass is composed of (from the outside in) the syncytiotrophoblast, an underlying *(152)* _____ _____ , loose connective tissue with reticular fibers, the basement membrane of the fetal capillary, and the *(153)* _____ lining of the capillary (Fig. 19-13).

152 *basement membrane*

153 *endothelial*

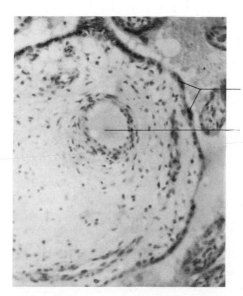

154 *syncytiotrophoblast*

155 *fetal capillary*

FIG. 19-13. Photomicrograph of a mature placental villus (original magnification ×125).

The part of the endometrium in contact with the pancakelike *(156)* _____ is called the junctional, composite, or penetration zone, and is part of the basilar layer. The cells in this layer become large and polygonal and have an abundant amount of glycogen and lipid in the cytoplasm.

156 placenta

Cervix

The cervix is the narrow inferior segment of the *(157)* _____. The mucous membrane is thrown into two large longitudinal folds, called raphes, which oppose each other. Numerous smaller folds radiate out from the longitudinal folds, or *(158)* _____. The mucous membrane is lined by mucus-secreting columnar glands that extend deep into the very *(159)* _____ *(fibrous, cellular)* lamina propria. The mucous membrane does not change much during the *(160)* _____ cycle; however, the secretion of mucus increases at the time of ovulation.

157 uterus

The inferior tip of the cervix, which extends into the *(161)* _____, is covered by a nonkeratinized stratified squamous epithelium. The transitional zone is the area in which the *(162)* _____ epithelium that covers most of the cervix merges with the epithelium of the inferior tip (Fig. 19-14). The

158 raphes

159 cellular
160 menstrual

161 vagina

162 columnar

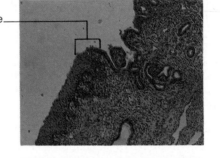

Transitional zone

FIG. 19-14. Photomicrograph of the transitional zone of the cervix, H and E stain (original magnification ×300).

wall of the cervix differs from that of the rest of the *(163)* _____ in that it is composed mostly of dense irregular connective tissue and not *(164)* _____ _____.

163 uterus

164 smooth muscle

Vagina

The mucous membrane of the vagina, like that of the cervix, is thrown into two *(165)* _____ *(longitudinal, horizontal)* folds with small folds called rugae radiating outward (Fig. 19-15). The mucous membrane is lined by *(166)* _____ _____ _____ epithelium. Are there glands present in the wall of the vagina? *(167)* _____. The lamina propria and submucosa appear *(168)* _____ *(cellular, fibrous)*, and the underlying layers contain loosely arranged bundles of *(169)* _____ _____. Numerous elastic fibers extend from the lamina propria through to the muscular layer.

165 longitudinal

166 nonkeratinized stratified squamous

167 no
168 fibrous
169 smooth muscle

Vagina

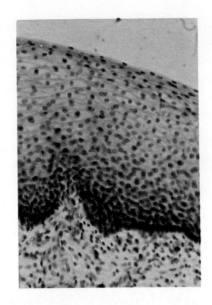

FIG. 19-15. Photomicrograph of the vagina, H and E stain (original magnification ×250).

Breast

The breast of a sexually mature female consists of superficial and deep structures. The nipple is a brownish pink cylindroconical structure; it is covered by keratinized stratified squamous epithelium. Supporting the nipple is dense irregularly connective tissue and circularly arranged smooth muscle. The areola is the skin located around this central *(170)* _____. Normally rosy in color, the areola becomes pigmented during pregnancy. Large *(171)* _____ (*apocrine, eccrine*) sweat glands found in the areola are called areolar glands of Montgomery.

170 nipple
171 apocrine

     The glandular tissue lies in the reticular layer of the *(172)* _____ (*epidermis, dermis*) and in the subcutaneous tissue. Large fiber bundles making up the interlobular connective tissue divide the glandular tissue into lobes and lobules. The larger of these fibers are referred to as suspensory ligaments of Cooper. The ducts of the glands, which develop from *(173)* _____ tissue, migrate downward, carrying cells of the papillary layer of the dermis with them. Thus, the ducts are covered by an outer layer of cellular connective tissue. The secretory portions secrete into intralobular ducts. The duct system, as it approaches the skin surface, expands into lactiferous sinuses, which then empty into lactiferous ducts, each of which opens separately at the base of the nipple.

172 dermis

173 epithelial

     The breast of a nonpregnant woman shows very little glandular tissue (Fig. 19-16). Single ducts, or clusters of ducts, are separated by dense irregular connective tissue, the *(174)* _____ connective tissue. The walls of the ducts contain two layers of epithelial cells. The connective tissue located directly around the ducts appears *(175)* _____ (*cellular, fibrous*) and originates from the *(176)* _____ layer of the dermis. This area, called intralobular connective tissue, may contain macrophages, lymphocytes, and antibody-producing *(177)* _____ cells. (You should finish #178–180 at this point.)

174 interlobular

175 cellular
176 papillary

177 plasma

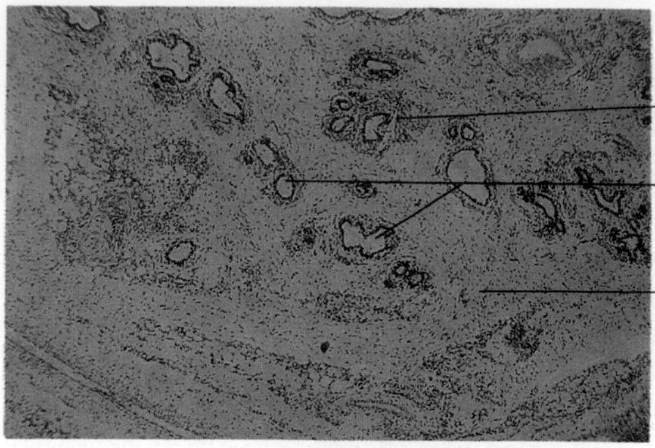

Female Reproductive System

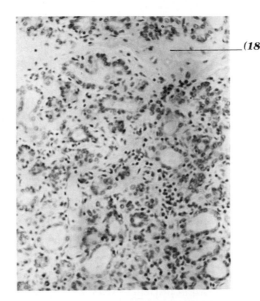

(179) _____

_____

_____

(180) _____

(178) _____

_____

_____

FIG. 19-16. Photomicrograph of a portion of the breast of a nonpregnant woman, H and E stain (original magnification ×30).

178 *interlobular connective tissue*

179 *intralobular connective tissue*

180 *ducts*

During pregnancy, there is proliferation of the duct system and development of the secretory alveoli (Fig. 19-17). The alveoli are lined by a single layer of *(181)* _____ epithelium, surrounded by a layer of contractile *(182)* _____ cells. As the alveoli secrete fluid (which is not milk until after the birth of the baby), the ducts and alveoli become distended. As a result, the *(183)* _____ connective tissue separating the lobules appears thinner. The hormones involved in this phase include the ovarian hormone *(184)* _____; the hormone produced by the corpus luteum, *(185)* _____; growth hormone; and prolactin.

181 *columnar*

182 *myoepithelial*

183 *interlobular*

184 *estrogen*

185 *progesterone*

(186) _____

_____

_____

186 *interlobular connective tissue*

FIG. 19-17. Photomicrograph of a portion of the breast of a pregnant woman (original magnification ×125).

Lactation, the production of milk, does not begin until after *(187)* _____ (Fig. 19-18). The most obvious features of the breast at this time are the secretory *(188)* _____, which appear extremely distended and full of secretory product of lactating breast, *(189)* _____. The contractile *(190)* _____ cells that surround the

187 *delivery (birth)*

188 *alveoli*

189 *milk*

190 *myoepithelial*

Breast

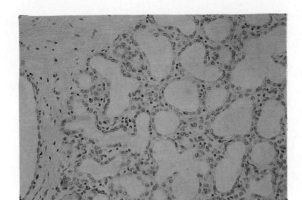

FIG. 19-18. Photomicrograph of a portion of a lactating breast, H and E stain (original magnification ×125).

(191) _____ are stimulated by nursing and oxytocin, a hormone produced by the *(192)* _____ _____ gland. As a result, milk is squeezed from the alveolar lumen into the *(193)* _____ sinuses. The production of milk is stimulated by prolactin, produced by *(194)* _____, cells of the *(195)* _____ pituitary gland. After lactation ceases, the breast regresses to the prepregnancy state in which only *(196)* _____ *(alveoli, ducts)* are seen, although some alveoli may be observed.

191 *alveoli (glands)*
192 *posterior pituitary*

193 *lactiferous*
194 *mammotrophs (lactotrophs or acidophils)*
195 *anterior*
196 *ducts*

Index

Page numbers followed by an *f* indicate illustrations.

A

M

S